A history of the Royal College of Nursing 1916–1990

C000183689

A voice for nurses

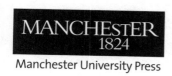

Manchester University Press

In Memory of Monica Baly
(1914–98)

A history of the Royal College of Nursing 1916–1990

A voice for nurses

Susan McGann, Anne Crowther and Rona Dougall

Manchester University Press

Manchester and New York

distributed in the United States exclusively by Palgrave Macmillan

Published by Manchester University Press
Oxford Road, Manchester M13 9NR, UK
and Room 400, 175 Fifth Avenue, New York, NY 10010, USA
www.manchesteruniversitypress.co.uk

Distributed in the United States exclusively by
Palgrave Macmillan, 175 Fifth Avenue, New York,
NY 10010, USA

Distributed in Canada exclusively by
UBC Press, University of British Columbia, 2029 West Mall,
Vancouver, BC, Canada V6T 1Z2

British Library Cataloguing-in-Publication Data
A catalogue record for this book is available from the British Library

Library of Congress Cataloging-in-Publication Data applied for

ISBN   978 0 7190 7795 1   *hardback*

ISBN   978 0 7190 7796 8   *paperback*

First published 2009

Typeset
by SNP Best-set Typesetter Ltd., Hong Kong
Printed in Great Britain
by CPI Antony Rowe Ltd, Chippenham, Wiltshire

Contents

List of illustrations   *page* vi

Acknowledgements   viii

List of abbreviations and definitions   ix

Introduction   1

1 Foundations   5

2 Consolidation   41

3 The struggle for influence, 1930–45   86

4 Nursing and the National Health Service, 1945–50   126

5 The work and training of a nurse   160

6 The 1960s: a decade of discontent   196

7 A professional union   239

8 Nurses, managers and politicians   284

Conclusion   325

Appendix 1: timechart   331

Appendix 2: RCN membership, 1916–2007   335

Appendix 3: structure of the College, 1932–49   336

Appendix 4: structure of the College, 1950–70   337

Appendix 5: structure of the College, 1970–77   338

Select bibliography   339

Index   348

List of illustrations

1.1 Dame Sarah Swift   *page* 6
1.2 Sir Arthur Stanley   10
1.3 Alicia Lloyd Still and Ethel Bedford Fenwick   19
1.4 Mary Rundle, College secretary, 1916–33   20
2.1 Opening of College building, Henrietta Place, 1926   43
2.2 College of Nursing, London   45
2.3 Private Nurses' Section, London, 1930s   51
2.4 College Council, 1926   67
3.1 Headquarters staff in Cavendish Square   88
3.2 Frances Goodall, general secretary, 1933–57   89
3.3 Annual general meeting, Sheffield, 1931   94
3.4 Nursing Reconstruction Committee (Horder), 1941   113
4.1 College of Nursing library, 1945   144
4.2 Princess Elizabeth, president of the Student Nurses
        Association, 1945   147
4.3 Student nurses' protest, London, 1948   150
5.1 Annual general meeting, London, 1950   162
5.2 Membership records staff, headquarters, 1952   164
5.3 Typing pool, headquarters, 1952   176
5.4 Heads of departments, 1952   181
6.1 Catherine Hall, general secretary, 1957–82   198
6.2 International students, 1960   204
6.3 Annual general meeting, golden jubilee, 1966   224
6.4 Catherine Hall addressing meeting in Manchester, 1969.
        Courtesy of the *Wigan Evening Post and Chronicle*   229
7.1 Catherine Hall, general secretary, and Winifred Prentice,
        president, 1974   243
7.2 M. E. (Betty) Newstead, head of the Labour Relations
        Department, *c.*1970   247
7.3 Pay campaign, 1979   252

7.4 Council meeting, 1975   255

8.1 Cartoon on the relationship between Mrs Thatcher and the
health service unions, 1988. Courtesy of Les Gibbard and
the British Cartoon Archive, University of Kent   287

8.2 Trevor Clay, general secretary, 1982–89   289

8.3 RCN newspaper advertisement commenting on the Griffiths
reforms, 1986
298

8.4 Congress, Glasgow, 1989   315

8.5 Christine Hancock, general secretary, 1989–2001   317

All illustrations, unless otherwise stated, are from the RCN Archives.

Acknowledgements

We gratefully acknowledge the financial assistance of the Wellcome Trust[1] and of the Royal College of Nursing, in supporting the research for this book.

Although the book was undertaken with the encouragement of the RCN, and of its then General Secretary, Beverly Malone, the views expressed in it are the authors' own, and no restrictions were placed on us. We were, however, greatly helped by a panel of discussants, to whom individual chapters were submitted. Their uninhibited comments have been very valuable to us, and special thanks are therefore due to Maura Buchanan, Jackie Cheeseborough, Celia Davies, Alison Kitson, Helen Sweet, Helen Thomas and Pat Thane. Additionally, we have greatly benefited from the advice of June Clark, Eleanor Gordon, Christine Hancock, Jim Phillips and Anne Marie Rafferty.

Special thanks to Edith Parker who, as Chair of the RCN History of Nursing Society, supported the project from its first inception. Thanks to Fiona Bourne, Assistant Archivist, who has given us invaluable help in the RCN archives in Edinburgh, particularly in the production of illustrations and tables.

We thank Les Gibbard for his permission to reproduce his *Guardian* cartoon of the RCN in the Thatcher years, and the *Wigan Evening Post* for permission to reproduce the photograph of Catherine Hall addressing the Manchester pay campaign meeting in 1969.

Barbara Mortimer has played a major part in research for this book, particularly in sifting the bulky minute books and annual reports of the RCN, and in undertaking a number of key interviews. We have greatly appreciated her assistance. Many members of the RCN have contributed in different ways, and a permanent record of their work and of their recollections of RCN history are kept in the RCN's extensive and growing oral history archive.

---

[1] Grant no. 072190/Z/03/Z.

List of abbreviations and definitions

Abbreviations

AR	Royal College of Nursing, *Annual Report*
BJN	*British Journal of Nursing*
BMA	British Medical Association
BMJ	*British Medical Journal*
CHANNEL	Centre of Help and Advice for Newcomers to Nursing Education and Life in the UK
CM	College [RCN] Council Minutes
CMB	Central Midwives Board
CNR	Civil Nursing Reserve
COHSE	Confederation of Health Service Employees
DES	Department of Education and Science
DHSS	Department of Health and Social Security
Ec.H.R.	*Economic History Review*
EEC	European Economic Community
GNC	General Nursing Council (1919–80)[1]
IANE	Institute of Advanced Nursing Education
ICN	International Council of Nurses
LCC	London County Council
MRC	Modern Records Centre, University of Warwick
NALGO	National Association of Local Government Officers
NASEN	National Association of State Enrolled Nurses
NCN	National Council of Nurses of Great Britain and Ireland (later Northern Ireland)
NCW	National Council of Women
NHS	National Health Service
NM	*Nursing Mirror*
NS	*Nursing Standard*

[1] There was one council for England and Wales, another for Scotland and, following the founding of the Free State, a Joint Nurses' and Midwives' Council for Northern Ireland.

NT	*Nursing Times*
NUPE	National Union of Public Employees
ODNB	*Oxford Dictionary of National Biography*
PRB	Pay Review Body
RBNA	Royal British Nurses' Association
RCN	Royal College of Nursing
RCNA	Royal College of Nursing Archives, Edinburgh. Individual references with the prefix RCN are from this archive
RRB	RCN Representative Body
SEN	state enrolled nurse (England and Wales only)
SMA	Socialist Medical Association
SNAC	Standing Nursing Advisory Committee
SRN	state registered nurse
TNA	The National Archives, Kew, London
TUC	Trades Union Congress
UKCC	United Kingdom Central Council for Nursing, Midwifery and Health Visiting
VADs	Voluntary Aid Detachment workers (Red Cross)
WSIHVA	Women Sanitary Inspectors and Health Visitors Association
WLAM	Wellcome Library, London, Archives and Manuscripts Collection
WHO	World Health Organization
WHR	*Women's History Review*

Definitions

A 'student' nurse is a person being prepared for the qualification of state registered nurse (SRN, RGN)

A 'pupil' nurse was a person being prepared for the second level qualification of enrolled nurse or state enrolled nurse (EN, SEN)

A 'pupil' midwife is a person being prepared for the qualification of registered midwife (SCM, RM)

Introduction

When the British media need an instant comment on any issue affecting nurses, from nurses' pay to violence against hospital staff, it will turn to the Royal College of Nursing (RCN), although the RCN is not the only organisation that can speak for nurses. From small beginnings in 1916, it is now firmly fixed in the public mind as the voice of the nursing profession, but it has often struggled to make that voice heard. The aim of the RCN was to establish nursing as a profession, with a distinct body of knowledge and skills, for which all nurses should be fully trained. Following the example of the prestigious royal colleges of the medical profession, it adopted the title of 'College' to signify its association with learning, but two major obstacles stood in the way of its ambitions.

Firstly, there was no agreement on the status of nursing as an occupation, or on the nature of nursing skills. Since the nineteenth century, nursing in Britain and many other countries was inevitably associated with the legacy of Florence Nightingale, who was given credit – perhaps too much credit – for reforming the discipline and training of nurses and raising them in social esteem. But nursing could still be variously defined as an instinctive female skill, a vocation, a craft learned through apprenticeship, or a profession. From its beginning, the RCN fought to establish the professional status of nurses, but many, even in its own ranks, continued to argue that nurses were born, not made; that only women could be effective nurses; and that too much theoretical education would create nurses who were unskilled and insubordinate. Many critics, particularly in the medical profession, contended that nurses were spoiled by too much theory, and that most of what they needed to know could be learned on the job. In days when medical equipment was relatively uncomplicated, it could also be argued that much nursing work was merely an extension of feminine 'instincts' for cleanliness, order and nurturing.

Secondly, for much of the period under discussion, nursing was an occupation largely for women, and specifically for young, unmarried women, who often saw it as a short-term expedient before marriage. The weight of gender stereotyping lay heavily upon it. Gender bias in nursing, and the transitory nature of many nursing careers, meant that this was a group difficult to organise and easy to exploit. With the exception of a core of matrons and senior nursing sisters, who were assumed to have deliberately chosen a celibate life, nursing could be dismissed as a kind of preparation for marriage, not requiring more than a minimum wage, and that the young women who made up such a large proportion of the nursing staff must be regimented both on and off duty.

As an organisation of nurses, the RCN developed in response to these challenges. Its first task was educational policy. It wished to define nursing as a skilled profession, which meant that education and training were at the heart of its activities. It began by offering systematic training courses to keep qualified nurses in touch with developments in their profession, and it still offers in-service training to today's nurses. It expected to be consulted in any official inquiry into nurse education; but over time it took a more active view in setting up its own inquiries into nursing education, with a view to influencing policy directly.

The second task was to improve the condition of nurses in the workplace. Very shortly after its foundation it began to act for nurses in negotiations with their employers, though at that stage it deliberately and vigorously denied that it was taking up the role of a trade union. This position could not be maintained, and the RCN is a professional association that finally accepted that it needed a legal basis for its employment negotiations, and so in 1977 reluctantly registered as a trade union. Its workplace concerns were in the early days described as 'professional organisation', and more straightforwardly from the 1960s as 'labour relations'. These always included negotiation with government, because after the Nurses Act of 1919 the government was directly involved in regulating nurse training, and in 1948, when the National Health Service (NHS) began, it became the largest employer of nurses in Britain.

The structure of this book tends to divide between these two major concerns of the RCN, though its founders saw the two as closely linked. They insisted that the respect given to nurses in the workplace would depend on their level of training and professional knowledge, and so labour relations could not be divorced from professional issues. They believed that it would be impossible to raise the status and pay of nurses until all were fully trained; hence, the standards of entry to the profession were always of major concern.

The history of the RCN is part of the history of the professions, of gender history and of labour history. Although men were admitted to membership in the 1960s, its role has been to negotiate for a largely female labour force in workplaces that were usually controlled by men. The RCN's history is therefore part of the history of women in modern British society, and the RCN has changed as women's expectations have altered. It began as a small organisation composed mainly of middle-class women, and we trace how it developed into a large and more inclusive body. Although the views of its leaders were undoubtedly influenced by changing climates of opinion, and shifts in social and gender relations, they were also active in contributing to some of these changes. The RCN also had to adjust to greater specialisation in medical knowledge and nursing work. We therefore describe the changing institutional framework of the RCN, giving due weight to the role of its leaders, not as a celebratory 'institutional history', but to explain how an organisation of this type survives, and how it adjusts to new circumstances.

The founders of the RCN quite deliberately called it a College of Nursing rather than a College of Nurses, and stressed that the advancement of nursing was its main priority. Unfortunately, this book cannot follow their precept, and it is a history of nursing only in that professional changes are obviously significant to the RCN's development. Most historians of nursing have, like us, concentrated on nurses rather than nursing. The history of nursing as a day-to-day activity, its technical advances, and the development of its growing number of specialties deserve more careful attention than this history of a single institution can give them.[1] We have also spent less time on the RCN's work in Scotland and Northern Ireland than we would have wished. The history of nursing in these areas differs in many ways from England and Wales, and their health systems and professional regulation vary from the English model. We have discussed their relations to the RCN in England, and their views on significant events, but their individual records are extensive and deserve separate attention.

Many of our chapters also deal with the public image of nurses, since few professions can have received such sentimental attention. Several historians have noted the disparity between high public esteem for nurses, and their relatively low pay. The press has been consistent, over a very long period, in presenting nurses as 'angels', and the arrival of a significant number of men in the profession has made very little difference to this. The RCN was more conscious of the importance of its public image than comparable professional bodies, and realised from an early date that public relations would be an important part of its activities. We have followed the development of management practices in the RCN to show how a large organisation with several functions has tried to satisfy its members' varied demands, while also maintaining a specific public profile.

The historian of any occupational group faces the problem of writing about organisations with lengthy titles that are usually reduced to their initials. We hope the reader will accept the abbreviated forms for organisations still in existence, or which appear frequently in this account. We use the common short forms for the British Medical Association (BMA), the Trades Union

Congress (TUC), and the Royal College of Nursing itself. But few readers today, even in the nursing profession, will recognise NASEN (National Association of State Enrolled Nurses) or NCN (National Council of Nurses of Great Britain and Ireland), while trade unions whose initials were once in everyday use, such as COHSE (Confederation of Health Service Employees) and NUPE (National Union of Public Employees) are fading from memory as unions regroup and rename themselves. This applies also to acronyms once well known to all nurses, such as GNC (General Nursing Council), or even SEN (state enrolled nurse) and SRN (state registered nurse). The acronym habit of professional and administrative bodies was pilloried in 1979 by community nurses, who christened their short-lived ginger group the Association for Community Nurses' Emoluments. Following this instructive warning, we have tried to avoid the short forms as far as possible. The RCN itself changed its full title twice in the twentieth century, as we describe in Chapter 5, and it appears as 'the College' in the first part of the book and 'RCN' in the second, for reasons explained in that section.

Note

1 Significant exceptions include, for example, Peter Nolan, *A History of Mental Health Nursing* (London: Chapman & Hall, 1994) and Helen Sweet and Rona Dougall, *Community Nursing and Primary Healthcare in Twentieth-Century Britain* (London: Routledge, 2008).

1

Foundations

On 25 February 1916, Rachael Cox-Davies, matron of the Royal Free Hospital, London, wrote a letter of congratulation to Sarah Swift, the matron-in-chief of the British Red Cross, and to Arthur Stanley, MP: 'by force of kindly good will' you have kept them all from 'scratching each others' eyes out'.[1] Cox-Davies was one of fifty hospital matrons who received a circular letter at the end of December 1915 setting out proposals for a College of Nursing and suggesting a meeting in February. Like many of her colleagues she was immediately sceptical but, out of curiosity, she went to the meeting at the offices of the British Red Cross Society in Pall Mall. Swift and Stanley were drawn together by their wartime work for the Red Cross, and well knew the problem of finding well-trained nurses in the chaotic conditions of British nursing at that time. Swift had retired from her position as matron of Guy's Hospital in 1909, but when war broke out she accepted the Red Cross post. Now in her early sixties, she was tiny and indomitable, an acknowledged expert in hospital administration. Like other leading matrons of her generation, she was unmarried, came from an upper-class family (in her case, landowners), and had many elite connections, reinforced by her war work. Arthur Stanley was the third son of the sixteenth Earl of Derby, and started his career as a professional diplomat before moving into politics. By 1916 he had been a Conservative MP for eighteen years and was well known for his work as chairman of the British Red Cross Society. A bachelor, and disabled after an attack of rheumatic fever in his youth, he devoted much time to voluntary work related to health and disability. His family background also included important nursing connections. As the wife of the Governor General of Canada, his mother founded the 'Lady Stanley Institute for Trained Nurses', the first training school for nurses in Ottawa in 1891, but perhaps more significantly, his grandfather, Lord Edward Stanley, was an ally of Florence Nightingale and supported her public health work. The alliance between Swift and Stanley, nurse and politician, echoed the well-known tactics of Florence Nightingale in her political campaigns. At this point, ventures on behalf of women were unlikely to attract much political attention without influential male support.

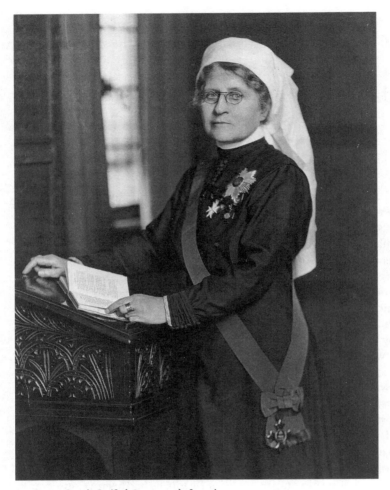

1.1 Dame Sarah Swift (1854–1937), founder.

In her letter to the two organisers, Rachael Cox-Davies was reflecting on the great divisions in British nursing, and Swift and Stanley knew they were entering a battlefield. Nursing was a largely unregulated occupation. The major British voluntary hospitals tried to guarantee their nurses' quality by training them in their own nursing schools, normally for three years. Such women, usually selected from the higher social classes, formed an elite to which Rachael Cox-Davies and Sarah Swift belonged. These hospitals did not lack middle-class applicants for training, thanks to the romantic legacy of Florence Nightingale and the absence of attractive careers for women. A shorter period of training, and much less prestigious, was offered by the larger poor law infirmaries in the cities, and by the municipal fever hospitals. The voluntary hospitals were supported by subscriptions and charitable dona- tions, and the poor law hospitals were supported by local taxation. Both were intended only for the poor, but the voluntary hospitals accepted mainly acute and surgical cases, and the poor law had to take the chronic sick, elderly and disabled. Their facilities, and the quality of their staff, reflected their different positions in social esteem and in funding, though with wide local variations. The central poor law authorities tried to lay down minimum educational requirements for nursing recruits, but literate and capable trainees were hard to find, given the poor pay and working conditions in poor law hospitals. An even more perfunctory training was offered to nursing attendants in mental hospitals, the only places outside the armed forces where male nurses were employed in any numbers. The sole branch of nursing that required an offi- cially sanctioned training was the specialised one of midwifery, where state registration was imposed from 1902, following a national panic over high rates of infantile mortality and a declining birth-rate, which seemed to threaten the nation's military and economic efficiency.[2] Any person could use the title of 'nurse', particularly in domestic nursing. Certain charities, such as the Queen Victoria's Jubilee Institute for Nurses, employed only well-trained nurses for domestic visits among the poor, but private agencies ('co-operations') were often less scrupulous about whom they employed, and there was no control over individual nursing entrepreneurs.

After the doctors achieved state regulation in 1858, many other professions, including teachers, dentists, engineers, pharmacists and accountants, aimed for similar professional protection. Legislation was the preferred route, or failing this, self-regulation through respected professional associations, like the long-standing practice of the legal profession.[3] The social argument for professional regulation seemed obvious: if unqualified people were prevented from offering their services, the public would be safeguarded from incompe- tents. Behind the social argument lay professional self-interest, for unquali- fied competitors would undercut professional incomes. While there was a growing number of prominent nurses in Britain who believed that only state registration could guarantee the quality of nurses and improve the standing of their occupation, nurses were not in the same position as other aspiring professions. Most of them were women, and for many, nursing was a short- term career that they left on marriage. In the 1911 census there were over 83,000 'nurses' (very loosely defined) in England and Wales, of whom 66 per cent were unmarried, and another 20 per cent widowed or divorced.[4] Married women, and widows with children, were more likely to work in midwifery or domiciliary nursing than in the hospitals with their long hours and fixed routines, and the census did not clarify whether they were in full-time work, or even in regular practice.[5]

Nursing also suffered from the handicap of gender stereotyping. Because their work was often seen as an extension of women's normal domestic duties, nurses were not classed as professionals, unlike women elementary school teachers, who were also struggling to establish their professional status, but who were more successful in their demands for two years' college training as an entry requirement.[6] By the end of the nineteenth century, there was still no representative professional body for nurses. Women doctors and teachers had their own associations, but men controlled their professions as a whole. Teachers fought their battles on a gender platform, but were largely concerned with discrimination from within their profession, manifest in unequal pay. Similarly, women doctors faced considerable hostility from medicine's male strongholds, and tended to be marginalised into areas regarded as suitable for their sex. The gender bias facing nurses was of a different character, because it did not come from within their own ranks. At best, nurses were regarded as brave and dedicated workers, exercising their womanly skills, at worst as glorified domestic labour, but being a woman was the primary qualification for the job. There was no internal competition with men in general nursing, but, like all women's occupations, its skills were therefore undervalued.

It was difficult to organise a profession with a high turnover, scattered among many different employers, but nurses were further divided by disputes among themselves. A 'profession' was usually defined by the nature of its training, which set it apart from outsiders. Academic training was more highly esteemed than apprenticeship, and the medical profession, in particular, successfully struggled during the nineteenth century to move away from its old apprenticeship system and into regulated training schools. Nursing was not perceived in the same way. Women were more acceptable as nurses than as doctors because they were thought to exercise practical skills that reflected their 'womanly' instincts.[7] The nineteenth-century exponents of nursing, both before and after Florence Nightingale, believed nursing to be a vocation. It could be learned only from practical experience and it required a hard apprenticeship to separate 'true nurses' from the half-hearted. In this framework theoretical study and examinations were not a priority. Florence Nightingale fervently believed that nursing was a vocation, and feared that many able women would be deterred from it if forced to pass examinations. She therefore resisted state registration for nurses. Nursing competence, she argued, relied on character rather than education, and her views reflected the experience of women like herself who were denied formal schooling.

Florence Nightingale died in 1910, and her influence was still strong in the profession when Swift and Stanley met to plan a College of Nursing. They knew they would have to become involved in the 'battle of the nurses'.[8] This was the campaign for state registration led by the formidable Ethel Bedford

Fenwick. A former matron of St Bartholomew's Hospital, she had retired
from nursing on her marriage to Dr Bedford Fenwick and from that point
directed her considerable energy into a personal mission to professionalise
nursing. She founded the British Nurses' Association in 1888 (Royal British
Nurses' Association (RBNA) from 1892), to develop professional awareness
among nurses and to promote state registration. This campaign became a
battle for registration that lasted thirty years, running parallel to the women's
suffrage campaign in Britain. The two campaigns had many similarities and,
while the nurses' campaign did not include an extreme militant voice like the
suffragettes, it encompassed many different shades of opinion on both sides
of the battle. Largely because of her early experience of the tactics of the
anti-registrationists, Bedford Fenwick became the most strident voice of the
registrationists. Having successfully launched the Royal British Nurses'
Association with the support of Princess Helena, Queen Victoria's daughter,
and of leading members of the medical profession, she soon encountered
opposition. Certain influential doctors suspected that registration would
allow nurses to challenge their authority, especially as many of the campaign-
ers came from the higher social classes. Hospital governors also feared that
registration would lead to organised, and hence more expensive, labour.
These influential groups captured the RBNA council and by 1899 it had
changed sides in the registration campaign. These events left a lasting impression on Bedford Fenwick and contributed to her enduring hostility to the
involvement of men, particularly doctors, in the affairs of nurses. Swift and
Stanley anticipated her opposition to the establishment of a College of
Nursing, because it did not emphasise state registration, because it would
include doctors and laymen like Stanley on its council, and because she would
have no control over it.

In 1915 opponents of the College argued that debates on the status and
training of nurses were peacetime issues, not appropriate during the war, but
the College's promoters persisted in their aim, even if the goal of registration
could not be achieved during the national emergency. Swift and Stanley
believed that the problems of war should not be an excuse for ignoring the
chaotic state of nurse training, for 'after the war the nurses would be faced
with a large and well-organised body of partially trained women. This competition would be very serious unless the nurses organised themselves to meet
it'.[9] A nursing college, while in sympathy with the goal of state registration,
would offer an alternative register until this could be achieved, and would
accept only trained nurses as members. Swift and Stanley valued well-trained
nurses, both for tending to the casualties of war, and for developing a healthy
nation in peacetime. They were astute negotiators, and no doubt appreciated
that public and political interest in nursing issues was more readily aroused
in war than in peace.

In her role as matron-in-chief of the Joint War Committee of the Red Cross and the Order of St John of Jerusalem, Swift well knew the problems created by unregulated nurse training. Thousands of women were volunteering to work as nurses with the Red Cross, which tried to assess their qualifications from their certificates of training. Yet any hospital, no matter how small or specialised, could establish a training school and set its own standards. Could two years' training at a large teaching hospital be compared with four years' experience in a small fever hospital? Previous attempts to organise nurses were based on associations, societies or unions, but Stanley and Swift rejected these tactics in favour of a College. Their model was a male preserve: the prestigious royal colleges of the medical profession. These had the power to examine entrants to the profession, and membership was open only to doctors of standing. The colleges offered many social and educational benefits, including the opportunity to keep abreast of medical knowledge after qualification. The title of 'College' suggested not only instruction and scholarship, but social status. It differentiated the new scheme from existing organisations, and implied a commitment to education and professional standards. Since a College needed a material symbol of its importance, a suitably impressive headquarters was also desirable. Stanley realised that the proposed College of Nursing must attract enough members to make it a national body, including

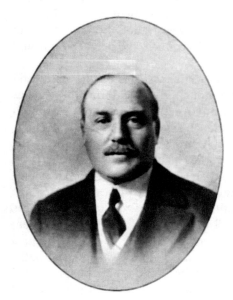

1.2 Sir Arthur Stanley (1869–1947), founder.

all types of nursing, and that it needed support from doctors and the hospital authorities. This support was not guaranteed, since many doctors preferred to see nurses as well-disciplined handmaids, rather than an independent profession.

Before the February meeting, Swift and Stanley discussed their scheme with a small group of influential hospital matrons and trusted medical advisers. Swift enlisted her old chief, Sir Cooper Perry, the medical superintendent of Guy's Hospital, who was also on the Army Medical Board, and well aware of the problem of supplying trained nurses during the emergency. Louisa Haughton, the current matron of Guy's, also responded enthusiastically, and assisted Swift by writing letters of encouragement to her own network of nursing colleagues. She urged Swift to gain the confidence of Rachael Cox-Davies and to include her as early as possible in any discussions – there was a general feeling that Miss Cox-Davies would cause trouble if she were not part of the inner circle. They also enlisted Alicia Lloyd Still, the matron of St Thomas' Hospital, and Annie Gill, matron of Edinburgh Royal Infirmary. They agreed on the need for 'a central controlling body' to standardise the education of nurses and work for state registration. Achieving this would be difficult, and Annie Gill thought they needed a 'Trade Union among nurses without the difficulties of Trade Unionism . . . an organised body of control with an organised council'.[10] Stanley had powerful contacts in the political world and among aristocratic hospital governors and the leaders of the medical profession. The matrons understood that influential men must be included in the plans, but behind the united front there was some disagreement. After one of the early meetings, Haughton wrote to Swift, 'it is difficult to get the men (even Sir Cooper) to see our side . . . how are we all going to do it?'[11] Male supporters, particularly the doctors, did not wish to set professional standards in nursing too high in case this discouraged recruits. Nevertheless, the nurses worked harmoniously with Stanley. Swift and Haughton canvassed for support among matrons of the voluntary hospitals, through letters and personal visits, while Stanley corresponded indefatigably with his extensive political and medical network.

At the end of December 1915 a letter outlining the new scheme was circulated to the governors of all the major hospitals in Britain and Ireland, inviting them to allow their matrons and 'such representatives of your Board as you may think advisable' to attend the February meeting.[12] A variety of replies came in, illustrating the wide spectrum of opinion among hospitals and their matrons on the need to organise nurses. The Royal Devon and Exeter Hospital did not think it an appropriate time for such a plan, but promised to consider it after the war; the Royal Berkshire Hospital wanted to wait until the College of Physicians gave its opinion; St Bartholomew's reserved judgement until the scheme was more definite, and the Mater Misericordiae Hospital in Dublin immediately offered a representative to assist in promoting the proposed College. Most hospitals were favourable, as were most hospital matrons, although protective of their own training systems. The matron of University College Hospital, London, wrote that she was willing to co-operate, but only on condition that three years' training in a general hospital of over 100 beds be enforced as the standard for a 'trained' nurse. But the proposed College also had numerous opponents, including Eva Luckes, the elderly and well-respected matron of the London Hospital, and disciple of Florence Nightingale. In January 1916, referring to the demands of war, Luckes wrote to Swift, arguing that this was not an opportune moment to 'raise controversial nursing questions'. She could not see how any matrons 'desirous of serving their country as well as their hospital' could spare time to worry about the organisation of nurses in 'normal' times.[13] The matrons, particularly in the London hospitals, were already in several camps over the question of registration. Haughton wrote to Sarah Swift, 'Miss Luckes throws a horrible shadow quite equal to her size!'[14]

One group of nurses was omitted from the list of participants. These were the nurses in poor law institutions, who, although less numerous than nurses in the voluntary hospitals, resented being excluded. The Vice-President of the Tynemouth poor law union wrote to Stanley on behalf of the poor law nursing service, complaining that poor law training schools were not invited to the original meeting, although they generally supported the College's aims. These schools, with their shorter period of training, did not meet the standards required by matrons in the voluntary hospitals, though the matrons in charge of the larger poor law training schools were themselves trained nurses. The letter was an early indication of the poor law nurses' sense of insecurity in the face of a professionalised service, but the College's founders continued to underestimate the need to win their support. The consequent hostility was to plague the College in future years. The College's founding matrons reflected the values of their own training in the voluntary hospitals. These usually recruited probationers in their early twenties, regarding nursing as a vocation for more mature women. Working-class girls in search of employment did not have the luxury of a long delay before training, for secondary education was not free or compulsory, and most of them left school at fourteen. The poor law hospitals could not afford to be too discriminating, and had to employ younger women with less education. The College founders' attitude to poor law hospitals reflected the class divide in nursing.

Diplomacy was never more essential than in the weeks after the February meeting. Stanley's letter invited comment and some of the replies also betrayed the different standards of training in the voluntary hospitals. Lord Knutsford, chairman of the London Hospital, wrote to Stanley supporting his matron, Eva Luckes, and her two-year nurse training system: 'I earnestly hope that you will not allow the matrons to make this College an attack on Miss Luckes' method of training nurses . . . the London Hospital nurse in England will rise up against it if it is done'. Miss Luckes was nearing the end of her life, and Knutsford did not wish to perturb her last days. He added that the London Hospital had already been asked to increase its period of nurse training from two to three years but that this was, in his opinion, quite unnecessary. 'We keep them [trained nurses] in the service of the hospital for four years but we send them out to nurse the King and other such patients (!) after two years . . . no-one can say that the London Hospital nurses are not properly trained'.[15] The general response of the London Hospital house committee was that this was a bad time for such a scheme, but they offered support on certain conditions: that the certificates of training schools should be accepted as entry to the College; that there should be no interference with individual training schools; that there should be no fixed length to the training period; and that the College should in no way support state registration. Although Lord Knutsford's conditions contradicted most of the aims of the proposed College, Stanley's reply was diplomatic: 'I see no reason why we should not be able to come to some agreement along the lines laid down in your letter'.[16]

To appease the hospitals, Stanley played down the training requirements for entry to the College, and claimed to have an open mind on registration, having been advised equally by registrationists and anti-registrationists. He did not underestimate the importance of state registration, but his attitude was much more relaxed than many of the matrons, and he believed that once the new College was established, registration would take care of itself. He reasoned that 'if after some years working it is felt that the certificates originated by the "College of Nursing" require state support there will be little difficulty obtaining it; if, on the other hand, it is generally felt that the certificates of the Society are strong enough without State support there will be no reason to ask for it.'[17] Such a measured view of the future was conciliatory, if not always consistent. In the same week, Stanley wrote to Comyns Berkeley, consultant at the Middlesex Hospital, and leading member of both the Royal British Nurses' Association, and the Central Committee for the State Registration of Trained Nurses, to say that the College scheme 'was in no way intended to delay State Registration of nurses'.[18] Stanley's cautious approach to the divisive registration question did not please the more militant matrons, who felt that he was putting too much weight on the educational function of the College at the expense of the professional role.

The meeting on 25 February was the first of three intended to win support for the College. Representatives of all the nursing associations, leagues and unions, who were curious to know more about this initiative, attended along with doctors, hospital governors and journalists. Predictably, there was much contention over state registration, and Ethel Bedford Fenwick had much to say. She wanted to know who sent out the invitations, who had drawn up the scheme and whom they represented; in short, why had she not been consulted? Now aged fifty-nine, internationally known as the founder of the International Council of Nurses (ICN) and the owner and editor of the influential *British Journal of Nursing (BJN)*, Bedford Fenwick was not known for her willingness to compromise.[19] Sarah Swift, who was also impatient of opposition, did not speak at the meeting, but left the main speech to Stanley, a man with a reputation for charming committees. Louisa Haughton outlined the aims of the College. She and Stanley spoke of 'state recognition' for nursing, by which they meant something more wide-ranging than state registration. The College aimed to advance nursing as a profession; introduce better educational standards through a recommended uniform curriculum, central examinations and qualifications; set up a register of members who were trained nurses; and establish a headquarters in London with educational facilities similar to the royal medical colleges. It would form a large consultative board comparable to the General Medical Council for the medical profession, and would be responsible for devising training schemes and approving nursing schools. Its examining board would ultimately offer national examinations for nurses and other women working in hospitals.

The audience at the February meeting included all shades of opinion in nursing politics. Among the supporters of state registration were many who could not be easily convinced that a voluntary system of registration would be effective. The sceptics were more worried about the intimate connection of Swift and Stanley with the Red Cross, and whether they intended to include the large numbers of Red Cross Voluntary Aid Detachment workers (VADs) within the proposed College of Nursing. The VADs held only first aid and home nursing certificates. The legally minded among the audience argued that they had to determine what 'trained' meant before the many partially trained nurses claimed this status at the end of the war, and that this must be done by legislation. 'You may talk as you like about the Nursing College, but the Nursing College will do absolutely nothing to meet this impending difficulty. It cannot. The Nursing College will be a voluntary institution'.[20] No-one, however, suggested that the College should include men in its membership. Male attendants in the forces, asylums, prisons and similar institutions were not considered on the same level as fully trained hospital nurses. Unspoken issues of social class lay behind this assumption. Although middle-class women were prepared to accept poor pay to follow their 'vocation' in the voluntary hospitals – and had few career alternatives – asylum posts, often associated with the use of physical force, were for working-class men.

With this exception, Stanley's vision was on a grand scale: a College that embraced all aspects of women's work in hospitals to include not only nurses but clerks and storekeepers.[21] He proposed four categories of affiliation:

Fellows (matrons or superintendents of recognised hospitals and others who had diplomas entitling them to the position); Members ('trained nurses' with a specified number of years training in a recognised hospital or holding appropriate diplomas); Associates (mainly to include VADs), and a fourth, undefined, class which might encompass other classes of hospital worker such as clerks and storekeepers. From such a body the partially trained VADs need not be excluded; rather, they would be accommodated within a system that would utilise their various skills, recognise their contribution to nursing and encourage them to take further training. Stanley's College would also have emphasised the distinction between nurses with a high level of formal training and those without it; and between nurses trained in the general hospitals and those with more specialised or limited experience. In this way, he seems to have foreseen a multi-skilled nursing workforce. Stanley's view of the College as democratically run and including all types of staff was considerably broader than that of his female colleagues, who wanted an exclusive body reserved for nurses with an approved training. Given the reputation of hospital matrons as the leaders of nursing, it was probably inconceivable to Stanley that the new college might elect anyone other than matrons to positions of power. This would bring all women hospital staff into the realm of nursing, under a regulating body managed by senior nurses. Stanley and Cooper Perry, both involved with the wartime medical services, did not wish to inhibit nursing recruits of any class, but the matrons hoped to raise the standards of the profession, and this meant excluding semi-trained women.

Not surprisingly, Stanley's proposed four-tiered structure did not appeal to the matrons, who argued for a much clearer distinction between trained and untrained nurses. They particularly objected to the proposal to include VADs. Many of these were from the upper middle class, and their social connections and elegance made them popular with the press and recruitment propagandists. Since the beginning of the war, trained nurses had witnessed the VADs being marketed as the image of nursing. The War Office, soldiers and the public responded to them as 'ministering angels'. This was particularly infuriating because VADs had only six weeks' training in first aid and were meant to work under the supervision of trained nurses.[22] Among nurses who had come through a tough three or four year training to earn their certificates, the popularity of the VADs aroused a stronger sense of professional awareness than any of Bedford Fenwick's pro-registration arguments had achieved. Stanley knew that the question of the VADs would have to be addressed at some point, but true to his diplomatic nature, and recognising the need to make progress, he quickly adapted his position and proceeded to more pressing matters. The broad church College that he envisaged disappeared, and the initial suggestion to make provision for VADs to gain certificates and enter a nursing career was put aside to be resolved at a later date.

The College founders were keen to obtain a royal charter for several reasons. It would underline their similarity to the royal medical colleges, but more importantly the College needed to be on an equal footing with the Royal British Nurses' Association. The RBNA had obtained a charter in 1893 on the grounds that it was concerned with nurses' welfare. The College founders hoped for a similar sign of royal approval, but on enquiry were told that the College was not eligible at this early stage. The founders required legal status in order to hold and manage property, and so they applied for incorporation as a limited company. The College of Nursing Ltd was incorporated on 27 March 1916, and placed under the direction of a College council. The application to the Board of Trade was signed by Stanley and the College's legal advisers. It contained no female names. Legal convention also dictated that members of the College were described in the Articles of Association as 'he', although it was taken for granted that the members would all be women apart from males elected to the council, who would automatically receive membership.[23] For an aspiring professional association, the implied connection with trade in a limited company was unappealing, and attracted fierce criticism, but it seemed the only way forward. The College's formal objectives were described largely as educational and professional, with specific reference to training courses and the compilation of a register of nurses. The only aims that offered openings for wider activity were indirect:

> To promote the advancement of nursing as a profession in all or any of its branches . . .

> To promote Bills in Parliament for any object connected with the interests of the nursing Profession . . .

The last of the twenty-five objectives in the Articles stated firmly: 'the College shall not do anything which would make it a Trade Union'.[24]

The nursing profession has traditionally been seen as beset by gender tensions, and there is no attempt here to minimise the force of discrimination. By the time the College was founded in 1916, the suffrage campaign was well under way. Two years later women over twenty-nine were given the vote. While a number of College members were supporters of this and other women's movements, they remained, in their working lives, bound within strictly gendered institutional hierarchies. The matrons who founded the College would have been puzzled by today's historical debates over the position of Victorian women, and whether they occupied 'separate spheres' from men. The matrons, products of a Victorian training, believed that nursing was a woman's occupation, and that it occupied a separate space in the hospitals from the work of men. But these matrons had considerable authority, not only over large teams of nurses and other hospital workers, but often over the medical staff and hospital governors as well. The College matrons undoubtedly fitted the conventional Nightingale image of celibate women dedicated to a vocation, but they were also career women who commanded respect, as Florence Nightingale had intended.

The College founders do not fit easily into vigorous feminist history. Excluded from the political process and conservative in social matters, they relied on influential men to take the public role while exerting influence from behind the scenes. But although Arthur Stanley's social position and skilful diplomacy played an essential part, it was the women's nursing expertise that allowed them to determine the shape of the College and define the educational standards that would underpin nursing's professional status. Bedford Fenwick's conception of nursing was more feminist, and she resented the continuing presence of men, even amenable ones, on the College council. By her standards, the College was not a self-governing society of nurses, although it was a unique professional organisation for women.

Early years

The first council was self-appointed from the College's supporters, but future councils would be elected by the membership. Inevitably, there was much conspiring to select a council that would work together harmoniously, a difficult task given the strong-minded constituency of matrons. Louisa Haughton and Sarah Swift compared notes on suitable candidates, and visited several London hospitals to persuade unwilling matrons to join the council, or at least to support the College venture.

> Miss Cox-Davies will be more manageable on the Council! [wrote Louisa Haughton to Sarah Swift] . . . I wish she would not worry Miss Lloyd Still who is very impressionable. Miss Musson will be a harder nut to crack! Miss Barton will be useful enough in her position as President of the Poor Law Association. Then there are only 5 more places for matrons or trained nurses and some of them must be from Ireland or the provinces.[25]

More controversially, the College council included interested parties – mainly men – who were not nurses. The twenty-five members of the first council consisted of thirteen matrons from the voluntary hospitals, including six from London, three poor law matrons – a number soon reduced to two, then one – and one leader each from the Red Cross (Sarah Swift) and Queen Victoria's Jubilee Institute for Nurses. There were eight non-nursing members. Sir Arthur Stanley, recently knighted for his war work, was the most prominent of these, but the council also included Sir Cooper Perry, Sir Comyns Berkeley, a leading gynaecologist and chairman of the Central Midwives Board (CMB), Colonel James Cantlie of the Army Medical Department, three other distinguished doctors, and a governor of St Thomas's Hospital. The council was expanded to thirty-six by the end of 1916, to include representatives from Scotland and Ireland in a similar configuration of matrons and medical men, though the naval nurses were also represented. Elections began in 1918, with the original unelected members due to retire in rotation over a three-year period. The elections made little difference to the nature of the council. The national groups had a fixed quota of representatives. Candidates did not have to be nurses, nor members of the College, but had to be nominated and seconded by College members. As a result, for much of the inter-war period the council fell into three groups: one-third hospital matrons, one-third other nursing posts (usually leaders of major nursing organisations), and one-third non-nursing members.

Unusually for a professional body, the College council included a substantial group who were not eligible for membership of the College by the normal route, since this was restricted to trained nurses. This aspect of the College proved a permanent obstacle to any amicable relationship with Bedford Fenwick. She was adamant that a nursing organisation should be run by nurses only, and its council should represent the various existing nursing associations. Since several of these were Bedford Fenwick's own creations – such as the National Council of Nurses (NCN) which she had founded in 1904 to enable British nurses to affiliate to the International Council of Nurses (which she had founded in 1899) – and small in size, the College resisted such a suggestion. She portrayed the College as a cabal of matrons, doctors and hospital governors, who reflected the views of employers rather than nurses. Although Bedford Fenwick was prone to exaggerate, the accusation that the College was an elite organisation, sponsored by aristocrats and hospital management, was not inaccurate, and was not shaken until well after the Second World War. Hospital governors, in particular, could see the point of supporting a body that specifically repudiated trade unionism.

Until membership subscriptions began to accumulate, the College needed some funding, and thanks to two substantial donations from members of the peerage, it began business. The council appointed Mary Rundle as College secretary in June 1916, and Gertrude Cowlin as her assistant. Miss Rundle, then in her early forties, was formerly Rachael Cox-Davies's assistant at the Royal Free Hospital, and then matron of the Royal Hospital for Diseases of the Chest. During the war, she became matron of a war hospital in London. She was released from this duty to take the College post, which suggests that the council was able to use some of its considerable influence in military circles. Mary Rundle and Gertrude Cowlin had trained together, and were lifelong companions who now dedicated the rest of their careers to the College for modest pay. Serious and deliberate in manner, Mary Rundle was efficient and conscientious, and valued also for her patience and tact. At this stage, the

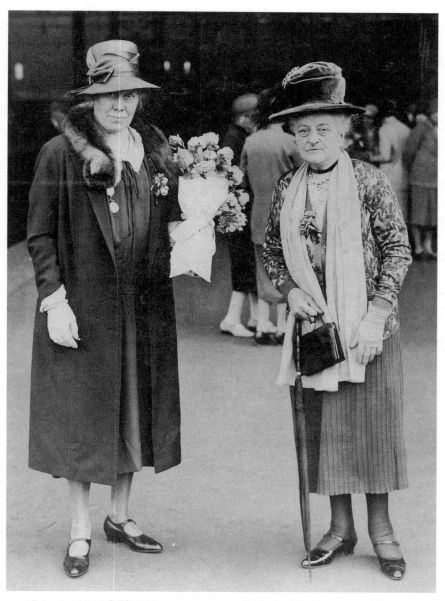

1.3 Alicia Lloyd Still (left), College supporter, and Ethel Bedford Fenwick, College opponent, 1929, at Waterloo station, en route to the meeting of the International Council of
Nurses in Montreal.

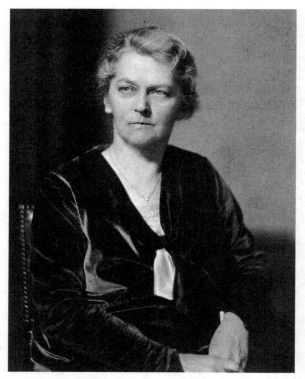

1.4 Mary Rundle, secretary of the College 1916–33.

secretarial role was fairly muted, and the College founders, rather than the secretary, took the day-to-day decisions. The College council met fortnightly during the early years, and the founders conducted most of the College business.

Stanley was able to use his wartime philanthropic connections to begin a national collection for the College, and this also helped to establish it in the public mind. This was the first of many such appeals, and gave the College a major advantage compared with its smaller rivals in nursing politics. In 1917 Stanley invited the British Women's Hospital Committee to collect money for a benevolent fund for nurses. The committee was formed at the start of the war by members of the Actresses' Franchise League, and was one of many such ventures by middle-class women.[26] Its leaders were Dame May Whitty and Lilian Braithwaite, actresses from genteel backgrounds who signalled that their own profession was improving its social status. These were women well connected in politics and the arts, and they brought the support of leading personalities, such as the popular novelist John Galsworthy and Sir Frederick

Treves, the King's surgeon.[27] The committee also included Annie Pearson, Lady Cowdray. Her husband, Weetman Pearson (who was created viscount in 1917), had amassed a fortune as a building engineer and oil magnate. He joined his wife in numerous philanthropic ventures and in supporting women's suffrage, and they became the most generous of the College's early benefactors.

The College knew that many nurses whose health had been damaged by war work were faced with no income or the minimum disablement grant from national health insurance. The British Women's Hospital Committee had raised a substantial sum for disabled soldiers at the beginning of the war, the Star and Garter Fund, and they now accepted the challenge of raising a similar fund for nurses. The appeal, the Nation's Fund for Nurses, was conceived as a thank-offering from the British Empire to British nurses. The central fund was to be divided into two parts: a tribute fund for the benefit of all nurses, and an endowment fund for the College of Nursing. The College council assisted in disbursing the tribute fund, and was given complete discretion over the endowment fund. Stanley and the other founders wished to provide the College with an impressive national headquarters in London, a suitable symbol for an aspiring profession. They knew that nurses could not contribute enough for this purpose, and they used this argument as the basis of the appeal. Leaflets advertising the Nation's Fund for Nurses compared it to the Nightingale Fund collected by a grateful nation for nurse training after the Crimean war. Treves wrote of the work of nurses in the war, dismissing the pictures of mincing ladies in nun-like dresses bending over the tidy beds of smiling soldiers: 'no picture can convey a sense of the riot and squalor of war, of the crowd of impatient ambulances, of the endless moaning tide of stretchers, of the piteous calls, of the ceaseless running to and fro'.[28] But although the campaign appealed to the public, it did not please some of the other nurses' organisations. Bedford Fenwick dismissed it as 'demoralising patronage by wealthy, leisured women', and accused the College of depriving nurses of their professional independence. The Fund's literature stated that although the College was striving to reorganise nursing so that nurses could command better pay, this would take time and there were many nurses who could not wait for help. At the College's annual meeting in 1919, Stanley referred to the 'virulent and disgraceful abuse' heaped on the women of the British Women's Hospital Committee:

> They have been told that they are insulting the nursing profession and that the nurses do not want charity. I wish those who use this language could have seen, as I have, some of the cases that have been brought before the Committee . . . Before we started this Nation's Fund there was practically no fund in existence that dealt with such cases.[29]

By 1920 the tribute fund reached £100,000 and the British Women's Hospital Committee transferred the work of the Nation's Fund to a council, composed of some of their own members, representatives of the College council, and other persons interested in the profession. It aimed to raise the same amount for the endowment fund, which at that time stood at £40,000.

Although the College nursed ambitious plans for a substantial headquarters, its first offices were in small rooms at separate addresses in Vere Street, lent free of charge by Sir James Boyton MP and Colonel James Cantlie. The council continued to meet in the Red Cross offices in Pall Mall. By the spring of 1919 the College could afford to rent premises at 7 Henrietta Street, part of which were used as club rooms by London members of the College, but these were not large enough for the College's projected programme of educational courses, meetings and social events. In 1920, 20 Cavendish Square, the home of the former Prime Minister, H. H. Asquith, was put up for sale. The College could not afford to buy such a property, but Mary Rundle went unofficially to see Lord and Lady Cowdray, hoping that they might buy the house and rent it to the College. The Cowdrays' response was munificent. Lady Cowdray, a strong believer in women's emancipation, wished to see nurses as part of a growing army of women professionals. She thought the town house unsuitable for offices, and offered to refurbish it as a club for professional women, a meeting place for different professions, and with hotel accommodation for professional women travelling alone. Lord Cowdray offered to build the College a new set of offices in the garden of the town house. The College thus acquired a magnificent headquarters in a prime location in central London, which, with various extensions, it still occupies. The foundation stone was laid in 1922, and the new buildings were opened by Queen Mary in May 1926. At the foundation ceremony, Lady Cowdray spoke of her long-standing wish to assist nurses, 'to lighten and enrich lives often darkened and depressed by the very nature of their services to humanity'.[30]

Through the nursing press, and encouraged by a network of supportive matrons, word of the College quickly spread to all sections of nursing throughout the country. In the first twelve months applications for membership proved overwhelming for an infant College with a handful of staff, and numbers continued to grow until by the end of March 1918 they stood at 7,962 and merited the employment of a full-time registrar. Although any estimate of the number of trained nurses eligible to join the College is hampered by deficient statistics, this figure probably represented upwards of 10 per cent of all women nurses in England and Wales.[31] Despite the dislocation caused by the war, new members came from many branches of nursing, including private nursing, voluntary hospitals, district nursing, the poor law hospitals, military nurses and nurses overseas. Senior nurses from the provinces became some of its most enthusiastic activists. Endorsed by influential and affluent patrons, the College promised higher professional status for nurses. But, although there were many expressions of hope and confidence in the new College, its original membership was largely concentrated on the nursing elite, and junior nurses were pressured to join by their matrons.

From the outset Stanley and Swift tried to attract national interest. Representatives from Scotland and Ireland were invited to the first meetings in 1915 and 1916. The Scottish and Irish contingents quickly sought to establish their own controlling boards within the College, independent from its London headquarters. As will be seen, political unrest in Ireland produced a particularly complex relationship between Irish nurses and the London centre. In Scotland the request for a separate board arose mainly from the difficulties of travel, since it was almost impossible for members from Scottish institutions to attend council meetings, given the problems of time and cost. Yet it is also clear that Scottish supporters of the College were worried that the council in London would lay down regulations that would aversely affect Scottish nurses. They believed that there were 'special conditions attached to the Nursing Schools in Scotland which could only be properly understood by those directly concerned', a comment probably referring to the large number of small training schools in Scotland. The Scottish contingent maintained that 'any organisations entirely managed from England would not be acceptable to Scotland' and that a separate Scottish administration was needed.[32] A meeting in Edinburgh in May 1916, attended by matrons, doctors and medical superintendents from all the leading Scottish institutions, proposed to set up a Scottish local board. A fortnight later the proposal was adopted and officials representing the five major Scottish cities were elected. With an initial £300 from the College in London, an office was taken in central Edinburgh and the Scottish Board established. The first Board had an even heavier concentration of medical men than the council in London. In the ensuing years it followed the model of the College council and engaged with all major College issues, though remaining in general agreement with the London headquarters. The Scottish Board raised questions, put forward resolutions and suggested amendments, but despite a few minor differences, supported rather than challenged the College council in London.

With the establishment of a national board in Scotland, followed by an Irish Board in 1917, and with membership in those areas of 831 and 268 respectively, the College could claim to represent the whole country. Nevertheless, its structure came under fire. Bedford Fenwick contended that lay members dominated the council, while poor law Guardians felt that their nurses were under-represented. To avoid accusations of being London-centred and exclusive, the College needed a system of communication with its members, and devised a scheme of local centres, each consisting of members who would hold regular meetings to discuss College policy. The first centres were formed in 1918 in Manchester, Birmingham, Bristol, Leicester, Liverpool and London. Manchester was the largest local centre, with a membership of almost 500. Most centres developed lecture programmes and provided educational and social activities for nurses. Through a mixed programme of lectures, dances, teas and outings, they allowed nurses to socialise and to form personal and professional networks beyond the walls of their own institution. In this, the College of Nursing came closer to the regional structure of the British Medical Association than to the centralised royal medical colleges, for although the College of Nursing coveted the prestige of the medical colleges, it could not be as exclusive as they were. It hoped to include all trained nurses, just as the BMA hoped to incorporate all qualified doctors, whatever their specialty.

The local centres were intended to encourage wider representation among all branches of nursing, though in practice it was hard to engage nurses working outside the hospitals. An important part of the future structure of the College was laid down when representatives of the first ten local centres met in London in June 1918 and agreed to form the Local Centres Standing Committee, which met officially for the first time the following month. Margaret Sparshott, matron of Manchester Royal Infirmary, was elected chairman. The Branches Standing Committee, as it became in 1926 when local centres were renamed 'branches', was the source of many proposals and resolutions over the years, not always in harmony with the College council. This pattern emerged as early as 1919 with representatives discussing the need to organise council elections on a regional basis to counteract the predominance of London hospitals. An organising secretary was appointed in 1919 to support the branches and stimulate recruitment.[33] Each centre appointed an honorary press secretary to keep the centres in touch with the press and with the editor of the *Bulletin*, the College's main newssheet. This was an early example of the College's sensitivity to public relations. Consequently, local papers often carried detailed accounts of the College's social activities, and fixed it in the public mind as an association far removed from trade unionism. Although readers of the local press might assume that the College's work consisted largely of bazaars and garden parties, the network of local centres was very effective in deflecting accusations of centralisation. However, in spite of good intentions, it was the senior hospital nurses, usually the matrons, who took the leading roles in the centres and College committees. Since the College recruited only trained women, it did not include a large proportion of the nursing workforce, and omitted the student nurses ('probationers') who were an essential part of nursing labour in the hospitals.

In the centres nurses could socialise with colleagues, develop professional interests through lectures and courses and voice their opinion on nursing issues. But attendance figures at centre meetings were variable, and returns in College referenda sent out to the centres were often disappointingly low.

Social evenings and lectures were well attended, but numbers were not high at regular meetings where the business of the College was discussed. In Bristol, for example, a centre was established in 1918 with a membership of 127, rising to 160 within two years. The centre's first lecture, on orthopaedics, attracted 150 nurses and attendance remained high for subsequent lectures in the series. Yet those attending general meetings averaged only thirty in 1921 and twenty-one in 1924. There are several possible explanations for the members' apparent lack of interest in the business of the College, but the reason usually given was that local matrons, who often chaired the meetings and put themselves forward to serve on College committees, dominated the centres.

With relatively low attendance at centre meetings, the influence of rank-and-file nurses on College policy was probably minimal. While some women were accustomed to involvement in social or political movements, the majority were neither well educated nor experienced in political activity. It must have seemed unlikely to the working nurse that her thoughts on such matters as the Hours of Employment Bill could affect College policy, far less that of the government. Also, in the hierarchy of their workplace, nurses were used to deferring to the authority of the matron, and would hesitate to challenge her at a public meeting. The failure to engage the majority of members did not escape Stanley's notice. In 1922, after local members failed to nominate many candidates for the new statutory body, the General Nursing Council, he wrote a sharp letter to Margaret Sparshott on the fundamental role of the centres:

> You know how anxious we are that the nursing profession should organise itself . . . The only way in which this organisation can really be effective is through the Centres, and if the Centres fail us then there is little can be done at Headquarters . . . urge upon them [the nurses] the very great importance to themselves and their profession of doing all they can to show that nurses are worthy and capable of self-government.[34]

Ireland

Another group that proved difficult to accommodate were the Irish nurses. In February 1917 Mary Rundle and Rachael Cox-Davies travelled to Ireland and addressed meetings in Dublin and Belfast about the aims of the College. They believed that there was sufficient support for an Irish Board, which was duly established in Dublin and held its first meeting in March. It had an office and a secretary, Vera Matheson, who outlined the main objectives: 'the College will do for nursing what chartered institutes and royal colleges have done for other professions. The headquarters in London will be the centre of nursing education, with examinations, lectures, library, and scholarships'.[35] Membership grew slowly but the Board believed that it could improve the position of nurses in Ireland, and in 1918 it collected statistics on their economic position. The figures showed not only that nurses in Ireland were paid less than those in England, but that the gap between them was dispro- portionate, even when the comparative poverty of Ireland was taken into consideration.

Inevitably, the Irish Board was affected by the political situation. The new Board aroused interest in the nursing question and provoked many previ- ously indifferent nurses into action. The Irish Matrons' Association and the Irish Nurses' Association, part of Bedford Fenwick's network of national associations, both objected to the formation of an Irish branch of the College.[36] With the support of the Royal College of Surgeons of Ireland, they set up an independent Irish Nursing Board in May 1917, in direct opposition to the College's Board. This independent Board, like the College, wanted to raise the standard of training of Irish nurses. It intended to grant certificates to nurses passing its examinations, and to place them on a voluntary register. The two boards competed for the support of Irish nurses. The College appealed to them to become part of the larger organisation of British and colonial nurses, but the independent Board drew support from Irish nurses who did not want to join a body with its headquarters in London. The royal medical colleges and other institutions of the protestant ruling class supported both the College and the independent board, but neither had much success in attracting Irish nurses. Wartime conditions had been propitious for founding a College in England, but there could hardly have been a worse time for seeking support in Ireland. After the 1918 general election, the victorious Sinn Fein declared an Irish Republic, and Dublin was in no mood to welcome an English-based nursing campaign.

Most Irish nurses were working-class Catholics, and had a different agenda from the nursing boards. This became clear when a trade union for nurses was launched in February 1919 at a large public meeting in Dublin. There was a good deal of public sympathy in Dublin for a nurses' union, and the Lord Mayor presided at the meeting, with many well-known persons on the plat- form and over 500 nurses in attendance.[37] The Irish Nurses' Union was led by Louie Bennett, the general secretary of the Irish Women Workers' Union. She argued that the only way for nurses to improve their situation was to join a union backed by the Labour Party:

[why] should we join an isolated organisation, backed by matrons and a group of benevolent people of the middle, or even the aristocratic class . . . who, when questions of higher salaries or shorter hours are raised, gently explain to us why the present time is not a suitable one to give them to us! If nurses choose the latter method of organisation they will retain the position of heroines whose mission it is to live in poverty.[38]

The Irish Board of the College realised that the union offered serious competition for the loyalty of Irish nurses, and were dismayed at the prospect of nursing being associated with trade unions and strikes. They published recommendations for minimum rates of pay and maximum working hours in all the daily papers, and appealed to Irish nurses to follow the professional road to reform.[39] But Irish nurses found unionism more attractive, and by the early 1920s the Irish Nurses' Union was the largest nursing organisation in Ireland.[40] The Irish Board of the College tried to defend itself, arguing that it was an Irish body working for Irish nurses. It published a programme for the future which emphasised improvements in nurses' economic conditions, protection of their professional interests, and higher educational standards. It contacted the other nursing organisations to suggest co-operation, but nothing concrete was achieved. In February 1921 the secretary of the Irish Board wrote to Mary Rundle, acknowledging the College's financial losses in Ireland, but pointing out that the Irish Board maintained its presence in the face of '1) keenest opposition within the profession. 2) Intense national feeling as regards English institutions. 3) A condition of affairs in the country generally which has amounted to a reign of terror'. She commented that one reason for the College's lack of support among Irish nurses was that 'Ireland's best nursing material either goes over to England to train, or as soon as trained transfers its energies and good influence to England because of the better material prospects there'.[41] A further deterrent was the establishment of the first Irish General Nursing Council in 1920, which many Irish nurses gave as one of the reasons why they did not need the College. The College had three representatives on the first appointed GNC for Ireland, and the rival Irish Nursing Board four.

Although the situation looked hopeless for the Irish Board in Dublin, a local centre was established in Belfast and, following the establishment of a separate parliament in Ulster, the Belfast centre became a College stronghold. The Irish Board believed that when peace and stability returned after the civil war, Irish nurses would begin to think about their professional development and would appreciate what the College offered. However, the College council in London refused to continue to underwrite the Irish Board and decided in 1923 that it should be dissolved. The Irish Board successfully pleaded for more time and continued its work for another two years, but in May 1925 it finally accepted defeat and voted for dissolution. After that, College activities were confined to Northern Ireland.

The division in nursing

Although Stanley had desired an inclusive nursing college, its first public discussions soon focused on the 'trained' nurse, as defined by the standards of the larger London teaching hospitals. A particularly divisive factor in the structure of the College was the stipulation in its Articles of Association that members should be general trained nurses. In 1916, when this condition was set down, the founders expected that when state registration was introduced it would be based on general nursing, and that training in specialist areas such as children's nursing, mental nursing and fever nursing, would become a post-basic training. It seemed to them appropriate to limit membership to general trained nurses, since specialist groups like the fever nurses had a shorter training and could not readily move into positions in general hospitals. The position of the poor law nurse also remained questionable. Some of the larger poor law infirmaries provided a full general training, but many of the smaller training schools were authorised to provide only one-year training for 'assistant nurses'. In many small rural institutions, the older staff often had no training at all. Hence, while many poor law nurses supported the professional aims of the College, they feared that they would be under-represented and marginalised. During the College's first year Stanley received a series of petitions from poor law nurses, with nearly 4,000 signatures. A small group from the College council then arranged to meet with delegates from the Association of Poor Law Unions to discuss representation of poor law nurses within the College. The council noticed that the signatories to the petitions were mainly assistant nurses and probationers, and so used the meeting to reinforce the College view that membership should be confined to trained nurses, as defined by themselves. The chairman emphasised that the council 'had no desire to differentiate between poor law trained nurses and those trained in the Voluntary Hospitals', and that this was a matter of standards, not of prejudice.[42] He noted that the present membership of 6,213 nurses included 1,874 with an acceptable training in poor law institutions. However, it was also conceded that, on the principle of proportional representation, poor law nurses were under-represented on the council and an additional seat on the council was promised, though in fact this never materialised.[43]

The case of the West Derby poor law union shows how some of the early enthusiasm for the College in the poor law unions diminished when confronted by assumptions that the voluntary hospitals would dominate in local affairs as well as on the College council. West Derby urged its qualified nurses to apply for membership without delay and even reassured them that their employers, the board of guardians, would reimburse their joining fee.

> There is now no room for doubt that the College of Nursing will materially raise the standard of the nursing profession both from the pecuniary point of view and that of proficiency, and it is much to be desired that the nurses of the West Derby Union should set the example in endeavouring to improve the status of the profession.[44]

Despite this co-operative spirit, the West Derby Union, like many others, suspected that the College would not effectively represent its nurses' interests. Its correspondent wrote to the College, apologising for his 'suspicious' reaction, but he feared that poor law nurses would be 'shouldered out' in the new local centre in Liverpool. 'You know how anxious we are to advance the college in every way we can, but I am afraid if the Liverpool Centre is to be a mere adjunct to the Royal Infirmary I shall feel I have not helped those poor law Nurses whom I have advised to register'.[45]

The matron of the West Derby Union also wrote to Stanley about the College's attitude to poor law nurses, for 'the recent meeting of Matrons held in Liverpool to which no poor law Matrons were summoned does not help me gain support for the College'. She feared that the College's opponents would 'capture' the poor law nurses.[46] In the face of such unease, Stanley tried to reaffirm the democratic nature of the College council, which would be elected directly from the membership rather than from nursing organisations. Therefore, if more poor law nurses joined the College, their share of the vote would be larger, and they would have more representation.[47] This reply was somewhat disingenuous. Although nurses were the most rapidly growing group of staff in poor law institutions, by 1920 there were only some 9,000 of them, including probationers, in England and Wales, and many of these were not trained to the standard required by the College.[48] The much larger numbers of nurses in the voluntary hospitals would inevitably outweigh them in College politics. The poor law nurses were in an unsettled and anxious state. There was much political discussion about dismantling the poor law, and they needed a powerful organisation to protect their interests if this should happen. The College did not appear to offer the kind of support they needed. Outside the poor law, municipal and county hospitals were also expanding, but these included many fever nurses and asylum nurses whose training also fell short of the College's required standard. At the end of the war, this division in nursing was further compounded by an influx of former military nurses seeking careers in civilian nursing. All nurses worked long hours, and their conditions of work, pay scales, pensions and bonus entitlements were at the discretion of individual employers. The College was not yet ready to accommodate these diverse interests.

Despite its achievement in recruiting nurses nationally, and its apparently democratic principles, the College could not quell what was now widely regarded as a state of chaos in nursing at the end of the war.[49] Who would represent the nurses whose 'inferior' training debarred them from College membership? Although the College wanted to empower nurses, its high standard of training divided them and its democratic structure had severe limitations. Even its supporters recognised that by limiting membership in this way, the College compromised its position with the rank and file nurses. The

Nursing Times concluded, 'If the nurses used the powers they already possess in their Local Centres of the College we believe they would not need any other organisation; but at present there are undoubtedly certain electoral difficulties in the way of dominant representation of the rank and file on the council, while probationers are, of course, not eligible to join at all'.[50]

State registration of nurses

While the College was establishing itself, the battle for state registration of nurses continued. Although Swift and Stanley were prepared to operate a voluntary system of registration, support for state registration was so high among nurses that the College was compelled to enter the political fray. The proposed strategy was to combine with other nurses' organisations to increase their negotiating power. From its beginning the College sought a Royal Charter and hoped at first to form some kind of alliance with the Royal British Nurses' Association in order to capitalise on its chartered status.[51] By the end of 1916, after twelve months of difficult negotiations, an agreement was drawn up between the two associations to amalgamate as the Royal British College of Nursing. All amendments to Royal Charters had to be agreed by the Privy Council, and when that Council insisted on certain changes to the RBNA charter if it merged with the College, the RBNA objected and withdrew from the process. The College was not dismayed. It was by this stage more confident in its growing membership and reputation, and replied to the RBNA that it no longer needed the alliance, 'the advantage to the College of amalgamation becomes less obvious ... I am instructed to ask your Council to refrain from incurring further expenditure ... and ... to regard negotiations as practically at an end'.[52]

The College also began separate negotiations with the Central Committee for the State Registration of Nurses, a body set up in 1909 to campaign for legislation, and which drew together all the groups in favour of registration at that time. The College wanted to present a joint Bill for state registration, but differences of opinion over representation on the proposed General Nursing Council made this impossible. Each organisation prepared a separate Bill, and in 1919 both Bills were before parliament. On this occasion, the political reaction was favourable. Lloyd George's government, which shared the national gratitude for nurses' wartime efforts, finally decided to pass the long-desired legislation, but refused to adopt either of the private Bills. Promising that the government would introduce its own Bill, the newly appointed Minister for Health, Dr Christopher Addison, asked the College and the Central Committee to withdraw their Bills. He hastily drew up a Bill largely based on that of the College, although its skeletal form left much to the discretion of the proposed GNC. The College's influence over the parliamentary process was largely due to Arthur Stanley. Appointed in 1917 as the Treasurer of St Thomas's Hospital, which provided him with a house, he bombarded his extensive political connections with letters on the College's Registration Bill, followed by meetings in London clubs and his own apartments. The Nurses Registration Acts were passed on 23 December 1919. They established three separate General Nursing Councils for England and Wales, Scotland, and Ireland, and among their duties was the responsibility to compile a register of qualified nurses.

Hailed by both Bedford Fenwick and the College as a measure of their own success, the GNC for England and Wales was beset with difficulties over representation. Its council members were to be elected in due course, but in the interim the Ministry of Health appointed a 'caretaker' council, and Bedford Fenwick's enthusiasm soon diminished when she and her supporters were outnumbered on it by the College faction. Perhaps in consolation, she was given a central role in the new structure as chairman of the registration committee, but she was so rigorous in her assessment of applications that progress towards compiling a register was painfully slow, the government became alarmed, and two-thirds of the council resigned in protest before she was asked to stand down. Despite several attempts to recover a position within the system she failed to do so. The continued influence of the College on the GNC aggravated her and she continued to criticise the GNC for several years. When the caretaker council was replaced by an elected one, College nominees routed the Bedford Fenwick camp, and the GNC included leading members of the College council such as Rachael Cox-Davies, Alicia Lloyd Still, Dame Ellen Musson and Margaret Sparshott, together with Gertrude Cowlin, the College's assistant secretary. The new register for nurses included 'supplementary parts' for nurses with specialised training, as distinct from general nurse training. During the 1920s, the only GNC members independent of the College were those drawn from the supplementary parts of the register. These were the fever nurses, male nurses, mental nurses and sick children's nurses, all from sections of the profession that were not eligible for College membership.

In the ensuing years the GNC was much criticised, not least by the nursing profession, but its hands were tied by frequent government interference to protect the hospital services from the professional ambitions of nurses. Bedford Fenwick's early attempts to achieve registration have been viewed as a 'female professional project', but it has also been claimed that the project ultimately failed.[53] Although nurses ran the GNC, the Ministry of Health consistently undermined its powers, and the official voice of nursing was rendered ineffective.[54] Under severe pressure from the government, the GNC was forced to lower its requirements for registration for nurses already in practice. A one-year training was accepted for registration as an 'existing nurse', and untrained nurses with long experience or certificates of good character from the medical profession were also admitted. The GNC was at one with the College on the need to exclude VADs from the register and, since these had less than a year's training, this was achieved. New entrants to the profession would be subject to examination, and had to undergo training in a school approved by the GNC. The new national examinations did not begin until 1925, but the government would not permit the GNC to impose a single national curriculum, fearing to discourage the small training schools and inhibit recruitment.[55] The *Nursing Times*, like the College, felt that qualified nurses should come from the educated classes, and therefore complained that the GNC was failing to improve the quality of nursing recruits. At this period, claims to social superiority were made without embarrassment:

> The institution of the GNC has had its desired effect in raising the educational standard, but has done nothing towards attracting the 'right class of women'. The richer and larger hospitals, where a full training can be obtained, have little difficulty in attracting the women they require, but the general army of hospital nurses will never reach a high average standard, so long as every cottage hospital in the kingdom is a recruiting station. Many changes will have to be made before nursing constitutes an attractive profession to girls whose fathers and brothers belong to what may be termed the officer class.[56]

Class distinction of this kind was a persistently divisive factor in nursing debates and clouded the arguments over education and training standards. From the College's point of view, improvement in standards was necessary to raise not only the quality of nursing practice, but also the professional status of nurses, their remuneration and their conditions of work. In order to bring this about, a high standard was set and the experience of existing nurses measured against it. But the imposition of high standards reinforced the supremacy of those already privileged by education and class and who could afford to train in the larger teaching hospitals. This presented the College with a conundrum from the beginning: how could it increase its membership and claim to represent the whole profession, when it demanded standards of training that would inevitably exclude many nurses? As will be seen in subsequent chapters, the slow changes in the College's position on this subject reflected much wider social changes in Britain, particularly in the education and employment of women.

Nurses' pay and conditions

Once the GNC assumed statutory responsibility for compiling the register and approving the training schools, the College was free to deal with other matters. The most pressing issue was the question of nurses' pay and conditions. The College was not complacent about the economic position of nurses, and it always championed any members who appealed for help against their employers. In response to complaints from nurses of the Royal Naval Hospital at Chatham, for example, the College wrote to the Royal Naval Nursing Service, drawing its attention to the demanding hours of duty worked by the sisters. Although the Surgeon Rear Admiral thought the nurses' grievances 'nothing but Bolshevism', within weeks they were given an eight-hour day.[57] But the College differed from the trade unions in both tactics and objectives. While it wanted to improve the conditions of nurses' employment, it was equally concerned with raising their standard of education, believing that these two aims were interdependent. Trade unionism was particularly worrying for the College when it was targeted at the probationers who formed an important part of the nursing workforce. The College believed that restricting membership to trained nurses was a necessary step in raising standards, but by excluding students it deepened the division between trained and untrained nurses. Student nurses had no representation in negotiations over pay and conditions, nor were they eligible for membership of local centres that could provide professional information and a social network.

Embedded in the differences between nurses trained in the voluntary hospitals and those in the poor law infirmaries was an ideology of class and professionalism that was bitterly contested in the arguments over trade unionism for nurses. The College council was drawn from a class that generally regarded trade unions with much suspicion. It believed that any hint of unionism would alienate supporters and undermine the College. The sub-text was that unionism would also lower the status of nurses by defining them as working class. Trade unions also implied a belief in strike action that was anathema to those seeking professional status and incompatible with their belief in the 'true spirit of nursing'. However, in the years following the war, trade union membership in Britain grew rapidly, rising from four million at the beginning of the war to over eight million in 1920, and labour relations were turbulent in the years leading up to the General Strike in 1926.[58] The growing impact of trade unionism could not be ignored, nor its implications for nurses. Mental nurses had already proved the effectiveness of a nurses' union in 1919. With the force of the National Asylum Workers' Union behind them, they achieved comprehensive improvements in pay and conditions, including an eight-hour day.[59] Unionism was an obvious alternative for nurses who were excluded from the College or refused to accept its principles.

Tensions foreshadowed in discussions with the West Derby Union grew deeper. In November 1919 Maude MacCallum, a vocal supporter of Bedford Fenwick, but also a member of the College, chaired a meeting of nurses and others to debate the formation of a 'professional' union of nurses. Notice of the meeting was published in *The Times*, with the claim that it was 'arousing widespread interest throughout the profession . . . for it is well known that nurses are anxious to promote an organisation of their own'. This union was originally conceived for nurses who worked in co-operations or a non-institutional setting.[60] As such, it highlighted the exclusive nature of the College, which principally targeted hospital nurses. The meeting would be attended not only by nurses but also by important physicians and surgeons.[61] Miss MacCallum was emphatic that the desire for a nurses' trade union originated in the 'ranks of working nurses' and that no existing society was responsible for the idea. This was undoubtedly a reference to nursing groups opposed to the College, but it might be argued that the College itself was indirectly responsible, since dissatisfaction with its procedures spurred some to look towards trade unionism. The meeting lasted almost three hours and set out nineteen objectives for a new trade union. Response was mixed and boisterous. Some pointed out that the College already fulfilled the role of a union, but criticism from the platform continued with Isabel Macdonald, secretary of the RBNA and a loyal supporter of Bedford Fenwick, branding Sir Arthur Stanley a 'great danger' to nursing because of his allegedly divided loyalties. She questioned whether, as chairman of the Red Cross, and responsible for VADs, he could further their interests while also, as chairman of the College of Nursing, achieve the seemingly contradictory task of raising the standards of nursing. The vexed question of a nurses' strike was addressed from the platform to reassure all present that this was not an inevitable consequence of unionising, for 'women would think a hundred times before striking'. The organisers argued that a trade union would negotiate better pay and conditions, and be the unifying force necessary to improve the lives of all nurses. They implied that the College had not concerned itself with such mundane affairs as nurses' pay and hours of work. In fact, the College had already conducted an inquiry into these issues throughout the UK and drawn up a scale of recommended salaries for all nurses, whether employed in an institution, privately or in the community. Maude MacCallum's meeting characterised matrons as employers' lackeys who misused their authority over nurses by pressuring them to join the College; while the College, through its involvement in the Nation's Fund for Nurses, 'dragged the nurses as a war charity before the public'. In short, those in favour of unionising accused the College of supporting the interests of employers, diminishing the ability of nurses to stand up for their rights, and obstructing the progress of state registration.

Accounts of this and a subsequent meeting were reported in the nursing press. Charlotte Seymour Yapp, matron of Ashton-under-Lyne Poor Law Infirmary and an active College member, conceded the benefit of 'industrial combination' but claimed that the College already offered the benefits of unionism while at the same time preserving the vocational spirit of nursing.[62] The *Nursing Mirror* published a response from Stanley in which he outlined the achievements of the College and its active concern for the economic conditions of its members.[63] However, the nursing press was not unbiased, since one of its major figures, Sir Henry Burdett, editor of the *Nursing Mirror* and *The Hospital*, was also a College supporter. The argument in the nursing press became so personal that Maude MacCallum took out a libel action against Burdett. He died before it was heard, and his publishers had to pay damages to her.[64]

At the same time as MacCallum was seeking support for her Professional Union of Trained Nurses, the Poor Law Workers' Trade Union, established in 1918, was writing to the nursing staffs of the poor law infirmaries urging them to join. Within months it claimed that 2,500 nurses had done so, a quarter of its total membership; but the majority of its members were general poor law workers and there was some resistance to it among poor law nurses who regarded themselves as nurses rather than poor law officers. The poor law was itself riven by factions, since the older Poor Law Officers' Association had long 'opposed Trade Unionism for persons engaged in the care of the sick and the aged poor'.[65] The Association was following now standard tactics of trying to raise its professional image by pressing for an approved training qualification for its members, and it had no wish to be bracketed as a trade union. It viewed with great disquiet the growing movement among Labour-controlled local authorities to insist that their employees be union members. The Association's most active members were men – the masters of institutions, and relieving officers – but it attempted to prevent the spread of trade unionism among poor law nurses by setting up a rival State Nurses' Guild, dedicated to protecting nurses' interests in the poor law unions. The secretary of the Poor Law Officers' Association wrote to the College to explain the reasons for the creation of the new Guild, and clearly implied that the College was not a suitable body to negotiate the complex pay and pension arrangements of this constituency of local authority nurses.[66]

It appeared that no single association could cater for the various needs of nurses. For those who subscribed to the vocational ideal of nursing, there was little to attract them into a general workers' union and so they looked towards the College. But even though the College was exclusively for nurses, many busy rank and file nurses could not identify with its privileged atmosphere. For many nurses who needed to earn a living, the vocational ideal must have faltered under the pressure of hard and ill-paid labour. Yet the trade unions were still mostly dominated by men, and ignorant of the specifics of nursing. A few senior nurses compromised, and it was noted throughout the College's subsequent history that some of its members were also members of trade unions, though wishing to take advantage of the educational, insurance and other benefits offered by the College. But, for most nurses, poorly paid as they were, membership of two organisations was not an option.

The College remained anxious about competition from the trade unions. As more poor law unions fell under the control of the Labour Party during the 1920s the trade unions began to present themselves as an alternative for poor law probationers. In October 1924, Dr Joseph Muir, Medical Superintendent of Whipps Cross Hospital, West Ham, wrote to Mary Rundle, to inform her that the hospital had recently required all its staff, including nurses, to be members of a trade union. Muir pointed out that there was no union designed to meet the needs of nurses, and while he believed that the hospital would accept College membership instead, this was of no use to student nurses as they were not eligible. Consequently student nurses were unable to meet the conditions of their employment. This concerned Muir primarily because it affected recruitment: 'So far no new probationers have signed on for training since the Trade Union clause was adopted. Very soon our waiting list will be exhausted and we shall have a terrible shortage of probationers. You know what that means to a hospital and Training School'.[67]

Rachael Cox-Davis had astutely perceived the danger of excluding students, and suggested as early as 1919 that they be admitted as 'associate' members of local centres. In this way they would be able to enjoy the educational and social advantages of the centres although they would not be admitted to members' meetings or be entitled to vote. She believed that if students were brought under the influence of the College while training they would be more likely to join when they qualified. Resistance to this idea was too strong on the council, who wanted the College to represent only the fully trained nurse. But in 1926, alarmed by the worsening shortage of nursing recruits, and faced with the menace of trade unionism, the College formed a Student Nurses' Association. Students had the social benefits of membership of the College, but could not take part in its policy-making. Although the College regularly took up the cause of probationers, its relations with this group were not always harmonious, as will be seen.

Conclusion

The College was founded by influential nurses during the First World War, in an effort to prevent a post-war influx of semi-trained women into the profession. It was unashamedly elitist in its approach to nursing, and restricted its membership firstly to nurses with substantial training, and then after the coming of state registration, to nurses qualified for the general register. Because it did not give priority to state registration, it antagonised other nursing organisations campaigning for this, but it rapidly became the largest of all nursing associations, and enjoyed solid financial support from wealthy patrons.

Why was the College so successful where other attempts to organise nurses had failed? Its refusal to campaign for state registration made it more acceptable politically, and it was pragmatic in its dealings with politicians, the medical profession, the hospitals and the public. It emphasised the need for trained nurses at a time when nursing standards were causing public anxiety during the war. It also appealed to hospital management at a time when trade union influence was rising. A body that offered to dampen any tendency towards trade unionism among nurses was likely to command official support. Anti-unionism, stated so firmly in its Articles of Association, would create future difficulties for the College, which wished to improve not only the education but also the working lives of nurses; but in its early years its distance from trade unions was an advantage in winning influential support.

The First World War, far from being an inappropriate time to organise nurses, as the College's opponents argued, was the most favourable time. Peers and politicians assisted the founders' efforts, a grateful nation donated to their cause, and leading matrons were showered with honours for their contribution to the national struggle, as the growing number of Dames on the College council attested.[68] The matrons were part of a wider group of forceful middle- and upper-class women who were finding positions of influence in society, regardless of whether they regarded themselves as 'feminists'.[69] This was both a strength and a weakness for the new College, providing it with finance and a permanent establishment, but perpetuating class division in nursing. Although it hoped to become a large national organisation, the College of Nursing deliberately excluded many working nurses who lacked the lengthy training required for membership. Nurses were divided by social class, epitomised in this period by two polarised stereotypes: the middle-class matron with her spirit of service, and the working-class poor law nurse agitating for higher wages and fewer hours. The College founders were of the former type, and in setting up the College they were not challenging the *status quo*. The ensuing history of the College proved to be a long struggle to cope with the consequences of this division.

Notes

1 RCN/1/1/1916/7 folder 3, R. Cox-Davies to S. Swift, 25 Feb. 1916.
2 Registration of midwives in Scotland began in 1915, and in Ireland in 1918.
3 See Harold Perkin, *The Rise of Professional Society: England Since 1880*, 1996 edn (London and New York: Routledge, 1989), especially the introduction, for an analysis and critique of these trends.
4 Figures from Brian Abel-Smith, *A History of the Nursing Profession* (London: Heinemann, 1960), p. 258. He notes the uncertainty of these figures, and it is not clear what proportion were working in hospitals.

5 For the domiciliary nurse, a largely unexplored subject, see Barbara Mortimer, 'The nurse in Edinburgh, c. 1760–1860: the impact of commerce and professionalism', PhD thesis, University of Edinburgh, 2002.

6 Dina M. Copelman, *London's Women Teachers, Gender, Class and Feminism 1870–1930* (London and New York: Routledge, 1996), pp. 144, and Alison Oram, *Women Teachers and Feminist Politics 1900–1939* (Manchester: Manchester University Press, 1996).

7 For a wider discussion, see Anne Hudson Jones (ed.), *Images of Nurses: Perspectives from History, Art and Literature* (Philadelphia: University of Pennsylvania Press, 1988).

8 For the history of the dispute, see Abel-Smith, *Nursing Profession*, p. 62 ff, and Susan McGann, *The Battle of the Nurses: a Study of Eight Women Who Influenced the Development of Professional Nursing, 1880–1930* (London: Scutari Press, 1992). For contemporary accounts of the campaign see, Sarah Tooley, *The History of Nursing in the British Empire* (London: S. H. Bousfield, 1906) and M. A. Nutting and L. Dock, *A History of Nursing: the Evolution of Nursing Systems from the Earliest Times to the Foundation of the First English and American Training Schools for Nurses* (New York and London: G. P. Putnam and Sons, 1907).

9 RCN/1/1/1915/4, account of early meeting addressed by Stanley, n.d.

10 RCN/1/1/1916/7 folder 1, draft proceedings at meeting of Committee held at 83 Pall Mall on 29 Nov. 1915.

11 RCN/1/1/1916/7 folder 2, L. Haughton to S. Swift, 2 Dec. 1915.

12 RCN/1/1/1916/7 folder 1, list of hospitals contacted, and comments on their response.

13 RCN/1/1/1916/7 folder 2, E. Luckes to S. Swift, 19 Jan. 1916.

14 RCN/1/1/1916/7 folder 2, L. Haughton to S. Swift, 2 Dec. 1915.

15 RCN/1/1/1916/7 folder 2, Lord Knutsford to A. Stanley, 16 Jan. 1916.

16 RCN/1/1/1916/7 folder 2, A. Stanley to Lord Knutsford, 18 Jan. 1916.

17 RCN/1/1/1916/7 folder 2, A. Stanley to H. Wade Deacon, 21 Jan. 1916.

18 RCN/1/1/1916/7 folder 2, Comyns Berkeley to A. Stanley, 26 Jan. 1916.

19 McGann, *Battle of the Nurses*, pp. 35–57.

20 RCN/1/1/1915/4, Major Chapple MP speaking at a meeting to consider the formation of the proposed College of Nursing, 24 March 1916.

21 RCN/1/1/1915/4, account of early meeting addressed by Stanley. n.d.

22 For accounts of VAD nursing see Diana Cooper, *The Rainbow Comes and Goes* (London: Century Publishing, 1984) and Vera Brittain, *Testament of Youth: an Autobiographical Story of the Years 1900–1925* (London: Arrow Books, 1960).

23 *Memorandum and Articles of Association of the College of Nursing, Limited* (London: Charles Russell, 1916), s. 6.

24 *Memorandum and Articles*, s. 3 (L), (W) and (Y).

25 RCN/1/1/ 1916 folder 3, L. Haughton to S. Swift, 27 March 1916.

26 Martin Pugh, *Women and the Women's Movement in Britain 1914–1959* (Basingstoke: Macmillan, 1992), pp. 7–8.

27 John Galsworthy, 'For the nurses', *The Observer* 28 Oct. 1917.

28 RCN/22/2/4, 'The British Women's Hospital Appeal in aid of the Nation's Fund for Nurses', leaflet, n.d. [1917].

29 RCN/22/2/4.

30 RCN/23/9.

31 Abel-Smith, *Nursing Profession*, appendix 1, shows the difficulty of calculating the numbers of 'trained' nurses from the census figures. The figure of 10 per cent is extrapolated from the censuses of 1911 and 1921 and is likely to be an underestimate.

32 RCN/1/1/1915/2, 'Minutes of a conference of those interested in the College of Nursing, May 11th 1916', p. 4.

33 Gertrude Cowlin held the post of organising secretary 1919–20 before she was appointed assistant director of the League of Red Cross Societies in Geneva. She was replaced by Edith Sheriff-MacGregor.

34 RCN/3/9/1, A. Stanley to M. Sparshott, 26 Oct. 1922.

35 RCN/IR/2/1, 'A nurses' talk to nurses', July 1917.

36 McGann, *Battle of the Nurses*, pp. 130–59.

37 *NT* 22 March 1919, p. 270.

38 *Irish Nurses' Union Gazette* 13, May 1925, p. 4.

39 RCN/IR/3/4 and RCN/IR/3/6.

40 By 1928 it was losing members and seceded from the Irish Women Workers' Union, changing its name to the Irish Nurses' Organisation in the belief that an independent nurses' organisation would be more attractive to nurses.

41 CM 3 March 1921, p. 192.

42 CM 26 July 1917, p. 143.

43 An additional seat was promised after an anticipated merger between the College and the RBNA, but this merger never took place.

44 RCN/1/1/1917/1 folder 4 S–Z, H. P. Cleaver to A. Stanley, Jan. 1918. At this stage, the College asked only for a one-off membership fee from new members, not annual subscriptions.

45 RCN /1/1/1917/1 folder 3, M–R, H. MacWilliams to A. Stanley, 9 Jan. 1918.

46 RCN/1/1/1917/1 folder 3, M–R, Mrs Roberts to A. Stanley, 30 Jan. 1918.

47 See RCN/1/1/1918/3, M. Rundle to the secretary of the National Poor Law Officers Association, 24 Oct. 1918.

48 M. A. Crowther, *The Workhouse System 1834–1929* (London: Methuen, 1983), p. 136.

49 See *NT* Oct.–Nov. 1919, where 'chaos' is used to describe the state of nursing.

50 'A nurses' union?', *NT* 25 Oct. 1919, p. 1103.

51 RCN/1/1/1916/7 folder 1, draft proceedings at meeting of committee held at 83 Pall Mall on 29 Nov. 1915.

52 *Hospital* 17 Nov. 1917, p. 142, quoted in Abel Smith, *Nursing Profession*, p. 91.

53 Anne Witz, *Professions and Patriarchy* (London: Routledge, 1992), pp. 128–67, and also Robert Dingwall, Anne Marie Rafferty and Charles Webster (eds), *An Introduction to the Social History of Nursing* (London: Routledge, 1988), p. 75.

54 For an opposing view, see E. J. C. Scott, 'The influence of the staff of the Ministry of Health on policies for nursing, 1919–1968', PhD thesis, London School of Economics, 1994.

55 Abel-Smith, *Nursing Profession*, pp. 110–12.
56 'GNC and the "Right Type"', *NT* 30 Jan. 1926, p. 108.
57 CM 19 Feb. 1920, p. 588, and CM 4 March 1920, p. 598, T. Lewin to M. Rundle.
58 Henry Pelling, *A History of British Trade Unionism*, 5th edn (Basingstoke: Macmillan, 1992), p. 261.
59 The National Asylum Workers' Union was established in 1910. See Christopher Hart, *Behind the Mask: Nurses, their Unions and Nursing Policy* (London: Baillière Tindall, 1994), pp. 39–41.
60 Anne Marie Rafferty, *The Politics of Nursing Knowledge* (London: Routledge, 1996), p. 87.
61 'A nurses' trade union. London meeting today', *The Times* 25 Oct. 1919, p. 9.
62 Charlotte Seymour Yapp, 'Trades unionism versus professional union', *NM* 22 Nov. 1919, p. 140.
63 Arthur Stanley, 'The College of Nursing', *NM* 22 Nov. 1919, p. 144.
64 After a brief hearing, they provided Miss MacCallum with a public apology and a settlement of £500. 'King's Bench Division. A nurse's libel action: £500 damages. MacCallum vs Burdett', *The Times* 24 Nov. 1920, p. 4.
65 RCN/1/1/1920/2.
66 RCN/1/1/1920/2, J. Simonds to M. Rundle, 18 Sept. 1920. For the development of 'white-collar' unions in this period, see P. Armstrong, *White Collar Workers, Trade Unions and Class* (London: Croom Helm, 1986); G. S. Bain, *The Growth of White-collar Unionism* (Oxford: Clarendon Press, 1970).
67 CM 16 Oct. 1924, pp. 64–6, J. C. Muir to M. Rundle, 3 Oct. 1924.
68 Early council members who were awarded Dame Commander and Dame Grand Cross Order of the British Empire included Sarah Swift, Alicia Lloyd Still, Ellen Musson, Sidney Browne and Maud McCarthy.
69 For an overview of this argument, see Pugh, *Women and the Women's Movement*, pp. 1–5.

2

Consolidation

'Reconstruction' was a word favoured by politicians as the war drew to a close, although it implied returning to pre-war values that not all shared. Women replaced men in many jobs during the war, and were expected to return to domesticity when it ended. After women over twenty-nine won the vote in 1918, the confrontational politics of the suffragettes were not revived, but few women were elected to parliament, and the impact of war on women's position in society has caused much historical debate.[1] War did not change women's lives dramatically, but it hastened trends already apparent in 1914. Women's participation in the workforce in 1921 was no higher than in 1911, but the types of work they did were changing. Domestic service was no longer the major occupation for young women, and as their standards of education improved, they moved into offices and retailing, though the 'marriage bar', whether formal or informal, restricted such work to unmarried women. These changes had many implications for nursing. Professional recognition, so long sought, was achieved at a time when white-collar occupations for women were expanding, and nursing had to compete with these for suitable recruits.

Recent studies have emphasised that, although women did not enter parliament in large numbers, they were politically active in other ways.[2] Many former suffragists realised that obtaining the vote was only the beginning of a struggle for greater social equality, and in the inter-war period many women's associations promoted women's issues through a 'patient, well-informed, well-targeted and organised lobbying for a variety of goals'.[3] These associations included the National Union of Societies for Equal Citizenship, the Mothers' Union, the Catholic Women's League, the National Council of Women (NCW) and the National Federation of Women's Institutes.[4] Some of these groups predated the war, but after it they became more prominent vehicles for women who wanted to achieve social improvement without emulating the contentious politics of the suffragettes. Some of the largest groups were non-feminist, but were politically engaged in specific areas. They took up issues identified as within the natural areas of women's expertise. By doing so, they exercised their responsibility as citizens, contributing to social reform, yet (with a few exceptions) remaining at a distance from national politics. Nurses of the post-war period are not seen as a politically minded group, but the College of Nursing fits the model of these non-feminist women's associations, often working behind the scenes and enlisting male MPs to make their case politically. As a professional body, the College was chiefly committed to an educational agenda, but it was increasingly drawn into the more controversial area of pay and working conditions, and also into social issues that affected its members as nurses and as women.

Within a few years of its foundation the College had an established status. By 1920 its membership was 17,336 and growing steadily. The initial recruitment of over 4,000 per annum began to slow down by 1925 to approximately 800. In 1927, when the College petitioned for a Royal Charter, counsel for the College estimated that there were 50–60,000 nurses on the nursing register of whom just under half were College members.[5] However, the growth rate continued to decline and the *Annual Report* of 1931 appealed to members to help recruitment by encouraging colleagues to join. Over 3,000 new nurses a year were placed on the state register, but less than a quarter of these were joining the College. Between 1932 and 1935 the membership fell slightly, and then crept up to around 30,000 in 1939.[6] Despite slowing growth, the College became the largest nursing organisation. Its impressive headquarters reflected its aspirations to lead the profession. The Cowdrays took a personal interest in the refurbishment of 20 Cavendish Square, and the club, a limited company registered as 'The Nation's Nurses & Professional Women's Club', was known as the Cowdray Club. In keeping with Lady Cowdray's desire to promote a professional community among women, the membership rules of the club stipulated that 55 per cent should be nurses, 35 per cent women professionals and 10 per cent other suitable women. Members who were not nurses paid a higher subscription. On 22 June 1922 the refurbished building was opened in a ceremony that included laying the foundation stone of the new College building in Henrietta Street.[7] The new premises had thirty bedrooms, advertised as having all the comforts of an up-to-date West End hotel, and extra ones were available after the new College building opened in 1926. The club was popular with nurses but it never made a large profit, mainly because most members were nurses, and paid a minimal subscription. In the inter-war period the membership stayed around 4,000 and in most years the club made a small loss. Lady Cowdray was chairman of the club council from its foundation until her death in 1933, when she was succeeded by her daughter. Although the College was favoured by high-class patronage from its inception, the patrons were not conservative in their ideas. Lady Cowdray supported women's suffrage and opening the professions to women; her daughter, Lady Denman, long-time chairman of the National Federation of Women's Institutes, was also active in the birth control movement.

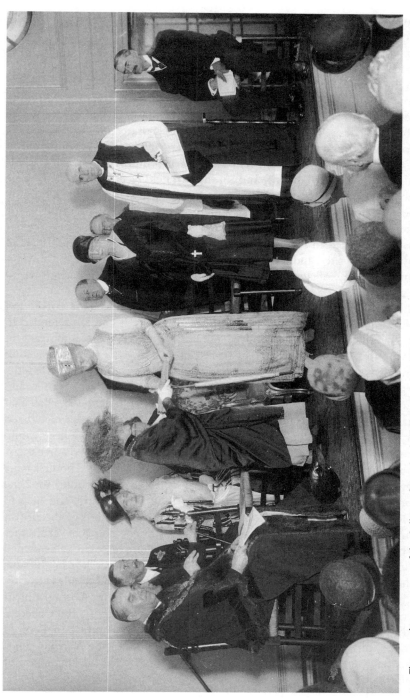

2.1 The opening ceremony of the College of Nursing building, Henrietta Place, London, May 1926 (from right to left): Neville Chamberlain, Minister of Health, the Archbishop of Canterbury, Viscountess Cowdray, Sir Arthur Stanley (behind), Queen Mary, Dame Sarah Swift, the Mayor of Marylebone (seated on left).

Queen Mary opened the main College building in May 1926, and was greeted by a guard of honour of nurses from all branches of the profession. The platform party indicated something of the College's social status, for it included the Minister of Health, Neville Chamberlain, the Archbishop of Canterbury, and the Mayor of St Marylebone. Dame Sarah Swift (as she became in 1919), President of the College, accepted the deeds of the building on behalf of the nursing profession and formally thanked the Cowdrays. The new building, designed by Sir Edwin Cooper, incorporated offices, classrooms, a laboratory, a library, meeting rooms and a large hall, and was connected to the Cowdray Club by a magnificent oak-panelled dining room. On the following two days Lady Cowdray and Sarah Swift held receptions at the College to encourage members to view their new headquarters. In 1930 the adjoining property at the corner of Cavendish Square and Henrietta Street came on the market. Lady Cowdray proposed that the College should buy the lease, for her husband, who died in 1927, had intended to extend the College and the club to cover the two sites, and the architect planned the building with this in view. By this date the College's educational and professional work had grown to such an extent that additional classrooms and offices were needed.[8]

Although the Cowdray Club was much appreciated by senior nurses and provincial matrons travelling to London for meetings, it hardly pretended to reach the whole profession. College publications were more important in achieving this, and the *Bulletin* was started in 1920 as a quarterly publication costing sixpence. In 1926 the Branches Standing Committee requested the College council to consider establishing a weekly nursing journal. Stanley and Sir Cooper Perry had 'conversations' with Sir Frederick Macmillan, chairman of Macmillan & Co., the publishers of *Nursing Times*. This journal, which dated from 1905, would become the official College journal, and the College would recommend it to members. In return, the *Nursing Times* published a free quarterly special edition of College news to supersede the *Bulletin*. The first issue under this arrangement was published on 4 December 1926. Stanley took the opportunity to appeal to members to support the new venture, and help to establish the College as 'the one great representative institution of the British nursing world'. This was probably a reference to the recent launch of yet another rival body by Ethel Bedford Fenwick: the British College of Nurses. She owned the *British Journal of Nursing*, which regularly criticised the College of Nursing, and her new college intended to award its own diplomas and to attract nurses who believed that a nursing college should be self-governing.[9] The agreement between Stanley and Macmillan was mutually beneficial, giving the College a weekly forum for its own view of nursing politics in contrast to Bedford Fenwick's, and guaranteeing the publisher a readership for the *Nursing Times*. At this stage, however, neither of these publications rivalled the circulation of the *Nursing Mirror*, which remained the best-selling journal among nurses.[10]

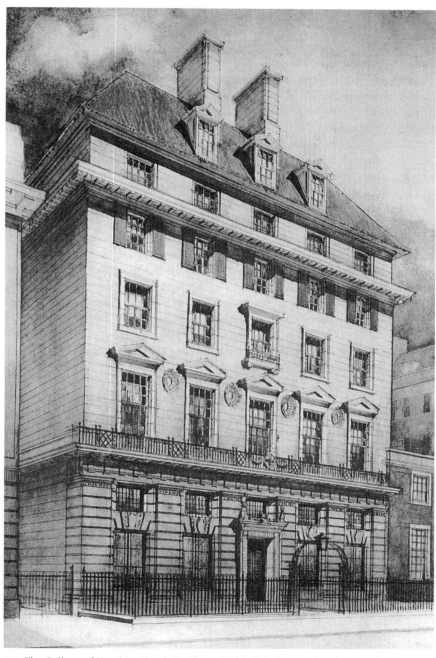

2.2 The College of Nursing, Henrietta Place, Cavendish Square, London, 1926.

In 1933, when the agreement over the *Nursing Times* came up for renewal, the College negotiated more advantageous terms, including a financial bonus for the College in proportion to the success of the journal. Two years later the College received the first cheque from Macmillan, and this paid for three months' free subscription to the *Nursing Times* for new members. The College had considerable influence over the content of the journal and the position of the editor had to be ratified by the College council. In the inter-war years the editors tended to be women who had held influential positions either on the College staff or among the membership. Following the practice in the *British Medical Journal*, the College also required that the journal not advertise nursing posts at wages below an approved minimum. Although this figure was less than the College's own recommended minimum, the policy did cause the journal some financial loss.

The College's elite status was embodied in its handsome headquarters and was consolidated shortly afterwards when Queen Mary agreed to become its patron. The Queen took much interest in nursing during the war, and the royal family was active in efforts to revive the fortunes of the voluntary hospitals after it. Thus began a tradition of royal patronage for the College that continues to the present. College events such as prize-giving and major fund-raising occasions were elaborate ceremonies, frequently in the presence of royalty, and attracted press attention. Within a year of the opening of the new building, the College founders were petitioning the Privy Council for a Royal Charter. This was the next step in their aim to position the College beside the royal medical colleges. A draft charter was prepared based on the Memorandum and Articles of Association of the College of Nursing Ltd, and this was approved by the members at an extraordinary general meeting in December 1926. However, when the proposals were sent to the Home Office, the Secretary of State replied that in the present stage of development of the College he could not properly recommend to His Majesty that the prefix 'Royal' be granted. Mary Rundle commented in a letter to Stanley, 'As I guessed, the Home Office was advised by the Ministry of Health – this is where our difficulty lies, as we have known for some time the Nursing Profession is not encouraged in its organisation in this Department'.[11] The reasons for this breach with the Ministry will be explained later, but the College's solicitors advised it to omit the prefix 'Royal' from the petition.

The College's application to the Privy Council immediately revealed divisions among the various bodies claiming to represent the nursing profession. Counter petitions were raised by the Professional Union of Trained Nurses, the Poor Law Officers' Association, the Royal British Nurses' Association, the Matrons' Council of Great Britain and Ireland, the Scottish Nurses' Association and the British College of Nurses. The Privy Council received letters in support of the College from over 200 voluntary and poor law nurses' training schools, as well as the Association of Hospital Matrons and the Poor Law Infirmary Matrons' Association. The Privy Council forwarded the petition and draft charter to the General Medical Council whose members declared their support for the College of Nursing. The hearing took place on 19 February 1928. Mitchell Banks KC represented the College. He cited its achievements, emphasising its educational work and referring to the £100,000 raised for the tribute fund, which was assisting hundreds of nurses suffering from ill health and misfortune. He referred to the College's role in, for example, improving nurses' salaries, free legal and medical advice for members, and the Federated Superannuation Scheme for Nurses and Hospital Officers. He dismissed the opposition as representing only small groups, in comparison with the College membership of 26,000, around half the nurses on the state register.

Gavin Simmonds KC, on behalf of the counter petitioners, argued that 'there is nothing which [the College] seek[s] to do which they cannot do under their present powers'. The College should be judged by its achievements measured against its original objectives, particularly the better education of nurses; and these achievements were 'simply trifling'.[12] A large proportion of its funds, he maintained, came from an 'emotional appeal' to the public, and very little was spent on education. He returned to a point much favoured by Bedford Fenwick, that the College had achieved rapid growth in membership by promising that those who paid its guinea membership fee would automatically be put on the state register when this was introduced, and then have their membership fee refunded. In defence, the College produced evidence that between 1921 and 1926 only 188 members had asked for their guinea back. The Professional Union of Trained Nurses argued that the College had been founded by the Treasurer of St Thomas' Hospital (Sir Arthur Stanley) with the support of matrons who regularly opposed any effort by nurses to improve their conditions of employment. The union believed that trade unionism was the only legal way for nurses to protect themselves in a working environment that kept them dependent on the goodwill and patronage of hospital authorities and matrons.

The Privy Council dismissed petitions from the smaller nursing bodies, such as the Professional Union of Trained Nurses with its 247 members, and the Matrons' Council with 125, but it paid more attention to the Royal British Nurses' Association and the British College of Nurses. It finally reported in favour of the College of Nursing, and on 13 June 1928 the King approved the granting of a charter. The College's case was probably assisted by its excellent social connections. The College of Nursing Ltd was wound up, and the first ordinary general meeting of the College of Nursing (incorporated by Royal Charter) took place on 19 June 1929. Stanley expressed 'a feeling of lingering regret . . . that the old company, under which such excellent work has been done, is now going to be definitely consigned to the grave. We started the old company with practically nothing except an abundant amount of hope; we are now starting this company incorporated by royal charter with very large assets, and a very great deal of good will'.[13] However, it was not until 1939 that the College received permission to use the prefix 'Royal', for in 1928 there were too many bodies which opposed its being singled out for preference.

Organisation

By 1939 there were 107 College branches around the country from Aberdeen to Truro (known as centres until 1925). They relied on the enthusiasm of local members and had to be self-supporting. Larger branches rented rooms, and some even had access to residential clubs, but most met on hospital premises. Branches were encouraged to hold their meetings in different parts of their area to give all members an opportunity to attend, since outside urban areas it could be difficult for members to travel to meetings. This led to a decision in 1925 to allow sub-branches where there were fewer than thirty members wishing to set up a branch. Branches came and went as new ones were formed and others were dissolved or went into abeyance. The Branches Standing Committee met quarterly, twice in London and twice in the provinces, and was an active agent for change. It stressed the importance of recruiting probationers, and this led to the formation of the Student Nurses' Association in 1926. The association was affiliated to the College and students could take part in activities for a reduced fee, but they did not have voting rights in elections or ballots.

The major social event of the College year was the Annual Meetings. Held over several days in late spring or early summer, and hosted by a different branch each year, the Annual Meetings offered both professional and social activities. They began with a religious service, followed by the annual general meetings of specialised sections, the Student Nurses' Association, the Branches Standing Committee and the AGM of the College. There was also a civic reception, a professional conference with invited speakers, and excursions to local hospitals and places of interest. The Annual Meetings were the forerunner of 'Congress', a more political occasion, which replaced them in the 1960s. Nurses plainly depended on the goodwill of their employers to release them for this lengthy event, and a period of freedom and sociability must have been particularly attractive to senior nurses who lived confined lives in hospital residences.

In the early 1930s, the membership in England was divided into four areas. An area organiser was appointed to each, based at Harrogate for the Northern Area, at Birmingham for the Midlands, at Bath for the Western Area, and an Eastern Area Organiser based at the College headquarters in London. They were to support the work of the branches, the units of the Student Nurses'

Association, and assist individual members within their area. Branch secretaries no longer collected the branch membership fee, which was amalgamated with the College membership subscription, and a per capita grant of 2s 6d was paid to each branch. To finance this new structure the annual subscription was raised from ten shillings to one pound, and new members paid a joining fee of one guinea. Although the College had 28,000 members, there were only 7,000 subscribing members, the others having taken advantage of various offers to become founder members, who joined before 1920 and did not have to pay an annual subscription, or compound members, who joined before 1931 and paid a life membership subscription of £5.[14] The four area organisers, the Branches Standing Committee and the branches were the basis of College organisation until the 1960s. Minor changes included the appointment of area organisers in Scotland and Northern Ireland in the 1940s, and the division of the old London branch into four separate branches in 1948.[15]

Before 1931, members of specialised sections held separate meetings in each branch, and each of these sectional committees appointed a representative to the executive committee of their branch. With the introduction of the area organisation scheme, the sections tended to hold area meetings instead of branch meetings. Resolutions from the Area Sectional Committees were referred to the executive committee of the branches and to the Central Sectional Committees at headquarters. The fourteen elected representatives who formed the Central Sectional Committee advised the council on professional matters in their own field. The system resembled the BMA, with representatives from specialist interests as well as general practitioners. It worked effectively for several decades, and proved flexible in accommodating the growth of new nursing specialties alongside the larger group of general nurses.

The educational work of the College

The College's original aim was to promote better education and training for nurses, through a uniform curriculum, approved training schools and central examinations. When the three General Nursing Councils took over these tasks, the College was free to pursue a different educational programme. Before the College was founded there was little provision for nurse education outside the hospital training schools. When a nurse qualified after three or four years' training, she could start work as a staff nurse in a hospital or as a private nurse on her own or with an agency. If she wished to continue her education, she could choose between midwifery, district nursing or public health nursing. The former required a year's training at a maternity hospital, while district nurses could obtain six months' training at the Queen Victoria's Jubilee Institute for Nurses. For public health nursing, which offered an increasing number of openings such as school nursing and health visiting, there was no required training, but some local authorities trained their own nurses. A few hospitals, realising the need for further training, set up in-house courses for their own nurses, particularly in areas of growing demand, such as theatre nursing and ophthalmic nursing. Mary Rundle, as matron of the Royal Hospital for Diseases of the Chest before the war, arranged a course on tuberculosis nursing.[16] These efforts were tentative, and the College's lectures filled a gap.

The College council encouraged members to take advantage of the many lectures offered in all College centres, and, as has been seen, these were much more popular than the routine meetings concerned with College business. As the only form of post-registration education available to nurses, the courses provided much-needed information on new treatments and techniques. Educational work developed in response to members' demands. Nurses preferred evening courses because most could not attend daytime lectures, and postal courses were also offered. For nurses, with their long working hours, the courses required considerable personal commitment. By 1930 over twenty courses were available, including applied anatomy and physiology, hospital administration, industrial legislation, public health, venereal diseases, tuberculosis nursing and public speaking. Most of the lectures were given by outside experts.

The College also developed more formal courses leading to recognised qualifications, and with the prestige of a university connection. The training of sister tutors was a major strategy to formalise and improve the standard of the teachers of nurses, and the networks of the College's founders were essential in achieving this.[17] Supported by the College's honorary secretary, Sir Cooper Perry, now Vice-Chancellor of the University of London, the College proposed a certificated course for sister tutors at King's College for Women.[18] Teaching began in 1918 and although the number of trained sister tutors remained a fraction of the total number of tutors required in the country, the course raised the aspirational standard of nurse teaching and influenced nursing schools throughout the country to employ sister tutors. The sister tutor course forged links between the College council and the University of London, and a second course, a Diploma in Nursing, was established in 1925.[19] This was an extra-mural course taught by the College of Nursing. There was already a model for such an arrangement, for an earlier Diploma in Nursing had been started at the University of Leeds in 1921, as a collaborative venture between that university and the General Infirmary, Leeds. Euphemia Innes, matron of the General Infirmary, who devised this course, had close connections with the College, being a member of the College council and its Education Committee.[20] In 1925 the Ministry of Health approved the College's six-month training course for health visitors, which involved lectures at Bedford College for Women and at the College of Nursing, together with practical work at the

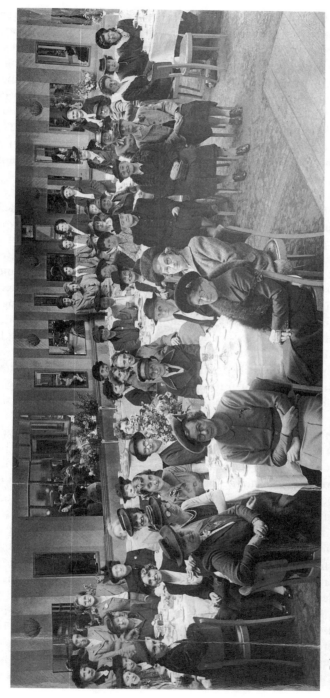

2.3 Private Nurses' Section study day, London, 1930s.

Women's University Settlement in Southwark. The College also offered evening lectures for practising health visitors, and these were also attended by nurses preparing for the University of London diploma. Bedford College and King's College for Women had been set up to cater for the small group of women who aspired to university education at the end of the nineteenth century. These women's colleges, which together with Royal Holloway became part of the University of London, had developed courses in 'women's sub-jects', such as household and domestic sciences. It was logical for the College of Nursing to approach them to develop higher education courses for nurses, for it anticipated a warmer response than from most of the more traditional universities.

Although these university contacts led to vocational diplomas, they were not part of the mainstream of university education. The College council knew that a university attachment would lend prestige to its educational work, but such courses were aimed at enhancing the status of a small group of nurses, and improving their knowledge, rather than a serious attempt to infiltrate the universities. In a period when even a secondary education for women was something of a luxury, there was little hope that nursing could become a university subject, though the council hoped that a Chair of Nursing might be established at the University of London in due course. To this end, in late 1919 the College appealed to local centres to commit regular donations to fund the chair. Although funds trickled in for many years, this ambition was not achieved. The first university department of nursing was not established until 1956, and the first chair of nursing fifteen years later.[21] This long gestation period emphasises the distance that had to be travelled before nursing was accepted as a suitable subject for university education.

The sister tutor courses led to a new arrangement that affected the future structure of the College and enabled it to accommodate specialist interests within a wider body. The sister tutors in the College wanted a forum for their own concerns, and a Sister Tutor Section of the College was set up in 1922, with membership restricted to College members in nurse teaching posts. The section defined its task as the theoretical education of the nurse in training, and aimed to standardise teaching throughout nursing schools in Britain. Section members saw themselves as pioneers of nurse education and defend-ers of British standards. As the most highly educated nurses within the profes-sion, the early sister tutors were its educational leadership, although their numbers were small. In 1927 membership of the section was 169, and grew to 376 by 1937. The sister tutors were the first to set up a specialised section within the College, followed by the public health nurses and private nurses. This laid the pattern for the professional structure of the College, with specialised inter-est operating alongside the general nurses. The section structure had two advantages: the section committees acted as specialist advisers to the College council, but also inhibited the tendency of specialist groups of nurses to form their own associations outside the College. The midwives, already possessing their own institute, never came within the College's structure, and in an age of growing specialisation, it was necessary to retain the loyalties of nurses with many different interests.

In the early 1920s the College also participated in limited but prestigious international plans for nurse training, reflecting the hopeful atmosphere of the time. The war stimulated international developments in public health, and, in the USA, the movement for university schools of nursing. Post-qualification education for nurses developed rapidly in North America, where courses in public health nursing were begun at several colleges.[22] Through this growing international public health movement the College of Nursing became involved in one of the first university courses for nurses. After the war the League of Red Cross Societies was established as a humanitarian counterpart to the League of Nations. Based in Paris, the League of Red Cross Societies sponsored nurse training in public health, to equip nurses for setting up new public health programmes in countries devastated by war. The courses empha-sised the importance of nurses in rebuilding Europe:

> The aim of this course is to prepare nurses for executive and teaching positions in all fields of public health nursing, that is visiting nursing, child welfare, school and TB nursing, prenatal and maternity nursing under state, municipal or Red Cross authorities. The functions of the public health nurse are those of health education, the prevention of disease through the early recognition of symptoms and defects and bedside care of the ill.[23]

The British Red Cross Society was one of the founders of the League, and the connection of Stanley and Swift with both the Red Cross and the College of Nursing ensured that London was chosen as the centre for these new public health courses. The Americans, who were the force and finance behind the League, were determined that international public health courses for nursing students should be based in a university. Here too, the College's links with King's College through Cooper Perry proved useful. The first course for international students, a one-year certificate offered jointly by the College and the League of Red Cross Societies, was held in 1920–21 at the Household and Social Science Department of King's College for Women.[24] Nineteen nurses from eighteen countries took the course, mainly from Europe, but including Canada, Japan, Mexico and New Zealand. The students received scholarships from their national Red Cross Societies and from the League, and were chosen because of their leadership qualities during their war service. The courses transferred to Bedford College for Women in 1921, where the international students could also attend some of the courses in the Social Sciences Department. In 1924 a second course for international students was

introduced for nurse administrators and nurse tutors, in response to demand
from several countries where Red Cross Societies were helping to set up nurse
training schools. In all, 350 students from forty-seven countries attended the
courses between 1920 and 1939. Many of these international students became
leaders of nursing in their own countries, establishing public health programmes and training schools. Although the camaraderie among these nurses
was shattered by the Second World War, several of them later became international leaders in the International Council of Nurses, the World Health
Organisation (WHO) and the United Nations Relief and Rehabilitation
Agency.[25]

As the College's role in running such courses became recognised, it took
part in an expanding range of educational activities, often at the request of
external bodies. For example, a five-day course was offered for nurses who
were taking on the inspection of nursing homes under new legislation. The
Colonial Office requested courses for their West African nursing staff, and the
BBC asked the College to nominate a member to broadcast health talks.[26] As
the work of the Education Department grew, the College's reputation as a
provider of post-registration courses became well established. It developed
new courses jointly with specialised institutions: on child guidance with the
London Child Guidance Council; on psychology with the Institute of Medical
Psychology; on occupational therapy with the Maudsley Hospital; and, at the
request of the CMB, a special course to prepare students for the midwife
teachers' examination in co-operation with the Midwives Institute. During
the 1930s the Education Department offered regular study tours for members
to European countries including Finland, Hungary and Russia. It also became
involved, at their request, in finding places for foreign nurses coming to
Britain for work experience.[27]

In the spring of 1927 Rachael Cox-Davies wrote a paper for the Education
Committee on future educational policy. Now that they had a new building
with classrooms, laboratories and a library, she believed that the time was
right to develop a more advanced programme. The College's application for
a Royal Charter would raise questions about its educational work. She believed
that the number of women entering nursing would increase to meet the
requirements of modern medicine, and that nurses would need a better and
more technical training. The General Nursing Councils had no power over
the economic or social conditions of the profession, nor could they assist in
post-registration training. The College was in a position to fill this gap, and
Cox-Davies had ambitious plans to attract grants from the Board of Education
similar to those given to other education authorities, by providing preliminary
training courses for probationers from the smaller training schools. She
proposed that the College should also develop its post-registration work,
including courses for international students, travelling scholarships, and the

establishment of a chair of nursing at a women's university. She assumed (wrongly, as it turned out), that it would probably take five or more years before a chair was founded. To fund this programme she recommended that the College set up an educational trust of at least £100,000.

The council accepted many of her suggestions, and appointed a full-time education officer in July 1927. Previously the post was part-time, held by officers such as Gertrude Cowlin, who was also College librarian. The first full-time officer was Ruth Hallowes, an Oxford graduate. She spent her first year on a Rockefeller Travelling Scholarship in the USA and Canada studying hospital administration and economics. At this time, British nurses referred to any post-registration course or qualification as 'post-graduate', although College courses were not post-graduate in the formal sense, since the students did not have a university degree. Nurses in North America, where nursing was taught in several universities by the late 1920s, did not consider this an appropriate description, but British universities would not accept nursing as a suitable subject for university education. Courses run by the College in conjunction with universities could not require the same entry standards as regular university courses, since there would be so few eligible applicants. Many British nurses who wanted to study nursing at university level went to the USA or Canada on travelling scholarships in the inter-war years.

Although post-registration courses were valuable in extending nurse training, keeping nurses abreast of new developments, and assisting in the creation of an important group of nurse educationalists, they were inevitably limited in scope. It was rare for even the most prestigious hospitals to fund their nurses to attend such courses, and most of the students either had to pay the fees themselves – taking an unpaid career break to do so, if their hospitals permitted – or to apply for one of a small number of scholarships offered by the College. Increasing the number of scholarships was a high priority for the College, and it drew on money from the endowment fund originally created by the Nation's Fund for Nurses, together with other bequests and donations. These now included a fund set up in memory of Lady Cowdray after her death in 1933. Although, as will be seen, the College eventually succeeded in winning government subsidies for its courses, it did not have resources to fund a national system of post-registration training. While its post-registration courses were available to all nurses and not just to members, in the inter-war years only the privileged few could afford the time and the relatively low fees. This reinforced the elitist image of the College among the rank-and-file nurses.

Conditions of work

As its negotiations over the Royal Charter showed, the College's relations with the Ministry of Health were not particularly cordial by 1928. This reflected nearly a decade of growing dissatisfaction with the Ministry's perceived failure to recognise the importance of nursing. Although the College's main priority was its educational work, it also assumed a responsibility for nurses' welfare, and this drew it inexorably into debate over their pay and conditions. Employment negotiations and educational courses were similar, however, in that they included nurses who were not necessarily College members. The College aimed to be a voice for the nursing profession, not only for its own members, and this brought it into confrontation with government agencies from an early period.

When the war ended, the College confronted a number of employment issues, including poor salaries, long working hours and the inclusion of nurses in the National Insurance scheme. This pushed it into the same area as the trade unions, even though many in the profession abhorred the idea of trade unionism among nurses. The College looked for allies among like-minded women's organisations, particularly the National Council of Women. The NCW had its origins in the National Union of Women Workers, dating back to the 1880s. Although its original name suggested a workers' union, it was in fact run by middle-class women who regarded their work, either paid or voluntary, as a vocation. The union concerned itself with the conditions of all women workers, and acted as a 'federation of all societies dealing with industrial, philanthropic and educational matters'.[28] Through its regular conferences and educative reading programme, it encouraged women to learn the conventions of committees, develop administrative skills and voice their opinions in public. Speakers addressed its branches on topics such as food reform, health insurance and maternity and child welfare. Although not an overtly political group, the NCW conducted enquiries and advised MPs in parliamentary debates concerning the working lives of women. The College sent delegates to NCW meetings and conferences, and the College council regularly discussed NCW resolutions. Hence the College commented on such subjects as the national and international traffic in women, women police patrols and working conditions for women, as well as on more domestic matters such as infant protection and family health. Through its links to women's organisations of this kind the College became part of a wider political debate while keeping itself at a distance from the confrontational trade unionism of the 1920s.

Relations with the NCW were nevertheless strained at the beginning of 1919 when the College and the NCW appointed separate committees to investigate the working conditions of nurses. In February 1919 the NCW invited the College to send representatives to a preliminary conference on how to reduce the long hours of probationers. The initiative for this conference came from Dr Herbert C. Crouch, who was medical adviser to the Nurses' Co-operation for many years, and saw many nurses suffering from chronic complaints that he believed were due to the hardships they experienced as probationers. He offered the NCW £500 to cover the committee's costs.[29] The College had already decided that the economic position of nurses must be a priority, and was setting up its own investigation. At first the two organisations agreed that it would be wasteful to have two committees deliberating on the same subject, and that they should work together; but it quickly became clear that co-operation would be difficult. The College was adamant that the committee should consist of women whose names would carry weight and should include only a small number of nurses, while the NCW proposed that its committee comprise two representatives from each nursing organisation. As these largely consisted of the various associations set up by Bedford Fenwick, all sharing a common membership and a common antipathy to the College, the College was not happy with this suggestion. After several meetings between Stanley and Dr Crouch and much correspondence, the College gave up its attempts to 'expose the hollowness of [Mrs Bedford Fenwick's] pretensions' and decided that the College Salaries Committee had already made such progress that a merger was impracticable.[30] The President of the NCW expressed her exasperation with the College in a letter to *The Times* but the College appreciated the importance of publicity and the value of involving public figures in its work.[31] Its ten-person committee consisted mainly of well-known women, former suffragists with a distinguished record of public service, including Sybil, Lady Brassey, Dame May Whitty, Rosa Barrett, Elizabeth Haldane and the author Janet E. Courtney.

The Special Committee on Salaries and Conditions of Employment of Nurses sent questionnaires to employers of nurses nationwide asking for details of salaries and conditions. It then drew up a report with a recommended scale of salaries, and circulated it to hospitals and other employers. The report favoured forty-eight hours as a maximum working week for all nurses.[32] This encouraged some hospitals and other institutions to reconsider their position, and several made efforts to improve the conditions of their trained nurses. Nurses were very popular during the war, and the College was able to exert moral pressure on hospital managers to reward them with higher pay. Nevertheless, salaries rarely rose to the figures recommended by the College, although council continued to intervene in specific cases at the request of individual nurses. Through the College Appointments Bureau, further pressure was applied on prospective employers to raise low salaries, and the council, as previously noted, persuaded the nursing press not to print advertisements for nursing posts at less than the recommended rates.[33] The scale recommended in the report was revised in 1920, and was cited by groups of nurses in local negotiations over pay. More importantly, the nursing shortage meant that hospitals had to make special efforts to recruit young nurses, and by adopting the College's scale of salaries they could demonstrate their superior working conditions.

In 1919–20 two contentious government measures, on hours of employment and on National Insurance, demanded a response from the College. The first aimed to regulate working hours for all employees.[34] During the war, the government tried to increase production at all costs, and pre-war legislation that limited the working hours of certain groups of workers was relaxed. Scientific studies showed that excessive working hours were counter-productive in industry, but long working hours were common during the war years. Some factory workers were on duty for up to 108 hours per week and shifts of twenty-nine hours were documented.[35] Nurses, already working long hours before the war, were under particular pressure to work whatever hours seemed necessary to deal with emergencies. Although the armistice lessened the urgency for high factory productivity, the war had altered workers' expectations, and the unions were not prepared to return to business as usual. At first, all parties were prepared to co-operate in legislation to reduce the hours of labour, seeing it as a 'debt of honour' to the workforce. The growing strength of the unions and the Labour Party also ensured that the conditions of workers would stay on the agenda. The government's first Bill in 1919 disintegrated because of the difficulty of adjusting it to the routines of agriculture and certain other occupations, but a further Hours of Employment Draft Bill in 1920 prescribed a maximum of forty eight hours per week with overtime to be paid as extra wages, and its promoters argued that in times of reconstruction it would benefit not only the workers but also productivity and the economy. In fact, most industries after the war honoured the forty-eight-hour week without legal compulsion, but nurses' average weekly hours could vary from fifty-two to seventy-one for daytime shifts and fifty-nine to eighty-four for night duty.[36] Hence nurses' hours were comparable to the unregulated work of domestic servants rather than to the restricted hours of women in industry.

The proposed Bill, supported by the trade unions, was intended to cover most occupations, but the possibility of exemptions was not ruled out, leaving the way open for much backstairs negotiation. While the College aimed for better conditions for nurses, and to negotiate on their behalf, it also wanted to uphold the professional status of nurses and did not wish to respond like a trade union.[37] Nurses' working hours were not a straightforward issue for the College, which sought for them the same self-regulation as other professions who were not public employees. But it knew that, in practice, nurses were exploited in the same way as many unregulated workers. Nurses were in a weak position compared with other professions. Schoolteachers' hours were defined by the school day, while most other white-collar occupations had fixed office hours. Doctors often worked long hours, but medicine was a profession with much higher rewards than nursing. Hospital nurses suffered from the double pressure of long hours set both by their employers, and by the hospital matrons, who would demand extra time from nurses whenever a ward was under pressure.

The College council knew that some poor law guardians had already implemented a forty-eight-hour week, that trade union activity had assured an eight-hour day for mental nurses, and that the Bill offered a degree of protection for many nurses. It appointed a committee to consider the Bill in January 1920, and was pleased when the Ministry of Labour requested an unofficial meeting with Mary Rundle to discuss nursing opinions on the Bill.[38] In March the College sent a delegation to discuss the redrafting of the Bill, but Sir David Shackleton, on behalf of the Ministry, was reluctant to make any amendments. He suggested, however, that nurses could be exempted from the Bill but that a Special Order should be inserted in the Bill making it possible for them to be included subsequently.[39] Many members of the College wrote indignantly to the council about the inclusion of nurses in the Bill, for they believed that hours of work should not be prescribed for an occupation that was 'founded upon a spirit of service'. Control of this kind would interfere with the nurse's power to give time to her patient as necessary. Nurses' flexible working hours were defended as a professional matter that would not benefit from state intervention. Although the College's report on nurses' salaries had favoured a forty-eight-hour week in 1919, in response to members' objections it now revised its recommendations, and raised the maximum number of hours from forty-eight to fifty-six per week. The salaries' report was produced by a committee of mainly lay people who assumed that nurses' hours should be similar to other occupations. The College council had originally accepted the committee's recommendation of forty-eight hours, but did not anticipate that this would be enforced by legislation. Members' reaction to the inclusion of nurses in the proposed Hours of Employment Bill showed that nurses who stressed the 'service' element of their work did not have a union view of working hours. The most vocal were, inevitably, matrons and senior nursing sisters. The nursing shortage in the hospitals was worsening, and many voluntary hospitals were in desperate financial straits. Hospital governors like Lord Knutsford feared that a forty-eight-hour week would force them to employ a much larger nursing staff.[40] The stand taken by matrons who wrote to the College to protest about the Bill was an early warning for the College of the tension between its labour relations role and the opinions of nurse managers among its members.

The College held a members' referendum on hours of work through its local centres. Feelings clearly ran high in the twenty-three centres that replied, but the level of response, as noted earlier, was disappointing. Brighton and Hove claimed its members to be 'most emphatic' that legislation on working hours for nurses would be 'putting the profession on the same basis as manual labour . . . in contradiction to the highest instincts of the profession'.[41] Leicester favoured the fifty-six-hour week over the forty-eight hours proposed in the Bill, but noted that its members were against inclusion in principle 'as savouring too much of trade unionism'. In Edinburgh, 50 per cent of voters favoured complete exemption of nurses from the Bill.[42] However, the majority who responded accepted the inclusion of nurses in the Bill, though somewhat reluctantly, and supported the College committee's recommendation of a fifty-six-hour week in preference to forty-eight hours. College members, of course, were hardly representative of all nurses. Most, either by choice or default, were unmarried, and their social lives often revolved around the hospital. The College also had an active membership among matrons and older nurses who expected to control the working hours of juniors as ward routine demanded. The GNC parted company with the College over the Bill, and Bedford Fenwick, supported by the GNC's poor law and private nurse members, ensured that it rejected the College's fifty-six hours in favour of forty-eight hours. The GNC, like the College, objected to the Ministry of Labour's intervention, and requested that the newly formed Ministry of Health draft its own Bill to regulate nurses' hours.[43] The College's reaction to the Bill might be compared with that of the Professional Union of Trained Nurses. This body, with a high proportion of poor law nurses, undertook its own survey and supported the forty-eight-hour week. The College council decided to petition for a Special Order allowing nurses exemption from the Bill, but in the event, the hostility of industrial employers caused the draft Bill to be dropped, to be revived again unsuccessfully in 1924.

The College was still in some disarray over working hours, and in 1927 it informally agreed with a forty-eight-hour week for nurses suggested by the Labour opposition.[44] In 1930 another Bill to regulate nurses' hours and salaries was presented to parliament by the Labour MP Fenner Brockway. It would have reduced nurses' hours to forty-four a week, except in life-threatening situations. Surprisingly, there were several points raised in this document, such as statutory meal breaks, that brought agreement between the Labour Party and the College. However, the Labour view was that nurses could achieve progress only through trade unionism, and the College would not accept this. Brockway's Bill was not well received generally and the College Parliamentary Committee's response was 'that it is not in the interest of the nursing profession or of the public that standards of hours of duty and salary should be enforced by legislation since experience has shown that these questions can best be settled by the nurses themselves acting through their professional organisation'.[45] This Bill also failed, but as in the matter of salaries, the College won some improvements by negotiating with individual hospital managements without committing itself to a national strategy. The issue was not resolved, being very divisive within the profession, and in 1937 it contributed to a peak of trade union activity among nurses that challenged the College's ability to speak for the majority of the profession.

Unemployment insurance

The second piece of legislation requiring the College's attention concerned unemployment insurance. During the war unemployment fell as men were conscripted into the services, and women took their place in many occupations. The government put resources into training women and in 1918 was unprepared for the return to peace. A brief post-war boom was followed by a slump and rising unemployment. Conditions worsened rapidly as the government was faced with growing industrial unrest and feared that unemployment would encourage the rise of 'Bolshevism'.[46] During the 1920s a series of Unemployment Acts were passed for reasons varying from the preservation of public order to the need for national economy, but one solution with obvious appeal to government was to bring a larger section of the workforce under the umbrella of compulsory unemployment insurance. Nurses, like certain other low-paid workers, were exempt from the 1911 National Insurance Act, but were included in an Unemployment Bill in 1920, and once more the College sought the views of its members through a referendum. Response was low, but a second referendum was held, and local centres were urged to encourage participation by their members. This time, forms sent out to all institutions and authorities employing nurses returned 35,000 signatures against the inclusion of nurses, arguing that the 'unemployment tax' was an unnecessary expense in a profession where salaries were too low to support insurance payments, and involuntary unemployment virtually unknown. The response was a reflection on the low pay of hospital nurses, who were mostly young women expecting to leave the profession on marriage, but it did not take into account the position of domiciliary nurses working on their own account, for whom unemployment was a regular problem. Rallied by the College, individual nurses as well as local centres lobbied their MPs and the Minister of Labour in support of an amendment making a special case for nurses. It was presented to parliament by the Conservative MP Leonard Lyle, a member of the College council. The amendment was successful and when the Act passed in April 1922, nurses were exempt. Such was the feeling of the members that a number donated the equivalent of one week's unemployment insurance contribution to the College as a mark of gratitude.[47]

Early state efforts at social insurance thus failed to reach the nursing profession, leaving them vulnerable to unemployment, long-term illness, and (if not supported by a husband) to poverty in an old age reliant on a state pension. Public sector employers did offer occupational pensions to nurses who worked until retirement age. The Local Government and Other Officers Superannuation Act (1922) allowed local authorities to provide a pension scheme to their public health nurses, although it was not compulsory for them to do so. This was based on a retirement age of sixty-five, which, Mary Rundle commented, was 'ten years longer than a woman can do justice to her hard, strenuous out-of-door duties'.[48] Public health nurses commonly retired at the age of fifty-five, having received a salary that made saving or contributing to a pension scheme very difficult. Private nurses led precarious lives financially, and invariably suffered intermittent periods of unemployment. Although they earned relatively high wages, the insecurity of the work left them fearful of the commitment involved in regular payments to pension or insurance schemes. Hospital nurses often postponed their retirement unduly for financial reasons, and if they moved from one hospital to another, or out of hospitals and into another branch of nursing, their pension entitlement was lost. Like other low-paid workers, they needed the security of national insurance and pension schemes, but lacked the income to fund them, while the schemes offered by most employers were unsatisfactory.

In 1922 the College appointed an actuary who drew up recommendations along the lines of the Federated Superannuation Scheme for Universities. Under this scheme, the employer's contribution would be 10 per cent and the nurse's 5 per cent; nurses could retire at fifty-five; and they could move freely from one post to another taking their policies with them. 'The scheme would cover the whole of the nurse's working life and it would remove a hardship that now deters many suitable women from taking up nursing'.[49] The College scheme was well received, and representatives of the British Hospitals Association, the Association of Hospital Officers and the College of Nursing formed a committee to agree its final terms. Known as the Federated Superannuation Scheme for Nurses and Hospital Officers, it extended to all nurses, including private nurses and hospital administrative and clerical staff, and was incorporated under the Companies Act in 1928. Despite support from the Ministry of Health, the proposed interchangeability between pension schemes of the voluntary and public services proved to be a problematic issue requiring government legislation. But the response was encouraging and established the scheme's popularity among nurses and their employers.[50] The retirement age was set at fifty-five, a clear indication of the exacting nature of the nursing profession.[51]

From its early days the College offered free legal advice as a service to members. Each year the *Annual Report* thanked its honorary solicitors, Charles Russell and Co., for their advice and assistance. It was assumed that hospital authorities accepted legal responsibility for the actions of their nursing staff, but by 1935 the council decided that the public was becoming more litigious, and that hospitals were not protecting the fully trained nurse, who was held personally liable. The council believed that nurses needed to insure themselves against risks incurred in their professional work, and negotiated an indemnity policy with an insurance company. Members were encouraged to avail themselves of this special policy, which cost six shillings per year for claims not exceeding £500, and seven shillings and sixpence for claims not exceeding £1000.[52] The indemnity policy, which was not offered by the trade unions at this time, was later incorporated into the membership fee, and became a major feature in the RCN's recruitment drives. It also included a 'Good Samaritan' clause, to protect nurses who came to the aid of the public in incidents outside the workplace.

The Ministry of Health and local authority nursing in the 1920s

The creation of the Ministry of Health in 1919, with a separate Board of Health in Scotland, followed many years of debate on the responsibilities of the state towards the nation's health. The Ministry's remit covered a wide range of public services, including housing and slum clearance, food regulation, health insurance, epidemiology and environment, and maternal and child welfare.[53] More problematically, it also took over responsibility for the poor law and its institutions. Supporters hoped it would be a major step towards a more integrated national health service, but political compromises necessary for its creation reduced its effectiveness. The Ministry is usually seen as weak, uneasily balancing central, local and private interests, including poor law authorities and the private insurance companies that managed most of the nation's statutory health insurance.[54] The voluntary hospitals remained independent of the Ministry and it lacked authority to effect change in the way its supporters hoped. The first Minister of Health, Dr Christopher Addison, began an ambitious and expensive programme of public housing, but his career was cut short when Lloyd George was forced to sack him, under much pressure from economy-minded Conservatives in the coalition government.[55] This early failure set the tone for the Ministry's future, as it became increasingly concerned with cost efficiency, and early hopes of radical intervention in the nation's health faded.

In the midst of post-war reconstruction, nursing did not feature prominently in public policy, and successive governments have been accused of merely responding to nursing shortages without establishing nursing as an integral and permanent part of the consultation process. The Ministry employed no nurses on its staff. However, Elizabeth Scott suggests that in its first years the Ministry of Health realised the potential of a co-operative relationship with nursing and sought to use this to its own advantage.[56] The Ministry's early relations with the College seem to support this argument. Nurses were generally less suspicious of the new Ministry than were the doctors, who were still coming to terms with the National Insurance Act of 1911 and their new role as panel doctors. The urban poor law infirmaries were expanding, and employing more nursing staff. In some areas their services were beginning to rival the voluntary hospitals, as they engaged consultants and conducted more surgical operations. A focus on nursing might improve the public image of the poor law, and an alliance with nursing might be convenient to the new Ministry. The Ministry began well, from a nursing perspective, through Addison's support for state registration for nurses in 1919.

The College courted the Ministry, using strategies that were distinctly conservative compared with the more militant rhetoric of the trade unions. In situations unfavourable to nursing it adopted a conciliatory approach. Unlike the unions, who were in confrontational mood after the war, the College negotiated towards a political allegiance with the Ministry, keeping it informed of nursing issues in the local authorities and seeking support for its own views. Although poor law nurses often felt excluded from the College, as noted in chapter 1, they still looked towards it as a defender of nursing interests, and the College received many letters from both members and non-members, complaining of working conditions. Although in individual cases the College could act only on behalf of its members, in collective grievances it was prepared to speak for all nurses. In 1921 the nurses of Plymouth Greenbank Infirmary wrote to the College council requesting a copy of the College's scale of salaries, and asked for support in fighting their board of guardians' recent reduction in bonuses by 50 per cent, bringing a charge nurse's salary to £59 per annum for a fifty-seven-hour working week.[57] The council agreed to write to the Ministry of Health on the reduction of bonuses in poor law hospitals and to send a copy to the Poor Law Officers' Association.[58]

The College persistently urged the Ministry to work with it in reviewing nurses' pay and conditions so that a 'voluntary professional organisation may prove to be the best medium for obtaining a high standard of Nursing Service'.[59] Nursing was affected by political changes at the local level. The Labour Party produced two short-lived governments in the inter-war period, but had much greater success in consolidating its hold on local administration in many areas. Advertisements requiring local authority and poor law nurses to belong to trade unions were becoming more frequent, a tactic used especially by Labour-controlled boards of guardians. In such cases Mary Rundle wrote not only to the editors of the relevant papers but also to the Ministry of Health: 'the [College] Council is confident that you will not sanction coercion of this nature, and has instructed me to draw your attention to this matter, in the hope that you will be able to ensure the appointment in question being thrown open to all nurses who are qualified for the post'.[60] In reality the Ministry had little power over local authorities but it co-operated with the College as far as possible. When the Borough of Bermondsey imposed a similar condition on its employees the Ministry intervened to prevent it at the College's request, by writing to the Bermondsey town clerk: 'the Ministry are of the opinion that a local authority should not make the terms of service of members of their staff depend upon such a condition, and they trust that the Borough Council will not insist upon it'.[61] The Ministry, of course, did not wish to encourage unionism that would lead to demands for higher salaries in the public services.

Boards of guardians who insisted that their nurses belong to a trade union were not exceeding their legal powers, and so the Ministry's power was limited. This was an issue that could be resolved only through negotiation. In June 1925, when the Stepney board of guardians imposed this condition on their nurses, the College asked them to accept College membership in lieu of membership of a trade union. At first this was refused, but after some reconsideration a representative from the College was allowed to attend the Stepney Board's finance committee, and in September a College delegate was permitted to address the Stepney nurses on the work of the College and its student nurses' association. In March 1926 the Stepney guardians agreed to accept membership of the College instead of a trade union among its nursing staff, and to refer to the College scale of salaries when revising its nurses' pay, but the College was still not accepted as an official negotiator.[62] Like the trade unions, the College was seeking improvements in nurses' pay and conditions, but it was anxious to be seen as a professional body, and not a union. By courting the Ministry it distanced itself from Labour local authorities as well as from the trade unions, while trying to protect its members. For the Ministry, the College's reputation and its support among some poor law nurses was a useful weapon against insubordinate local authorities. After a series of clashes with some famously militant local councils, and the collapse of the General Strike in 1926, Baldwin's Conservative government passed a Trade Disputes and Trade Unions Act in 1927, preventing local authorities from forcing their employees to join a union. This temporarily solved the College's difficulties with local government, but the subject of compulsory union membership resurfaced after the Second World War.

During the 1920s the co-operative relationship between the Ministry and the College deteriorated, probably because the Ministry was proving less effective than the College hoped. The College had gained considerable confidence, which it now expressed on behalf of all nurses, but the Ministry saw this as intrusion, for the College did not confine itself to strictly professional matters. Its intervention on behalf of nurses in public hospitals challenged the Ministry's own position, but also threatened to increase local authority spending at a time of severe retrenchment. In its various appeals to the Ministry the College aimed at official recognition of its claim to represent the profession, but this could easily be construed as another form of unionism, like the pressure applied by the BMA on behalf of doctors in the public service. As a persistent agitator on nursing matters, and regardless of how diplomatic and non-political it sought to be, the College implicitly commented on government policy. Its leaders came from upper middle-class families, had trained at prestigious hospitals, and regarded themselves as career nurses. They were prepared to exert as much political influence as they could through their extensive social connections. Above all, they were passionate about their profession, outspoken in their views, and linked to a wider network of middle-class women concerned to effect social change. The College established a foothold among sympathetic MPs and members of the peerage, and the Ministry began to see it as an irritant rather than an ally. This was most evident in 1926 during the negotiations over the Royal Charter, when the Ministry apparently resisted the College's attempt to place itself on the same footing as the royal medical colleges. The College was trying to secure its right to be heard on nursing matters, and it was a measure of its growing influence that the Ministry now tried to curtail it.

Public health

From the mid-nineteenth century, public health began to occupy a more significant place in national policy, and the new Ministry of Health concentrated much of its effort in this area. In the early twentieth century, emphasis shifted from sanitation to personal health, including better access to medical care, in response to anxiety about the nation's fitness for war. Hospital provision was in disarray, but change was not possible without major reform. Hospitals were distributed according to historical circumstance rather than the needs of the population, and some were poorly equipped. While hospital finance remained in the hands of cash-strapped charities or fragmented local authorities, improvements would depend on local initiative.[63] By contrast, public health was focusing on the maintenance of individual health rather than the treatment of illness.[64] Health promotion concentrating on nutrition and hygiene was now to form a central part of the government's health strategy, for the population should be taught how to take care of itself. From the government point of view, this was a less expensive option than tackling the fundamental causes of ill health, such as low wages and squalid housing. More expensive strategies were ruled out in the financial constraints of the time, while the rising numbers of unemployed consumed an increasing amount of the welfare budget. A programme that addressed individual practices was perhaps a diversionary tactic, but it was also attractive because of its presumed moral effect. It was cheaper, for example, to endorse a voluntary district nursing service than to extend national health insurance to the wives and children of working men. But final responsibility for the success of public health initiatives was given to women: as home visitors they implemented government policy by educating other women and monitoring family health practices; and as mothers they were useful scapegoats, held to account for the

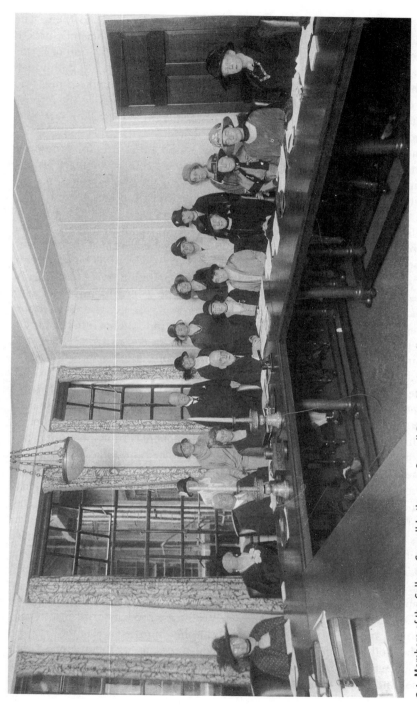

2.4 Members of the College Council in the new Council Room, May 1926 (from left, seated): Dame Sarah Swift, Viscountess Cowdray, Sir Arthur Stanley, Mary Rundle (secretary), Sir Cooper Perry, Ellen Musson, unidentified, Alicia Lloyd Still, Dame Maud McCarthy, Rachael Cox-Davies, unidentified.

health of their children regardless of the resources available to them. The medical inspection of schoolchildren began in 1905 and further measures to improve children's health were implemented under the Notification of Births Acts (1907 and 1915) and the Maternity and Child Welfare Act (1918).[65] Although much health surveillance of this kind was undertaken through schools and local clinics rather than overt intrusion into the family, it stressed the responsibility of mothers for the future health of the nation.[66] The lesson was reinforced in domestic science classes for schoolgirls.

The government gave modest subsidies to local authorities for promoting maternal and child health. Mothercraft classes were run by voluntary groups, and infant feeding became a preoccupation among the health professions and charitable workers. The whole project seemed progressive, achievable and virtuous. As the Labour Minister of Health Arthur Greenwood said to a group of health visitors in 1929: 'you can inspire the people to care for cleanliness of living and purity of life. It is a tremendous responsibility. I believe that in the Health Service of the future there is going to be a great centre which will radiate benefit on the lives of the people'.[67] For any voluntary organisation trying to further its cause with the government, there was much to be gained by involvement in public health. More local authorities began to employ health visitors as educators and reformers of family health. Between 1914 and 1918 the number of full-time health visitors in England and Wales rose from 600 to 2,577.[68] Many had nursing experience, although this was not mandatory. Local Medical Officers of Health supported the employment of nurses in this role, arguing that in such matters, nursing knowledge was more relevant than medical knowledge. Doctors claimed that their own professional skills would not be fully utilised in such work, and health visiting was clearly demarcated as a women's occupation.

Throughout the 1920s the College received frequent complaints from health visitors about variations in salary and poor pay. They also lacked standardised training. A survey in 1926 showed that 1,974 health visitors held between them twenty-two different kinds of certificates or varieties of experience, in eighty-eight combinations, with some possessing as many as five separate certificates. But the most common qualifications among health visitors were three years of general nurse training together with the Central Midwives' Board Certificate.[69] Hence many health visitors were eligible for College membership. To an organisation keen to prove its credentials as the voice of the trained nurse, and needing substantial membership figures to do so, this was an untapped source of support. The expansion of public health nursing gave the College an opportunity to raise its profile as an educator of health professionals and to improve its standing with the Ministry of Health.

The College initially looked to hospital nurses as its main support, but district nurses, tuberculosis nurses, private nurses, industrial nurses, school nurses and health visitors also became members and contacted the College for advice and information. In 1921 it formed a Public Health Advisory Committee to discuss strategies for improving co-operation between health visitors, local authorities and district nursing associations, and to advise the council on matters concerning public health work. The following year, two members of the committee presented papers at the Royal Sanitary Institute Congress. Each emphasised the importance of the general trained nurse in public health, and was well received by the audience. But, many public health nurses did not belong to any association and their salaries and conditions suffered through lack of organised action. Mary Rundle wrote to the Ministry of Education, the Ministry of Health and the Society of Medical Officers of Health recommending a minimum salary of £200 for all qualified public health nurses, in particular health visitors and school nurses, who were the worst paid of all trained nurses. She argued that the nursing profession was unable to recruit the 'right type' of nurse, and that this caused 'serious difficulties in hospitals throughout the country'. Furthermore, 'parents do not encourage their daughters to enter this profession because of the very low rate of salaries offered on completion of training', particularly in preventive work. At this time the nursing press advertised salaries of only £130–£155 plus £10 uniform allowance for health visitors, despite their specialised qualifications, which could take at least five years, 'under strenuous conditions of work, and at considerable cost'.[70] The College began a steady pressure on local authorities that advertised for nurses at less than £200 a year.

The College council needed to improve its own communication with public health nurses, and in 1923, with the approval of the district nursing associations, Medical Officers of Health and the Royal Sanitary Institute, it established a Public Health Section. For an additional annual subscription of 2s 6d, College members in public health could join the new section, linking them to a network of nurses with similar skills and interests. The section believed that public health nursing should be undertaken only by qualified nurses with special training, and aimed to improve salaries for all public health nurses. The section made the College more accessible to nurses outside the hospitals, and was less prone to the allegations of elitism sometimes aimed at the College council. It targeted particular groups, such as the London County Council (LCC) Nursing Service. These posts, closely involved with some of the poorest districts in London, tended to attract more politically radical women.[71] Like many trained nurses, the LCC nurses' chief loyalty was to their training hospitals and, although some joined the College, the group had largely resisted it. To combat this, the Public Health Section held a series of informal meetings ('at homes') in the College. This proved a successful public relations exercise, and the first gathering attracted thirty women, many of whom promised to become members.[72] The section also took up the question of their salaries with the London boroughs.

This widening of College interests took place at a time when more women workers were joining unions, and several groups were trying to establish themselves as the nurses' representatives. Health visitors could join the National Association of Local Government Officers (NALGO). The other body particularly interested in appropriating public health nursing was the Women Sanitary Inspectors and Health Visitors Association (WSIHVA). This body, established in 1902, changed its name in 1915 on opening its membership to health visitors, but it did not give them voting rights, because, unlike the sanitary inspectors, they did not have a training approved by the Royal Sanitary Institute.[73] Resenting this, some health visitors formed local independent associations. By 1917, realising that they could lose their health visitor members completely, the WSIHVA revised its membership policy to include not only health visitors but also superintendents of maternity and child welfare centres, and tuberculosis visitors. In 1921 membership was extended to 'suitably qualified' school nurses, clinic nurses, municipal midwives and infant life protection visitors – the same public health workers that the College listed as eligible for membership of its Public Health Section two years later.

The WSIHVA became known as a champion of women in public health, and had support from several women's social and political organisations. In 1908 it affiliated to the National Union of Women Workers. The WSIHVA was viewed as a radical group, with members activated by the poverty they encountered in their work. But like the College, it was torn between its responsibility as a professional association and the need to improve its members' pay and conditions. Ultimately it chose the trade union role. It supported the Women's Trade Union League, to which it affiliated in 1918 after deciding to register as a trade union. When the WSIHVA applied for affiliation to the Trades Union Congress in 1924, the tension between unions and the College of Nursing was further exposed. Its application was at first rejected, but was accepted the following year. The deciding factor seems to have been the forceful personality of a leading WSIHVA member with notable trade union credentials, but also 'a letter from the Association pointing out that the College of Nursing, which was not a trade union, could undermine the activities of the Association whose aim was to organise all women in the public health service on trade union lines'.[74] Again the College found itself in competition with trade unions over representing nurses, and the possibility of trained nurses being attracted to yet another trade union spurred it into claiming health visiting as a nursing specialty.

In 1923 when the Ministry of Health undercut the salaries suggested by the LCC for health visitors and sanitary inspectors in London, the Consultative Committee of Women's Organisations (of which the WSIHVA was a member) passed a resolution stating that the Ministry had launched 'a direct attack upon the principle of collective bargaining'. At this point the College and the WSIHVA decided to sink their differences in the face of a common threat.

The College's Public Health Section met with the WSIHVA to discuss the low salaries of health visitors. They agreed that salaries might be improved by standardising health visitors' training in line with general nursing principles and raising their professional status. After a joint meeting with the nursing press, a draft training scheme for health visitors was drawn up for government approval, recognising the College as the official training centre for health visitors. The Public Health Section continued to negotiate with the Ministry on training and qualifications but simultaneously offered training weeks in health visiting that proved very popular with nurses.[75]

Throughout the 1920s the Public Health Section fought on two platforms: health visitors' training and the salaries of all public health nurses. In 1924 it joined a College delegation to the Ministry to discuss salaries. The Ministry offered nothing more than sympathy, but in response to a College suggestion that only general trained nurses be allowed to qualify as health visitors, it issued a circular outlining a six-month hospital training for health visitors. This was to be undertaken in a general, fever or children's hospital and was to complement the requirement from 1925 that all health visitors pass the examination of the Royal Sanitary Institute. In contrast to the College's proposal, six months' hospital experience undertaken in nursing situations as variable as fever or children's work would not ensure a high professional nursing standard, nor any uniformity of training. The Public Health Section continued to argue that all health visitors should have three years' training in general nursing, and appealed to the Association of Hospital Matrons for its support, urging them to promote public health work among trained nurses and to encourage them to pursue it as a career. At the same time, the section urged the College to organise a course of lectures and demonstrations for trained nurses who wished to work as health visitors. This scheme, approved by the Board of Education, became the basic preparation for the Royal Sanitary Institute certificate that was now a requirement for practice.

The College did not win the battle to make health visiting a branch of nursing, but it continued to represent its health visitor members and wrote regularly to local councils, reminding them of the College salary scale. Although by 1928 more health visitors were earning between £150 and £200 a year, the Public Health Section pressed the Ministry to undertake a survey of salaries, and was prepared to do this itself in conjunction with the WSIHVA if necessary.[76] Recognising the explicit discrimination in public health salaries, in 1929 the College agreed to join with the London and National Society for Women's Service and other groups in a letter to the Minister of Health on the subject of unequal pay for men and women doing the same work for local authorities. In this way, rather than through openly political or trade union tactics, women's organisations worked behind the scenes to improve the conditions of working women, but progress was slow.

Health visiting was the most prominent issue for the College's Public Health Section, but throughout the inter-war period it pressed for compulsory general training for all public health nurses. During these years the section became very influential within the College, its membership grew to 1,559 by 1939, and it included many of the profession's most radical thinkers.[77] In 1928 its representatives attended joint discussions with the Industrial Welfare Society and the Institute of Industrial Welfare Workers to debate the place of the trained nurse in industry. During the war a Health and Munitions Workers' Committee had recommended that all factories provide dressing stations or surgeries, and, wherever possible, a trained nurse for their workers, and since then a number of nurses had been employed in industry.[78] These nurses were isolated from nursing colleagues and had no voice in negotiations over pay and conditions unless they joined a general union. The 1928 discussion included the pay and status of the trained nurse in industry, the additional training required, the scope of industrial nursing and its possible extension into preventive medicine, and the advisability of combining industrial welfare work with industrial nursing in smaller factories. The average salary of a trained nurse in industry was at that time £3 a week.[79]

Early the following year, College members were invited to attend a conference run by the Institute of Industrial Welfare Workers, where Dr Overton, Medical Officer of Health for the Factory Department of the Home Office, spoke on the 'Effect of industry on the health of the nation'. Evidently, the College included members who worked in industry, but it knew little about this branch of nursing. The Public Health Section tried to find out more about nurses in industry by appealing to members for information, but there was little response. However, in 1930 they asked the College's Education Department to offer a course for nurses employed in industrial welfare. From 1932 industrial nurses were encouraged to join the Public Health Section and discussions began on setting up special training in industrial nursing for new entrants to the service. In 1934 the Education Department offered two courses on industrial nursing in conjunction with Bedford College, a full-time course and a part-time course for those already working in industry. The courses were thinly attended because most nurses working in industry were not on the register, and the title was sometimes given to a worker with a minimal training in first aid. The College organised two bursaries for the industrial courses, but even so only one student took the full-time course in the first year, and this course was later reduced to six months.[80] In 1935 the University of Birmingham established a Department of Industrial Hygiene and Medicine aimed at doctors, nurses and welfare workers, and developed a one-year course for industrial nurses. This department had a close relationship with the College, and an executive member of the Public Health Section, Irene Charley, became a member of the university's advisory board. Charley believed that the industrial nurse was now 'stepping on the first rung of the ladder towards professional recognition', though in most fields of public health nursing, employers could hire nurses with far less training than the College thought acceptable. The College was not prepared to lower its own standards of admission, and held that for work of this type a fully trained nurse was essential.

Private nurses

The College was expanding its interests beyond hospitals and institutions, but private nurses were difficult to reach. In the 1920s the private nurse was still an integral part of health care, but often worked in isolated conditions. While hospitals and infirmaries offered free medical treatment for the working class, wealthier families often paid for private treatment at home, in nursing homes or in a small number of private clinics and hospital wards. Private nursing could offer reasonable rewards. Sometimes self-employed, advertising their services commercially or by word of mouth, private nurses might also be members of a nursing co-operation that operated like an agency, or were employed by a hospital to staff its private beds. But, as in other branches of nursing, wages or fees were unregulated, working conditions varied greatly, and wealthier towns tended to provide better conditions for nurses than the rural areas.[81] Working in the most itinerant branch of nursing, private nurses were often cut off from the support of family and colleagues, and trade unionism was almost impossible. Unlike nurses employed under local authority or hospital contracts, some were exploited by unscrupulous co-operations that charged high fees but did not pass them on to the nurse. Private nurses could also suffer sudden loss of income: for example, they might be booked for a maternity case where the patient went into hospital at the last minute – one nurse recorded that this meant a loss of eleven guineas. They were even disenfranchised if they failed to live in their constituency for three months. Judging from the many letters received by the College, private nurses were generally unsure of their contractual rights, what conditions they should expect, and what fees they could rightfully charge. They looked to the College for advice.

Early in 1931 the College appointed a Private Nurses' Committee 'to consider and report upon the position of private nurses, more particularly as regards conditions of employment, professional status, their organisation, economic position, housing, ethical standard and uniform'.[82] One of the most influential members of this committee was Amy Coward (aunt of the famous playwright), who ran a private nurses' agency for many years and was also a member of the council of the Cowdray Club. She proposed that the College set up a scheme with the co-operation of the matrons of the large general hospitals to 'create a real future for the private nurse'.[83] The scheme was to form a central organisation with branches, to regulate the fees for private nurses, administer their casework, and provide them with residential homes or clubs. Amy Coward wanted to see this branch of nursing under regulations approved by the College. The committee considered a scheme for a Professional Nurses' Advisory and Appointments Bureau, and investigated the cost of providing a club for private nurses in London. They decided that it would be more economical to accommodate private nurses in the extension to the Cowdray Club and to include a registry bureau. More pressing was the question of unemployment. Since employment figures were unavailable, the College mounted its own survey to determine the extent of the problem. A questionnaire went out to thirty-nine hospitals and 630 private nurse co-operations. The replies were a fairly small sample (twenty-three from the former and 129 from the latter); nevertheless, they revealed significant unemployment among private nurses working through co-operations. The main reason given for this was the economic depression, and this rather undercut the College's view that nurses did not need unemployment insurance. The rising cost of medical care, and improved medical techniques in the hospitals, led many middle-class patients to seek treatment in the pay beds of voluntary hospitals, and reduced demand for private nursing at home. Hospitals now employed private nurses to staff their pay beds, and on occasion these were nurses who had left the hospital's employ, but were then re-hired privately at a better rate of pay.

The results of this survey raised a number of questions about the supply and demand for nurses in the community, and the College held a conference on the subject in December 1933. Under the chairmanship of Arthur Stanley, delegates from the BMA, the British Hospitals Association and medical examiners for the state nursing examination, as well as matrons of voluntary hospitals, superintendents of private hospitals, private nurses, district nurses, public health nurses and sister tutors attended. When College representatives recommended legislation to regulate the domiciliary nursing service, including 'a voluntary register of ethical co-operating bodies', and put this before the BMA for its support, they received little encouragement.[84] At this stage, the self-employed nurse proved the most difficult of all the members of this varied profession to bring under the College's remit. In 1932 the Private Nurses' Committee distributed a schedule of recommended conditions of employment for private nurses, and in 1937 the College began a voluntary roll of approved nursing agencies. Conditions for approval included management by a general registered nurse, employment of registered nurses only, a minimum salary of £70 with uniform allowance, and board, lodging and laundry between cases, and, if the agency took a percentage of the nurse's fee, this should not exceed 7.5 per cent. But, out of ninety-one applications from agencies, only twenty-six were satisfactory, while many agencies employed unregistered nurses and made no allowance for off-duty times.[85] Response to the voluntary roll was slow, and in 1939 the College set up a Private Nurses Section. Within six months the section's membership was 500, although with the outbreak of war and the coming of the National Health Service, the private nurse had an uncertain future.

The *Lancet* Commission

Although its charter emphasised the College's educational role, much of the College's time in the inter-war period was devoted to investigations into the pay and conditions of trained nurses, and to negotiating improvements. Christopher Addison's most dynamic successor as Minister of Health was Neville Chamberlain, who chose to remain in this post during the 1920s in order to supervise his major programme of local government reform.[86] This complex planning, which resulted in the Local Government Act of 1929, had many implications for nurses. The Act began a slow process of removing health administration from public assistance. The independent boards of guardians, who had managed both, were replaced by public assistance committees of the local councils, while the county and borough councils were to take direct control of poor law infirmaries once they were brought up to an adequate standard, as part of an integrated local health system. Local government finances would be made more equitable through a redistributive government grant. Local councils would be large-scale employers of nurses in hospitals, sanatoria, schools, clinics and in the community. As the scope and size of local government grew, so the organisations representing their employees expanded, with NALGO becoming one of the most substantial national trade unions.[87]

During the 1920s, the concept of 'municipal medicine' was much favoured. Government had no intention of taking command of the health services, preferring to leave them to reinvigorated local government, but it offered incentives to improve them. Nurses were important to these new schemes, but their working conditions varied considerably from one area to another. In spite of the growth of unions and professional bodies, including the College itself, the position of nurses in the workplace remained weak. By 1930 a shortage of candidates for nursing was reported throughout the country, although it was felt most keenly in the smaller hospitals. At this stage the larger, more prestigious hospitals complained rather of a shortage of 'suitable' candidates, by which they meant women of superior social class and education. Middle-class parents were encouraging their daughters into less strenuous and better-paid white-collar occupations.

Without consulting the College (which was also investigating the problem), certain members of the medical profession, under the auspices of *The Lancet*, carried out their own investigation of the nursing shortage. It is not clear what motivated *The Lancet* to appoint a commission on nursing although it did have a history of intervention in this area.[88] Two women were particularly active in this investigation: the assistant editor of *The Lancet*, Dr Marguerite Kettle, and the medical superintendent of the Berkshire and Buckinghamshire Joint Sanatorium, Dr Esther Carling. Marguerite Kettle qualified in medicine in 1918 and joined the staff of *The Lancet*, where she discovered a natural talent for journalism and found 'an unexpected vocation'. Described as enterprising and insightful, she was also a member of the GNC. Esther Carling was respected as a pioneer woman doctor and was particularly interested in the treatment of tuberculosis and the development of sanatoria. Both women had been active in the suffragette movement.

Confronted by acute staffing shortages in TB sanatoria, which in some cases relied on the employment of ex-patients, Esther Carling alerted the medical profession to the 'approaching crisis' in a letter to *The Lancet* in October 1930. She focused on working conditions as the main reason for the lack of staff, and predicted that 'more and more the doctor depends on the nurse; less and less will he find her'.[89] This letter attracted sympathetic replies from doctors, spurring *The Lancet* into action. Kettle also discussed, over lunch with Gertrude Cowlin, the College's intention to investigate the nursing shortage. But, by the time Kettle returned to her office, notification of the *Lancet* inquiry had gone to press. The *Lancet* Commission was appointed in December 1930 'to enquire into the reasons for the shortage of candidates, trained and untrained, for nursing the sick in general and special hospitals throughout the country, and to offer suggestions for making the service more attractive to women suitable for this necessary work'.[90] Despite Esther Carling's rousing letter, the *Lancet* Commission was largely the creation of Marguerite Kettle, although her name is not disclosed in the final report.[91] She remained in close contact with the College through her friendship with Ruth Derbyshire, matron of University College Hospital. Derbyshire, an executive member of the College, was appointed to the *Lancet* Commission, linking the College and the Commission during the investigation.[92]

The Commission sent out questionnaires to 686 hospitals, inquiring into the conditions of service of nearly 44,000 nursing staff. In preparing its evidence the College contacted many more hospitals, organisations and individuals, and included information from Scotland and Ireland, and on nursing outside the hospitals.[93] The final report applied only to England and Wales and only to female nurses. It confirmed the nursing shortage and estimated that just under half the hospitals had difficulty in attracting suitable candidates for training. It noted that advertisements in the nursing journals for vacant nursing posts in voluntary hospitals or local authorities were sometimes repeated over weeks or months, while advertisements from state registered nurses seeking positions were few. The shortage was so acute that some hospitals admitted that they would take any candidate who could 'read, write and spell', and the LCC reported that of 8,000 applicants for probationer posts, 6,000 were rejected, mainly on the grounds of lack of education, even although a secondary education was not required.[94]

In a lengthy passage, the Commission's report outlined the contemporary perception of nurse training as 'excessively hard', where the young student was subjected to long hours of drudgery and 'cut off from her friends, her games, and her social amusements, will be always overtired physically, and often snubbed and reproved'.[95] Although dismissing many of these criticisms as misconceptions, the report nevertheless laid some blame at the matrons' door for valuing nursing apprenticeship on the wards over theoretical study, and for regarding long hours and hard routine as necessary for the development of the vocational spirit.

> Women in other professions are apt to regard such long hours of routine work, the restrictions on liberty when off duty, in short, the scanty opportunity given to the nurse in training to lead a normal social life and to cultivate interests apart from her work, as being associated with the desire of hospitals to econo- mise at the expense of their staff. They criticise senior nurses for acquiescing without protest in a system which admits of the exploitation of student labour.[96]

As a result, even the educated young nurse soon 'puts on the blinkers' and perpetuated the old traditions. The report argued that socially aware senior nurses were trying to bring hospital training into line with other forms of train- ing, but they too were 'hampered by the conservative attitude of valued members of their senior staffs'.[97] On the restrictions imposed on off-duty nurses – not only on probationers but also on qualified nurses – the report called for a change of attitude. If the nurse were trusted to conduct her social life sensibly, this 'might serve to secure the cooperation of all sections of the community in attempts to restore nursing to its former position in the esteem of educated women'.[98] In effect, the Commission was criticising the Nightingale tradition, which enabled matrons to impose heavy duties on subordinate nurses, and encouraged them to act as moral guardians to their staff. Yet in the matrons' defence it might be added that their own working hours were usually extremely long, and that they imposed similar conditions on their nurses because employ- ers would not take on enough staff to reduce the length of nursing shifts.

In its efforts to identify the reasons for the shortage of nurses the Commission was as much concerned about the gap between school and hospital training as it was about the harsh conditions of a nurse's life. Most girls left school between the ages of fourteen and sixteen and could not start nurse training until eigh- teen; indeed in some of the more popular voluntary hospitals the recruitment age was as high as twenty-one. This was seen as one of the main deterrents to a nursing career. The various groups who gave evidence to the Commission all agreed that the gap should be filled by pre-nursing courses, which would include lectures on anatomy, physiology and hygiene and relieve some of the pressure on probationers when they started general training. Organisations outside the nursing profession, such as the Association of Headmistresses and the National Council of Women, proposed that such courses be similar to the pre-medical examination and should exempt girls who had completed them from the theoretical part of the Preliminary State Examination at the end of the first year of nurse training. This suggestion, which would divide the practical from the theoretical section of first-year training, became known as 'splitting the prelim', and was very controversial within the profession. To allow girls to take part of their professional training before they entered a hospital ward seemed to threaten the authority of the hospital training schools. The more conservative matrons believed that these lectures should be taken in conjunction with nursing practice and not as pure theory. This was the opinion of Rachael Cox-Davies and Ellen Musson, who voted against the recommendation when it was discussed in a College committee appointed to respond to the *Lancet* report. The College nevertheless accepted the recommendation, as did the GNC for Scotland; but the GNC for England and Wales debated the issue for six years before it was finally introduced.[99]

The College welcomed the *Lancet* report, and the council wrote to its proprietors thanking them for a comprehensive report of great value to the profession. Many of the report's suggestions were in line with existing College policy. By 1931 the College had again shifted its position over working hours, in the face of the nursing shortage and challenges from the trade unions, and accepted a forty-eight-hour week. It also agreed with *The Lancet* on improving nurses' salaries, making the Federated Superannuation Scheme for Nurses and Hospital Officers available to all and fully interchangeable, allowing longer holidays and structured off-duty time. It agreed with suggestions to raise the standard of nurses' education, particularly the need for a higher proportion of sister tutors to student nurses (one to sixty was the recommended figure), they accepted that matrons should not be able to dismiss probationers without appeal to a hospital committee, and that discipline might be relaxed in the nurses' homes. Neither the College nor *The Lancet* envisaged any relaxation of senior nurses' control over hospital wards: the matrons might relinquish some of their discipline over the nurses' homes, but in the wards they were unchallenged. The aim of all these proposals was to make nursing as attractive as other professions for women, and to allay the anxieties of parents who were reluctant to let their daughters enter it.

Despite the report's harsh criticisms of some aspects of the nursing establishment, the *Nursing Times* reflected the College's gratitude for this attention to nursing.

The book [report] . . . is to be had from the Lancet . . . It rings so true; it is so human, so real in its understanding of *us nurses* and our problems, that no commentary, no series of extracts, however carefully selected, could take the place of the original. It should be on the desk of every matron, every sister-tutor, in short, every leader of the nursing profession . . . We have found it so absorbing in this office that even the most strong-minded of us did no more work till she had read it from cover to cover, and we laid it down with the satisfied feeling that here were our own personal convictions on the nature of the nursing reforms so urgently required, but expressed infinitely better than it has hitherto been in our power to do.[100]

The Lancet was concerned mainly with solving the nursing shortage, but within a year an editorial of the *Nursing Times* was concerned over an over-supply of trained nurses. The shortage had disappeared chiefly because of the financial depression. Girls had to take any available work, and there was no lack of student nurses. When hospitals could get cheap student labour they did not want to employ the more expensive staff nurse. As one matron said: 'We *can't* take them on at staff nurse status, because who is going to do the cleaning?'[101] Although grateful for the *Lancet* report, the College stressed that the problem was not one of shortage but of quality and deployment. In the following years, it repeatedly called for an official inquiry into the nursing services, but this did not come until 1937, in the form of the Interdepartmental Committee on Nursing Services known as the Athlone Committee. Although the *Lancet*'s suggestions on hospital discipline could probably have been introduced at little cost, complaints about old-fashioned ways continued for many years. Increased pay and shorter working hours were subjects that hospitals would consider only if finances permitted, which was rarely the case.

Conclusion

The period after the war was one of expansion for the College. Reflecting a general feeling of optimism for the future, it looked to the newly formed General Nursing Councils to take on the administrative responsibilities of registration, freeing it to develop a reputation as the professional body for nursing. The College tried to combine the professional status of the royal colleges of medicine with the more democratic and representative structure of the British Medical Association. It tried to set standards for nursing by admitting to membership only those on the GNC's register. Although this left many nurses ineligible for membership, it laid down a principle that would inform debates on nurse training in subsequent decades. Viewed by many as elitist, the College did not attract the majority of nurses, and it could never claim to speak for all. Nevertheless, membership during the first ten years grew steadily and a network of local centres/branches spread throughout the country. By the mid-1920s the College was the largest and most vocal nursing organisation in Britain. Through the branches it could collect information on nursing conditions and discuss resolutions on a range of issues. In establishing courses for sister tutors the College developed one of its key educational aims that would have a lasting effect on nurse education. It tried to foster a co-operative relationship with the Ministry of Health, and located itself in the established order, eventually gaining full recognition in the award of a Royal Charter.

College leaders, nationally and locally, tended to be the hospital matrons. While this may have restricted the College's appeal, their social position and connections gave the College a ready access to politics. As middle-class women they were in the main conservative, but they were not necessarily apolitical. The College became part of a network of women's organisations, and gave nurses a voice on social issues. Seeking to encompass all branches of nursing, and encouraged by a growing interest in public health and health education, the College extended its professional interests to include nursing outside the institutions. By the end of the 1930s its three specialised sections for sister tutors, public health nurses and private nurses enabled it to keep in touch with specialised interest groups in the profession. This was a strategic and successful manoeuvre in attracting new members. But it also begs a number of questions. Health provision in the community was mainly directed at the poor, and in particular at the working-class mother. Did the College feel it could take on a professional nursing role more easily if it concentrated on the lives of women? In moving into public health, the women who led the College reflected the values of their sex and class. Whether at the League of Nations, or Westminster, politically active women were often restricted to family health and welfare issues in the gendered political arena.[102]

Although ostensibly an educational body, the College from its earliest days began to feel a division of interests. As soon as it became involved in nurses' pay and conditions of work, it was entering the territory of trade unions that represented nurses, particularly those excluded from College membership. Nursing questions were becoming political, and despite its attempts to remain outside party politics, the College had to engage with them. Increasingly, it tried to speak for all nurses in the workplace, whether or not they were members of the College. Broadly speaking, the unions and the College shared the same goals for their nurse members, though the College insisted that the chief issue was the standard of nurses' training. If nurses were better educated and more highly trained, then improvements in their economic conditions must surely follow. The unions, realistically appreciating that working-class women who left school at fourteen were not in a position to share the College's ambitions for nursing education, were able to recruit more widely. This perpetuated divisions in British nursing that would present many difficulties for the future.

Notes

1 For general surveys, see Deirdre Beddoe, *Back to Home and Duty: Women Between the Wars 1918–1939* (London: Pandora, 1989), pp. 132–47; Sue Bruley, *Women in Britain Since 1900* (Basingstoke: Macmillan, 1999), pp. 59–91; Pugh, *Women and the Women's Movement*, pp. 43–70.

2 See Catriona Beaumont, 'Women's citizenship: a study of non-feminist women's societies and the women's movement in England, 1928–1950', PhD thesis, University of Warwick, 1996; Sue Innes, 'Constructing women's citizenship in the interwar period: the Edinburgh Women Citizen's Association', *WHR* 13: 4 (2004), 621–47.

3 Pat Thane, 'What difference did the vote make? Women in public and private life in Britain since 1918', *Historical Research* 76 (2003), 271.

4 Catriona Beaumont, 'Citizens not feminists: the boundary negotiated between citizenship and feminism by mainstream women's organisations in England, 1928–39', *WHR* 9: 2 (2000), 411–29.

5 RCN/1/2/1/1, papers concerning the petition for a Royal Charter, 1917–28.

6 For full membership statistics of the RCN, see Appendix 2.

7 RCN/23/9.

8 When the building alterations were complete, surplus offices were sub-let to organisations closely associated with the College, such as the Nation's Fund for Nurses, the 1930 Fund for District Nurses and the Federated Superannuated Scheme for Nurses and Hospital Officers.

9 McGann, *Battle of the Nurses*, p. 51.

10 The *Nursing Mirror* had a circulation of 31,000 in 1919, CM 20 Nov. 1919, p. 524.

11 RCN/1/2/1/2, M. Rundle to A. Stanley, 21 Jan. 1927; RCN/1/2/3/3, 18 Feb 1927.

12 RCN/1/2/1/1, Proceedings of Privy Council.

13 RCN/1/2/1/2.

14 After 1932 life membership was still offered at an increasing fee of £20, £40, £63 or £105 depending upon the date on which the fee was paid. In 1963 the names of over 3,000 founder members with whom the College had lost touch were removed from the membership roll causing a blip in the membership figures.

15 The former London branch office became the Central Co-ordinating Office for the four metropolitan branches.

16 Mary Rundle obituary, *NT* 20 March 1937, pp. 273–4.

17 The position of sister tutor was first introduced in St Thomas's Hospital before the First World War and in the inter-war years spread to other teaching hospitals. Around 1946, with the advent of men into general nursing and nurse education, the title male tutor was used alongside sister tutor. By 1950 the generic title nurse tutor was more common although sister tutor continued in use until the beginning of the 1960s.

18 This College, set up as a separate institution before King's College became co-educational, retained a separate legal identity for some years after the education of women was integrated into the university curriculum.

19 Rafferty, *Politics of Nursing Knowledge*, p. 115.

20 See J. Brookes, 'Visiting rights only: the early experience of nurses in higher education, 1918–1960', PhD thesis, London School of Hygiene and Tropical Medicine, 2005.

21 The first university Department of Nursing in the United Kingdom was established in 1956 at the University of Edinburgh. The first chair of nursing was
   established in Edinburgh in 1972. The University of Manchester established a
   chair of nursing in 1974.
22 I. M. Stewart, *The Education of Nurses: Historical Foundations and Modern Trends*
   (New York: Macmillan, 1944), pp. 194–5.
23 RCN/7/11/1, Syllabus 1926–27.
24 The Department of Household and Social Science became King's College for
   Household and Social Science in 1928.
25 NLD [Nan Dorsey] and MMK [Marjorie Kilby], *The Lamp Radiant, the Story of
   an Association of Nurses from Many Lands, by Two of Its Members* (London: privately published, 1955); Susan McGann, 'Collaboration and conflict in international nursing 1920–1939', *Nursing History Review* 16 (2008), 29–57. See also Anne
   Marie Rafferty, 'Internationalising nurse education', in Paul Weindling (ed.),
   International Health Organisations and Movements 1918–1939 (Cambridge:
   Cambridge University Press, 1995), pp. 266–82.
26 RCN/7/1/1/1, Education Committee minutes, 24 Jan. 1929, p. 136; RCN/7/1/1/2,
   Education Committee minutes, 28 Sept. 1931, p. 99; RCN/7/1/1/2, Education
   Committee minutes, 9 Nov. 1928, p. 130.
27 RCN/7/1/1/3, Education Committee minutes, 'Conditions under which the College
   of Nursing is prepared to assist nurses from foreign countries to obtain post-
   graduate work in England', 1 July 1936, p. 384.
28 Diary of Beatrice Webb, 15 Oct. 1895, cited in Daphne Glick, *The National Council
   of Women of Great Britain. The First One Hundred Years* (London: NCW, 1995),
   p. 8.
29 RCN/1/1/1919/1, Correspondence of Arthur Stanley, March 1919.
30 RCN/1/1/1919/1, Correspondence between Cooper Perry and Stanley, 10 March
   1919, and between Mary Rundle, and M. M. Gordon, 31 March 1919.
31 M. M. Ogilvie Gordon, 'Nurses' hours and pay', *The Times* 25 March 1919, p. 10.
32 RCN/4/1919/1, Report of the Salaries Committee on Salaries & Conditions of
   Employment of Nurses, 1919, p. 6; also, '48 hours a week for nurses', *The Times* 11
   June 1919, p. 9.
33 In 1918 the College set up an Appointments Bureau to help find posts for demo-
   bilised nurses. In 1920 it became an enquiry and information service. Gerald
   Bowman, *The Lamp and the Book: the Story of the Rcn, 1916–1966* (London: Queen
   Anne Press, 1967), pp. 75–7.
34 See Rodney Lowe, 'Hours of labour: negotiating industrial legislation in Britain
   1919–39', *Ec.H.R.* 35: 2 (1982), 254–72.
35 Helen Jones, *Health and Society in Twentieth Century Britain* (New York: Longman,
   1994), p. 45.
36 Abel-Smith, *Nursing Profession*, p. 137.
37 See Rafferty, *Politics of Nursing Knowledge*, pp. 139–41 for further details.
38 CM 22 Jan. 1920, pp. 570–1.
39 CM 18 March 1920, pp. 611–12.
40 'Nurses' new hours and training', *The Times* 4 Dec. 1919, p. 11.

41 CM 20 May 1920, p. 39.
42 CM 20 May 1920, p. 36.
43 *BJN* 18 Dec. 1920, pp. 338–9.
44 RCN/13/H/1, 'The Labour Party Draft Report on the Nursing Profession' prepared by a sub-committee of the standing joint committee of industrial women's organisations and the Labour Party's advisory committee on public health, 1927.
45 CM 5 Jan. 1931, pp. 7–8.
46 For a detailed account, see Alan Deacon, *In Search of the Scrounger: the Administration of Unemployment Insurance in Britain, 1920–1931* (London: Bell, 1976).
47 *AR* 1923, p. 3.
48 Mary Rundle, 'Pensions for nurses. Contributory scheme prepared', *The Times* 7 May 1924, p. 10.
49 'Pensions for nurses. Scheme for hospital staffs', *The Times* 10 Dec. 1925, p. 18.
50 Within one year of its operation, 255 hospitals were participating in the Federated Superannuation Scheme for Nurses and Hospital Officers.
51 Pat Thane, *Old Age in English History: Past Experiences, Present Issues* (Oxford: Oxford University Press, 2000), p. 285.
52 *AR* 1936, pp. 8–9.
53 Scott, 'Influence of the staff of the Ministry of Health', p. 31.
54 Bentley B. Gilbert, *British Social Policy 1914–1939* (London: Batsford, 1970), pp. 98–161.
55 Kenneth O. Morgan and Jane Morgan, *Portrait of a Progressive: the Political Career of Christopher, Viscount Addison* (Oxford: Clarendon Press, 1980), pp. 120–48.
56 Scott, 'Influence of the staff of the Ministry of Health', pp. 32–3.
57 This assumed board and lodging provided by the local authority.
58 CM 29 April 1921, pp. 10–11, and 21 July 1921, pp. 39–40.
59 CM 8 Jan. 1920, p. 556, 'Resolution from the Yorkshire Centre of the College of Nursing'.
60 CM 29 April 1920, pp. 25–6.
61 CM 20 May 1920, p. 35.
62 See RCN/13/EE/1 for papers relating to trade unions and the Stepney case.
63 See Martin Gorsky, John Mohan and Martin Powell, 'British voluntary hospitals, 1871–1938: the geography of provision and utilisation', *Journal of Historical Geography* 25: 4 (1999), 463–82; and also 'The financial health of voluntary hospitals in interwar Britain', *Ec.H.R.* 55: 3 (2002), 533–57.
64 Anne Hardy, *Health and Medicine in Britain Since 1860* (Basingstoke: Palgrave 2001), pp. 77–189.
65 This last Act did not apply to Scotland, where similar provisions were made under other legislation.
66 For a general account, see Jane Lewis, *The Politics of Motherhood: Child and Maternal Welfare in England, 1900–1939* (London: Croom Helm, 1980).
67 WLMA SA/HVA/D.4/1, 'A chance for every child. From the inaugural address given at the Women Sanitary Inspectors and Health Visitors Association Ninth Winter School, 1929–30 given by the Right Honourable Arthur Greenwood, M.P., Minister of Health'.

68 Deborah Dwork, *War Is Good for Babies and Other Young Children: a History of the Infant and Child Welfare Movement in England 1898–1918* (London and New York: Tavistock, 1987), p. 211.

69 WLAM SA/HVA/D.2, *Memorandum on matters connected with the administration of the Maternity and Child Welfare and other Acts directly concerning the work of Health Visitors*, 1926.

70 RCN/4, Public Health Advisory Committee minutes, 26 April 1926. Copy of letter from M. Rundle to N. Chamberlain, 14 April 1923.

71 For a full account, see S. Kirby, 'The London County Council Nursing Service 1929–1948', PhD thesis, University of Nottingham, 2000.

72 RCN/6/1/1, 1923–25, Public Health Section minutes, 29 Nov. 1924.

73 The Sanitary Inspectors' Association was formed 1883 but was for men only. When women sanitary inspectors were first appointed in 1896 they were denied entry because they would 'lower the status of the profession' and so had to form their own association. Jennifer Smith, *1896–1996: a History in Health. Health Visitors' Association 100 Years* (London: Health Visitors' Association, 1996). See also Dingwall et al., *Introduction to the Social History of Nursing*, pp. 184 ff.

74 Smith, *A History in Health*, p. 20.

75 After the first 'postgraduate week' in June 1924 it was noted that 'the average attendance at each lecture was 160 and the proceeds had covered the cost'. RCN/6/1/1, Public Health Section minutes, 27 June 1924.

76 RCN/6/1/2, Public Health Section minutes, 1 Dec. 1928.

77 For example, Olive Baggallay, Irene Charley, Mary Davis, Marjorie Simpson, Florence Udell and Alice Woodman.

78 Irene Charley, *The Birth of Industrial Nursing: its History and Development in Great Britain* (London: Baillière, Tindall & Cox, 1954), p. 61. See also Ronald Johnston and Arthur McIvor, *Lethal Work* (East Linton: Tuckwell Press, 2000), p. 50.

79 Charley, *Birth of Industrial Nursing*, p. 102.

80 RCN/7/1/1/3, Education Committee minutes, 7 Feb. 1934, p. 210, 2 May 1934, p. 220, 3 Oct. 1934, p. 245.

81 'Private nursing', *NT* 11 Nov. 1933, p. 1073.

82 RCN/6/3/1, Private Nurses' Committee minutes, 9 Jan. 1931.

83 RCN/6/3/1, Private Nurses' Committee minutes, letter from Amy Coward, 9 Jan. 1931.

84 RCN/4/1938/1–8, Athlone Committee. British Medical Association, 'Nursing problems: report on questions raised by the College of Nursing', April 1937.

85 RCN/6/3/1, Private Nurses' Committee minutes, 1937.

86 For a full discussion of this legislation, see Jonathan Paul Bradbury, 'The 1929 Local Government Act: the formulation and implementation of the Poor Law (Health Care) and Exchequer Grant Reforms for England and Wales', PhD thesis, University of Bristol 1990. Scotland had a separate Local Government Act that similarly consolidated local authorities into larger units.

87 For a full history, see Alec Spoor, *White-collar Union: Sixty Years of NALGO* (London: Heinemann 1967).

88 The history of the *Lancet* investigations into nursing was summarised in 'The position of nursing. Past and present', *The Lancet* 15 Nov. 1930, p. 1090.

89 E. Carling, 'Recruitment for nursing', *The Lancet* 11 Oct. 1930, p. 826.

90 Supplement to *NT* 6 Dec. 1930. Also quoted in preface to *The Lancet Commission on Nursing Final Report* (London: *The Lancet*, 1932), p. 7.

91 *Lancet Commission on Nursing*, p. 10.

92 See RCN/4/1931 for correspondence between the College and the *Lancet* Commission.

93 For more detailed information on the methods used by the *Lancet* Commission see Rafferty, *Politics of Nursing Knowledge*, pp. 146–8. See also RCN/4/1931, draft memorandum by the College of Nursing Salaries and Superannuation Committee.

94 *Lancet Commission on Nursing*, p. 34.

95 Ibid., pp. 27–8.

96 Ibid., p. 29.

97 Ibid., p. 30.

98 Ibid., p. 32.

99 Eve Bendall and Elizabeth Raybould, *A History of the General Nursing Council for England and Wales 1919–1969* (London: H. K. Lewis & Co. Ltd, 1969), pp. 101–3.

100 *NT* 20 Feb. 1932, p. 178.

101 'The paradox', *NT* 20 May 1933, p. 483.

102 See Carol Anne Miller, 'Lobbying the League: women's international organisations and the League of Nations', PhD thesis, University of Oxford, 1992.

3

The struggle for influence, 1930–45

The *Lancet* report of 1932 highlighted difficulties in recruiting nurses, but this was only one of many problems. The College wished to review the whole system of nursing, and throughout the 1930s it persistently demanded a full government inquiry. This was finally granted in 1937, in a committee chaired by the Earl of Athlone, but its work was ended by the war. Yet the Second World War, like the first, brought nursing into the limelight. Civilian resources and health services were the subject of surreptitious government planning some years before war broke out, and nursing organisations gained in importance. In recognition of this, in 1939 the College of Nursing was granted the coveted prefix 'Royal'. This gratified its patron, Queen Mary, but also enhanced the College's prestige.

During the 1930s the national governments of Baldwin and Chamberlain hoped that reformed local government would improve the standards of public hospitals, and they encouraged regional co-operation between voluntary and public health services.[1] The future of nursing became a matter of public and political anxiety as the supply of trained nurses could not expand fast enough to meet the growing demand for both hospital and community nurses. The College of Nursing was one of many bodies struggling to gain the government's attention on nursing policy, and by the end of the decade the government had to respond, knowing that nursing would soon be essential to the war effort. Although the College was still relatively small, with membership restricted to nurses on the general register, it was nevertheless the largest nursing organisation, and its resolutely non-union stance was attractive to conservative governments. Debates over nurses' pay and conditions exposed ideological differences between the College and trade unions with nurse members, and the College could not speak for all in the profession. Although these differences were put aside during the war, they appeared again when it ended.

The story of this important period in British health policy struggles to emerge from the bureaucratic paperwork that records it. It was dominated by official and unofficial inquiries, the findings of each scrutinised and debated at length by the College. The College performed several different functions: offering specialised training, negotiating on behalf of individual members, and engaging in public and private debate with government ministers and Whitehall officials. It had to maintain a high public profile, for which forceful advocacy was essential, and the duties of the College secretary expanded as a result. Although its relations with government officials were often strained, it was becoming a body that governments found hard to ignore.

New management

As the original founders of the College gave way to the next generation, the College needed an executive secretary to act rapidly on its behalf, and to negotiate effectively with government. In 1928, before these responsibilities were anticipated, the council appointed Frances Goodall as assistant secretary at the age of thirty-five, and in 1933 she succeeded Mary Rundle as secretary. In this crucial period, much responsibility rested with her. Goodall, the daughter of a bank clerk, was educated at home with her two brothers. Medical connections in her extended family introduced her to hospital work, and she began her nurse training at Guy's Hospital in 1916.[2] She gained experience as a private nurse, a theatre nurse, a night superintendent, a sister in a children's ward and outpatient sister at Moorfields Eye Hospital. When she applied for the post of assistant secretary, the council was much impressed by her natural charm, and her credentials were declared 'much superior' to the other candidates'.[3] As assistant to Mary Rundle, Goodall proved highly efficient and she was an obvious choice as secretary in due course.

The leaders of the RCN in each generation naturally adopted the tactics available to women in public life, circumscribed as they were by gender expectations. Dame Sarah Swift, daughter of a substantial landowner, was not of Florence Nightingale's high social status, but could call on the support of aristocratic patrons in launching the College, as Nightingale had done for her own projects. Nightingale and Swift both relied on private means and personal connections, and assumed that powerful men must be co-opted into their campaigns. Frances Goodall was akin to the new, and still very small, band of professional career women who entered administrative posts in the First World War and – if not evicted by the marriage bar – remained in them, rising to positions of authority in a masculine world where charm was a considerable asset. Goodall had to deal effectively with a wide range of people, from royal patrons to the press, and skill in personal relations was essential. She was a very elegant woman whose appearance was always immaculate. She travelled extensively, and made svelte appearances at branch meetings throughout the country. She was keenly intelligent, not easily intimidated and

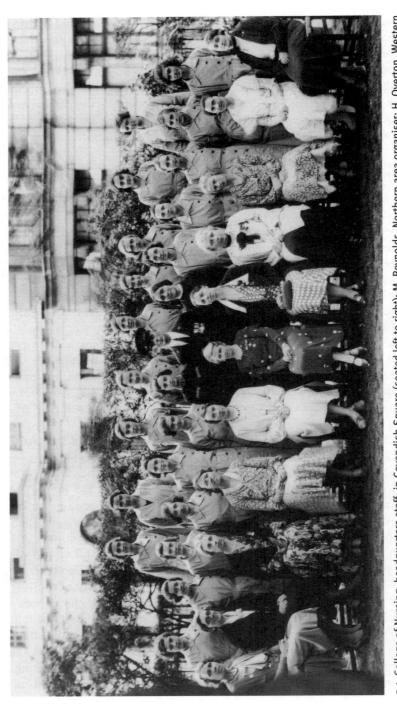

3.1 College of Nursing, headquarters staff, in Cavendish Square (seated left to right): M. Reynolds, Northern area organiser; H. Overton, Western area organiser; H. Heaton [Mrs Blair Fish], editor *Nursing Times*; H. Parsons, director, Education Division; F. Goodall, assistant secretary; M. Rundle, secretary; G. Cowlin, librarian; M. Barrett, financial secretary; M. McEwen, tutor; F. Udell, secretary, Public Health Section; R. Pecker, Midland area organiser; clerical and other staff behind, 1933.

was outspoken or diplomatic as the situation demanded, qualities she attributed to 'having been trained to think like a man'.[4] She was adept in cultivating good relationships with people of importance, and often invited them to speak at the College and its conferences.

In contrast to Mary Rundle, who was reticent by nature, Frances Goodall wanted to take the College into the world, and closer to politics. By courting sympathetic MPs, particularly Irene Ward and other female politicians, Goodall was alerted to any questions relating to nursing as soon as they were raised in parliament. From an early date the College hired a press-cutting agency, and monitored its own public image. The cuttings, from the national press and a very wide range of local papers, show the impressive publicity Frances Goodall achieved as she commented on government policy and reported the College's views. In the letters columns of the press, criticisms of the College, which had several rivals for the loyalty of nurses, were usually met by an efficient early version of the 'rapid rebuttal' technique.[5] Although she did not encourage the prospect of College membership for male nurses,

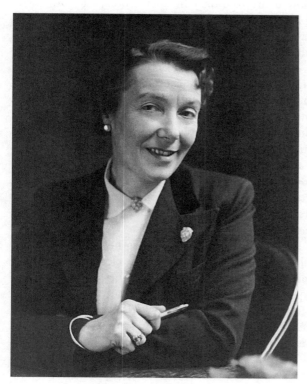

3.2 Frances Goodall, general secretary 1933–57.

she nevertheless advised them to form their own association as a first step towards inclusion. Her commitment to her work was unstinting, and during the war she spent most nights in a basement storeroom in the College, which she converted into a bedroom, reinforced against air raids.

Within the College, Goodall was an admired if somewhat awe-inspiring figure, but her reputation was not always positive. As a devoted advocate of the College she worked hard to make contacts within the government but, as will be seen, was not able to avoid disagreements with the Ministry of Health, which regarded her with some suspicion. She took part in numerous deputations to the Ministry, and lobbied Ministers of Health at every opportunity, often with the backing of the press. Her diplomatic skills could not disguise the College's opposition to government views on the place of nursing.

The training and regulation of nurses

Although the College's ambition was a fully trained nursing service, this looked even less likely in 1939 than in the College's early years. A resurgence of charitable funding allowed the voluntary hospitals to expand, but many had serious financial problems by the late 1930s, especially in areas of high unemployment. This was reflected in very variable standards of service.[6] Employers with constrained budgets fell back on staffing the wards with untrained women, who were cheaper than registered nurses. This was less common in larger teaching hospitals treating acute cases and able to attract highly trained nurses, but municipal hospitals and institutions had many chronic or elderly patients. In these institutions there was a rapid turnover of nurses, and hospital authorities had to choose between the costly solution of using supply nurses from an agency, or the cheaper alternative of employing unqualified nurses. An argument stemming from the days of workhouse nursing was often employed as a defence: that patients with chronic or terminal conditions did not need highly trained nurses, but merely a good standard of personal care.[7] For this, a 'motherly woman', the assistant nurse, might be preferred to the trained nurse.

Student nurses had a rigorous training, worked long hours in the wards, and many hospitals still expected them to undertake cleaning and other domestic chores. They earned little more than pocket money as students, and low salaries when they qualified. They had to live in residences of variable quality provided by the hospitals, and their personal lives were often strictly controlled. In the circumstances, the College feared that some students would give up training to take assistant nurse posts, and the same choice beckoned to students who had difficulty passing their examinations. The College did not support a working wage for probationers, regarding them not as workers but students undergoing a professional training. An assistant nurse could start earning full wages at an earlier age than a registered nurse, though she could not expect promotion to a more responsible position. In fact, many experienced assistant nurses did the job of a trained nurse, though in theory they had to be supervised by a trained superior. Some local authorities accepted this, and tried to formalise the position of assistant nurses. In 1935 the public health department of the county of Essex, 'driven by dire necessity', developed a two-year scheme of training for their 'assistant probationers' to bring them 'into the general fold of nurses'.[8] The scheme offered a modified training, fitting the probationer to nurse the 'chronic sick', but she would not qualify for registration. The Essex scheme received much publicity, but despite appeals to the Ministry of Health and the GNC for recognition, and requests for a separate register for assistant nurses, it was not accepted as nurse training. Essentially, the scheme would have created another tier of nursing, which the College would bitterly resist for some years.

Similar arguments arose over private nurses. Middle-class clients might pay high fees to nursing agencies, but since anyone could call herself a 'nurse', agencies did not have to provide trained nurses. Working-class families with national insurance sometimes had the services of a nurse as part of their insurance policy, but home nursing for poor patients varied greatly from one district to another. The district nursing service supplied by Queen Victoria's Jubilee Institute was well respected, but it could operate effectively only in communities capable of supporting it, or where local government was prepared to give a subsidy from the poor law funds.[9] The independent MP Eleanor Rathbone and others introduced a private members' Bill on domiciliary nursing services in 1934. It aimed to give local authorities much wider powers to run a home nursing service but, opposed by the County Councils' Association and without government support, the Bill failed. The College urged the pressing need for such legislation on the Minister of Health and stressed the inadequacies of the existing service. With Rachael Cox-Davies heading a College deputation, the subject was debated in full at the Ministry of Health, but no action was taken. The Ministry, much beset by alarming official reports on maternal mortality, was preoccupied with legislation for a salaried district midwifery service. This, it stated, must take precedence over any other public health legislation.[10] Frustrated, the College council appealed again for a review but extended its request to a full examination of the whole system of nurse training and supply. The Ministry was not responsive.

Preparing its case in the hope of an inquiry, in April 1936 the College documented the principal issues affecting the recruitment of hospital nurses and provision of nursing in the community. It contended that, for many women, work as an untrained assistant nurse was more immediately rewarding than the arduous life and very low pay of a probationer. The College considered financial impediments, not only in pay, but in pensions, which were not transferable between public and voluntary nursing posts. It concentrated on posts where less trained, or untrained, women were regularly employed. The College noted the lack of any regulation of domestic nurses, the limited training of many midwives, and the problems of finding trained nurses for the chronic sick, the elderly, and patients with tuberculosis. TB sanatoria were particularly difficult to staff, because many nurses saw the work as isolated, monotonous and possibly dangerous. The College looked to the BMA for support, since they agreed on most of these issues.[11] The College's views also reflected its own interest in capturing the areas of nursing least subject to regulation, and staffed with nurses who were unlikely to be College members. In particular, it wanted a major expansion of nursing services in the community. The College did not desire a state-funded district nursing service at this stage, for it believed (as did the BMA), that patients who could pay for medical services should do so. But it argued that domestic nursing should be removed from commercial agencies with no medical credentials, and that 'co-operations' should be regulated to ensure that they hired only trained nurses.

The College and the trade unions

Meanwhile, other bodies claimed to represent nurses in less favoured areas of nursing. In 1934 NALGO produced its own response to the *Lancet* Commission, agreeing with most of the conclusions about nurses' working conditions, but making a stronger case for nurses in public hospitals, particularly probationers and male nurses. The College had no interest in recruiting male nurses who, although their numbers were slowly expanding, were restricted mainly to work in asylums or with venereal patients. NALGO, which also saw itself as a professional body and not a trade union, claimed at this time to have more nursing staff among its members than any other organisation.[12] As an association for local government workers, including nurses who were not state registered, it was in many respects more appealing to public health and poor law hospital staff, and better placed to speak for them, than the professionally minded College. It had already attracted a number of matrons who brought their staff with them. NALGO recommended an improved scale of salaries for institutional staff. It made more headway over salaries and working hours with local government than the College achieved in the voluntary hospitals, and the scramble to represent nurses continued.

By 1935 the College's position on nurses' pay and conditions was being attacked by the trade unions and the press. A typical incident occurred when Cardiff City Council proposed to reduce the salary of its probationer nurses from £35 to £25 per annum, while raising the salary of trained nurses.[13] It justified this action by referring to the College's argument that probationers should not be paid at a rate out of proportion to trained nurses. It was College policy, accepted by the *Lancet* Commission, that the salaries of trained nurses should be improved, and it tended to sacrifice the interests of probationers, arguing that they were receiving valuable training to prepare them for elite status in the profession, and that their problems would appear less serious if they could look forward to a decent salary when they qualified. Frances Goodall and her officers were well aware of the growing unrest among nurses, and considered liaising with the Trades Union Congress over salaries, though they were apprehensive that such discussions might 'taint' the College with allegations of political bias or trade unionism. In February 1937 Goodall wrote to the secretary of the BMA, G. C. Anderson, asking about the BMA's relations with the TUC. Anderson assured her that 'you will find no danger of political contamination'.[14] In the years that followed, the College was more conciliatory to the TUC. Delegates from both sat on numerous official committees and inquiries, and made common ground against the Ministry of Health over nurses' pay and working hours.

The nursing shortage was discussed widely in the newspapers and many local papers carried letters from nurses exposing the out-of-date culture of the hospitals and the humiliating treatment of some probationers. The College responded by circulating a letter to over 2,000 hospitals and institutions. It stated the College's position on salaries, and recommended a ninety-six-hour working fortnight for nurses. But the government's refusal to respond to the College's requests for a full inquiry into nursing played into the hands of the TUC. Growing dissatisfaction among nurses gave the unions an opportunity to recruit them, and 1937 proved to be a significant year in the relationship between nurses and organised labour.

In 1937 the TUC appointed an Advisory Committee on Nursing, which represented the Transport and General Workers' Union, the National Union of County Officers, the Mental Hospital and Institutional Workers' Union, the National Union of Public Employees, the Women Public Health Officers' Association and the National Union of General and Municipal Workers, and it delegated some of its members to produce a nurses' charter. The union movement was reviving after a lengthy period in the doldrums after the 1926 General Strike, particularly in white-collar occupations, and women workers represented an opportunity for recruitment. One of the College's main objections to general unions was that the voice of nurses would not be heard in bodies recruited from several occupations, and with a predominantly male leadership. The TUC's committee was intended to counter such arguments, and its importance was emphasised by the involvement of Ernest Bevin, general secretary of the Transport and General Workers' Union, and one of the most powerful figures in British trade unionism.[15] Bevin was a driving force behind the nurses' charter, which demanded a ninety-six-hour working

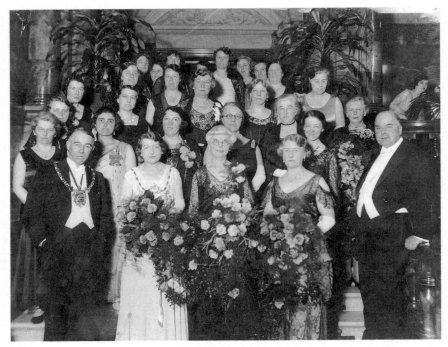

3.3 Annual general meeting, Sheffield, office holders and staff, including Margaret Sparshott, president (centre), 1931.

fortnight for nurses; one month's holiday with pay; overtime pay; super-annuation rights throughout the nursing services; free post-qualification courses; compulsory preliminary training schools; arbitration bodies (Whitley Councils) to standardise salaries and working conditions; and opportunities for trained nurses to live outside the hospitals.[16] Unlike most other workers, nursing organisations wished to negotiate a working fortnight rather than a working week in the hospitals. They accepted that if there was a problem on the ward, the matron might call on them to work a longer day at very short notice, and flexibility over a two-week period seemed appropriate. But the extra time worked was rarely compensated by free time later, and there was no overtime pay. The charter's aims were not much different from those of the College, but they were to be achieved through unionisation. Bevin was challenging the College's claim to speak for the nursing profession; but their relationship was to become closer than either could have expected.

The TUC followed the publication of its charter with a recruitment campaign, and distributed an attractive pamphlet entitled 'Off Duty', with illustrations of nurses enjoying social activities. It aimed to associate trade unions with the struggle for better conditions. This appeal to nurses' longing for leisure was shrewd, since nurses had little free time. The pamphlet asked, 'Doctors have their trade union – why not nurses?' and included a message from the much-admired actress Sybil Thorndike, warning nurses that, like actors, they could easily be exploited if they did not join a union. At the TUC Congress in September, the nurses' charter was debated. Delegates heard that the shortage of nurses was so serious that the voluntary hospital system was on the verge of a breakdown, while the collective income of the voluntary hospitals exceeded their total expenditure by over a million pounds. This calculation was reached by amalgamating the incomes of all the hospitals, though any pooling of the voluntary hospitals' resources would have required major government intervention. George Gibson, general secretary of the Mental Hospital and Institutional Workers' Union, attacked the College's social pretensions and vocational ideals: 'the rising generation is not prepared to give their services for nothing . . . a close-up of a duchess is not sufficient to balance the demerits of the profession'.[17] The TUC was told that nurses were difficult to organise because 'they have a superiority complex' and 'believe that they have a status which will be affected by joining a trade union'.[18] While agreeing that to allow five or six unions to recruit nurses was undesirable, the TUC decided not to encourage a new union for nurses only. Nevertheless, a union of this kind was already being established.

Thora Silverthorne, a young staff nurse, decided to set up the Association of Nurses as a trade union for nurses. She was a communist, and had recently returned from Spain after volunteering her services to the Socialist Medical Association (SMA) ambulance unit with the International Brigade. She nursed at the front in Aragon, and married the unit's Commandant 'to the sound of guns'.[19] She wanted all hospitals to adopt the TUC charter and, while acknowledging the efforts of the existing unions, hoped to prevent nurses being split between several unions alongside workers who did not share their professional interests. She accused the hospitals of exploiting nurses, arguing that if all hospital surpluses and deficits were pooled, there would be enough to implement the ninety-six-hour working fortnight and improve nurses' salaries. The apparent success of the Association of Nurses, which boasted of having received nearly 2,000 applications for membership within a month, demonstrated the attraction of a trade union run by nurses.[20] Branches of the Association were quickly formed in several of the large London hospitals, including St Thomas' and University College Hospital, and at Sheffield, Cardiff, Worcester and Leicester. Silverthorne wanted the Association to have the same position in the nursing world as the British Medical Association among doctors.[21]

All these events received much press and radio coverage and caused anxious debate in the profession. Newspapers printed articles and letters about conditions in their local hospitals. Many nurses, members and non-members, wrote to the College asking for a public response, and begging it to save nursing from trade unionism, which they believed would endanger the professional ideal. Matrons requested College area organisers to come to their hospitals and speak to the nursing staff. The College advised the organisers not to speak against trade unionism but in favour of professional organisation. Florence Udell, the area organiser in Scotland, addressed meetings in the Glasgow municipal hospitals, where the matrons were mounting a counter propaganda campaign against the unions.[22] The College also wrote to matrons and 'kindred organisations', including the BMA, the Institute of Hospital Almoners, the Chartered Society of Massage and Medical Gymnastics, the Medical Women's Federation, the National Council of Women, the Society of Medical Officers of Health and the Midwives' Institute, outlining its policies and asking for support. All these status-conscious associations were sympathetic to the College and agreed that nurses should join a professional association and not a trade union. The response from these middle-class bodies probably confirmed the TUC's suspicion that nurses were afflicted by a superiority complex.

In September 1937, the *Nursing Times* printed a supplement comparing the College's policy to the TUC charter, arguing that the College had been working on several of the charter's aims for years (though this was hardly an advertisement for the College's effectiveness). The supplement assessed the advantages of trade unions and professional organisations and appealed for loyalty to the College. It compared the College to the BMA and NALGO, non-political bodies with large memberships, which were not registered as trade unions. It set out the issues where the College had been striving for reform: working hours, annual leave and off-duty periods, sick pay, nurses' homes, superannuation, personal restrictions, salaries, the proportion of nurses to patients, and the need for a central arbitration machinery for nurses and their employers. On this last point it quoted the College's submission to the Voluntary Hospitals Commission in 1936:

> The College has constantly felt the need of some body composed of members of the boards of management of the hospitals, on which nursing as well as other hospital departments could be represented, both centrally and regionally, through their associations. Too often nurses' needs and nursing matters are discussed, and conclusions arrived at, in the absence of any nursing expert and in ignorance of many importance factors. This manner of dealing with nursing affairs is short sighted and contrary to modern ideas . . . The College would welcome the formation of a really representative body with which nursing problems could be discussed and possibly solved.[23]

The journal reminded its readers that the College had for the last two years been asking for a full government inquiry into nursing. The request was repeated in July 1937, and Kingsley Wood, the Minister of Health, had agreed to receive another deputation from the College on 3 November. But before the *Nursing Times* supplement appeared, the Minister, while opening a new municipal clinic at South Shields on 22 September, announced that he was setting up an inter-departmental committee of inquiry into nursing. The College was taken aback, but was informed, in strict confidence, that the political position was such that the Minister was forced to make his announcement in this way because he did not wish to seem overly influenced by any particular group.[24]

News of the inquiry intensified the trade unions' scramble to recruit nurses. In October the National Union of County Officers renamed its nursing section the Guild of Nurses and appointed a photogenic nurse, Mrs Iris Brook, as its national organiser. Her speeches emphasised that nurses should enjoy a normal private life that included romance.[25] The inaugural meeting of the Guild was held at St Pancras town hall on 26 November, and the Labour leader, George Lansbury, addressed over 500 nurses. The Guild particularly targeted the London County Council as a large employer of nurses, and kept up a vigorous campaign for a ninety-six-hour fortnight in LCC hospitals. In April 1938 it staged a dramatic demonstration in London when a small number of its members took part in a protest march in their white uniforms, wearing black masks to prevent victimisation.[26] Although this protest made no impression in the nursing press, it was most unusual for nurses to take this kind of action, and it received wide coverage in the national newspapers. The LCC, a Labour-controlled body, bowed to the pressure, at a time when a number of other local authorities were also conceding the ninety-six-hour fortnight.

The nursing shortage and government intervention

The nursing services had become a highly political matter. Conditions for nurses remained undeniably poor and were still founded on hospital custom and the disciplinary habits of individual matrons. These varied from one institution to another, which encouraged intervention in individual cases and undoubtedly stimulated trade union membership. By the late 1930s the traditional superiority of the voluntary hospitals was being undermined by the inability of some to pay staff an acceptable wage or to employ enough nurses to reduce the strain of long hours. By this time, municipal hospitals had greatly increased their nursing staff under the stimulus of the 1929 Local Government Act. Some began a programme of hospital investment, assisted by the government grant, and provided better working conditions, shorter hours and higher pay than the voluntary hospitals.[27] Turnover of staff in all hospitals was high, partly due to the rigours of training, but also because young women left when they married. The Association of Nurses claimed in 1938 that 'of every 100 girls who enter the profession, 38 leave in their first year while only 50 complete their training'.[28] Modern improvements in medical treatment and expansion of hospitals and local authority services such as maternity clinics brought a further demand for nurses. The nursing shortage was acute, and those who entered the profession were not always of the educational standard that the College thought desirable – it still hankered after an 'officer class'. Recruitment was a major issue, but future prospects were also discouraging. Despite the College's recommended pay scale, nurses' pay was not keeping pace with comparable jobs for women. A College survey taken in 1938 compared nurses' salaries with those of teachers and civil servants, assuming that they had a secondary education and were 'in each case an average worker, not brilliant'. Nurses did not fare well. During the first ten years of their working lives, qualified nurses earned £1,522, taking board and lodging into account; teachers £1,509; clerical civil servants £1,217, and executive civil servants £1,695. The nurses' apparently favourable position was because they received some salary and emoluments during training, and the other professions did not: 'in the case of the teacher for two years, and in the case of the civil servant for one year – and during that time they are paying for tuition'. However, the same comparisons over the subsequent ten-year period showed that nurses received in cash and kind, £2,175; teachers £2,835, and clerical civil servants £2,500. The other occupations, of course, did not subject their students to the gruelling domestic work of the probationer nurse. Nurses continued to fall behind because their annual increments were not as high as in the other services.[29]

With the agenda for the College's deputation now changed by the Minister's announcement, the Minister asked the College to outline a strategy for the government inquiry. In consultation with other health service organisations the council drew up a list of five topics: recruitment, staffing and planning of hospitals, education, economic conditions, and nursing the chronic sick.[30] The most pressing of these was recruitment. In 1932 the *Lancet* Commission tried to address the problem by suggesting reforms in the nursing service, but the economic crisis of the early 1930s then brought an influx of recruits, as women who could not afford training in other professions signed up for nursing. A probationer nurse was at least guaranteed board and lodging, an assistant nurse a basic salary, and the situation was reversed so that it briefly appeared that the profession would have no difficulty in finding recruits. This period of high recruitment coincided with the first attempts of Jewish women from Germany to apply for nurse training in Britain, leading to a regrettable decision by the College to protest to the Ministry of Labour against the training of foreign refugees because they would compete with British nurses for training places.[31]

The *Lancet*'s recommendations on how to solve the nursing shortage became redundant, but only temporarily. In 1934 the Employment Committee of the Association of Headmistresses of Public Secondary Schools experienced a period of unprecedented activity. After a series of addresses on careers given by professional and business experts and attended by over 700 school-leavers, the number of girls finding employment through the committee rose to 1,782, 75 per cent more than the previous year. Careers suggested for girls included salesmanship, nursery nursing, chartered accountancy, social work, librarianship, scientific research and domestic science. Nursing featured too, but as the service sector in Britain expanded, white-collar positions for women increased, and offered more attractive alternatives. The following year the committee dealt with even more applications. By the end of the decade, as the economy recovered, there was growing demand for junior office staff. Girls with a secondary education were sought after and sometimes encouraged by training bursaries, particularly for clerical and secretarial posts. This expansion of career options for educated girls affected nursing, and it soon lost any advantage it had gained.[32] The public image of nursing was badly tarnished by press criticism of nurses' poor working conditions, and the better-educated girl and her parents were now less likely to consider it an attractive career. Nevertheless, Abel-Smith's magisterial account of the profession contends that nursing was holding its own among girls with a secondary education in this period, and the proportion choosing the nursing profession was fairly constant.[33] The College's emphasis on the professional nature of nursing was an effective strategy for capturing the middle-class women that it chiefly targeted. The main problem was the slow expansion of secondary education in this period, and the gap between leaving school and entering nurse training at the minimum age of eighteen. Since most girls left school at fourteen, the pool of potential recruits was much restricted.

The inter-departmental committee met under the chairmanship of the Earl of Athlone, the King's brother-in-law. Its twenty members were not meant to represent different interests in nursing, but were selected from matrons, local authorities, mental services, medical officers of health, voluntary hospitals, doctors, the teaching profession, the GNC, sister tutors and district nursing.[34] Four nurses on the general register were included: Dame Ellen Musson, Gertrude Cowlin, Dorothy M. Smith and Frances Wakeford. At the age of seventy, Musson was one of the elder 'statesmen' of the profession and was nominated by the GNC. She was a founder of the College and an elected member of its council from 1916 to 1939, chairman of the GNC from 1926 to 1944, and Honorary Treasurer of the International Council of Nurses from 1925 to 1947.[35] Cowlin, who was at that time a visitor for the Central Council of District Nursing in London, was more obviously a College nominee, having been at various times area organiser, librarian and education officer. Dorothy Smith was matron of the Middlesex Hospital, and a member of the Association of Hospital Matrons, a body close to the College in membership and outlook. Wakeford, in her early thirties, was a staff nurse at the Kingston and District

Hospital in Surrey. She claimed many years later that her matron nominated her for the committee 'for her own glorification'. She was supposed to represent the ordinary nurse, but admitted that she had been timid and overawed by the senior nurses.[36] All four nurses were members of the College, to the disgust of Thora Silverthorne and Ethel Bedford Fenwick.[37]

With the long-awaited inquiry under way, the problems of the nursing profession continued to attract press attention. Throughout the autumn, newspapers printed damning articles on the conditions endured by nurses and reflected old tensions between the College and the unions. The *Daily Mirror* invited nurses to send in stories of their appalling working conditions (anonymity guaranteed), while other papers featured headlines such as 'Wanted: As slaves for hospitals. Sad story behind shortage of nurses', and 'Nurses may be ministering angels to the sick but their life is cheap labour slavery. What they urgently need is a trade union'.[38] Even advertisements reinforced the message. Johnson and Johnson ran a cartoon strip of a stern matron criticising a probationer's efforts to polish the floor. Aided by Johnson's Wax, the probationer's task was eased and she received fulsome praise from the matron, but the implications of domestic servitude were not well received by the College. This spate of criticism culminated in an article by the popular novelist and doctor A. J. Cronin, under the headline, 'The myth of Florence Nightingale is dead. To invoke it now in the cause of SWEATED LABOUR is sheer hypocrisy'.[39] Goodall wrote indignantly to Cronin, inviting him to 'put aside a little time to come here and find what nurses themselves are asking of the community they serve'.[40]

The College's response to the trade unions' attack may not have won it many new supporters, but it rallied some dormant members. Ruth Pecker, registrar of the General Nursing Council for Scotland, wrote to Goodall, 'It's a very great temptation that I am resisting today in not writing to the press to say "Thank you TUC"! In Edinburgh this week we really should feel grateful to the TUC for rousing the nursing profession to sit up and take interest in the College of Nursing'.[41] One of the key College speakers at the time was Florence Udell, who believed passionately that if nurses joined trade unions their professional interests would be swamped:

> [the] unions are enrolling all kinds of nurses, including those in training, trained nurses, and nurses who will never be trained, all on the same basis. This is bound to lower the standard of the state registered nurse, for which the College has fought for years and now jealously guards.[42]

The weekly review *Time and Tide* ran a series of four articles in early 1938 under the heading 'Do nurses get a square deal?' that aimed 'to acquaint readers ... with existing nursing conditions and possible reforms', from different viewpoints. The paper's founder and editor, Margaret Haig Thomas,

Lady Rhondda, was a vehement supporter of women's rights. She claimed a seat in the House of Lords after her father's death but, after much legal wrangling, was denied the place. Her magazine aimed to inform women on political issues, and she featured articles by prominent feminists. The readership was small, though contributors included the reforming and literary elite of the day. The series was very critical of the College, and editorials implied that the College was reactionary and even hypocritical. The first article expressed the views of the militant Association of Nurses. Balancing this was a second article the following week from the College's point of view. The third was by Harold Balme, a former medical missionary in China, and a member of the College council. He had already published a criticism of nursing education, claiming that the hospital training system reduced nursing to a craft.[43] In *Time and Tide* he also implicitly criticised the College by suggesting that the leaders of nurses had 'failed to adjust themselves to modern conditions and demands' by clinging to the inspiring but outmoded ideal of 'service, devotion, obedience, and personal self-sacrifice'.[44] But Balme was fundamentally on the side of the College, and defended nursing as a profession that required a high level of training.[45] He also accepted that much of the more menial work done by nurses could be delegated to other grades of worker.

Lady Rhondda seized on the notion of failure of leadership in nursing and wrote the final article herself. She described the nursing shortage as a form of strike against poor conditions:

> The College of Nursing . . . with a Council headed by the Treasurer of St Thomas's Hospital and composed largely of medical men and Matrons of hospitals, has failed, on its own showing . . . For twenty years it has held the field as the great nurses' organisation, and now, at the end of that twenty years, the position of nurses, economically, educational and socially, is so bad that we are facing a crisis of the gravest nature. So, far from the best type of women being attracted into nursing, no type at all is attracted.[46]

She argued that the College had failed because its officers were not 'rank and file nurses but the employers of nurses', such as the council's chairman, Sir Arthur Stanley. It was anomalous that the College was promoting the ninety-six-hour fortnight, while its chair was treasurer of a hospital that allegedly worked its nurses for 140 hours per fortnight. Such criticisms must have seemed unfair to the College council, which had spent much time trying to achieve a complete review of nursing services, but its position on working hours was easy to attack. The College was not against modernisation, but still regarded flexible hours as a sign of professional status, and the matrons who led the College wanted to keep control over nurses' hours.

The College prepared its evidence for the Athlone Committee in January 1938.[47] It dealt with recruitment, education, the supply and conditions of nurses in general hospitals (the largest group of registered nurses), private and domiciliary nurses (the second largest group), public health nurses and sister tutors. It argued that the nursing shortage was caused by the 'phenomenal expansion of the health services of the country' and through wastage by marriage, since there was no decline in the actual number of recruits.[48] It asked for a survey to determine the number of nurses required for an adequate national nursing service in Britain, modelled on a Canadian survey of 1930. The two major areas of reform should be staffing levels in the hospitals, and the salaries of every grade of nurse, particularly the staff nurse and ward sister. The College recommended a wider training to prepare nurses for all fields of nursing, that central training schools for groups of hospitals should be established with the aid of state grants, and that the Board of Education provide grants for nurses on post-registration courses. The College believed that nursing was out of step with other professions in allowing unqualified tutors to hold teaching positions, and the College offered to establish its own roll of qualified sister tutors. It wanted an assessment of the number of public health nurses and health visitors required for present and future needs, and noted that, because of the cost of training, health visitors in rural areas often had no specialist qualifications. The College again demanded regulation of private co-operations and nursing agencies.

Comparable evidence was presented to the Athlone Committee by thirty-six other associations and individuals. The Student Nurses' Association, while reiterating College policy on salaries and conditions, wanted improved facilities for study, better clinical instruction in the wards, well qualified sister tutors, access to good libraries, refresher courses after graduation and the opportunity to take post-qualification courses, aided by scholarships. The opinions of two student nurses were added in an appendix, and although these were not included as the Association's view, they showed that some of the younger generation of nurses had a positive approach to state intervention in nurse training.[49] They wanted to be recognised as students, not cheap labour, to close training schools not approved by the GNC, to separate the training schools' finances from those of the hospitals, and asked for state aid for the schools, and bursaries and scholarships for students. They believed that such reforms would in time solve the problems of recruitment.

The Athlone Committee heard evidence from all the major organisations concerned with the employment of nurses, including the College and the trade unions. In response to widespread anxiety about the nursing shortage in the face of imminent war, the committee produced an interim report in December 1938.[50] Welcomed by the College, the report was debated at length within its professional sections and branches, and the council's reactions were published in the Nursing Times.[51] The council agreed with almost all of the report's findings, and particularly its basic premise that the state, the public and the hospital authorities should treat nursing as a service of outstanding national importance to encourage the flow of recruits. Conditions of service, salaries and pensions should be determined nationally, so that nursing could compete with other types of employment for women, and the ninety-six-hour fortnight must be introduced in all hospitals. The committee recommended state grants to voluntary hospitals unable to meet the increased cost of these reforms, and further grants for all hospitals that were recognised as nurse training schools.

But the College council 'deplored' the report's assumption that a large proportion of nurses must be recruited from elementary rather than from secondary schools. The Athlone report called for pre-nursing courses for girls too young to begin nurse training, but the College believed that such courses would be too demanding for elementary school leavers and unappealing to the better-educated girl who was the College's main target. The College agreed that a more co-ordinated system of recruitment was needed, and would consider establishing a central bureau itself. Athlone's desire for nursing committees to regulate nurses' salaries was in line with College policy, but the College did not want a centralised body like the Burnham Committee for teachers, concerned only with salaries. Rather, it continued to press for its own scheme of regional and national committees to deal with wider nursing issues. Crucially, the College compromised over Athlone's recommendation that the GNC establish an official roll of assistant nurses. The status of the untrained nurse had long exercised the College, and although it believed that formal recognition of this group might undermine the professional status of nursing, it accepted that in a national crisis there was little room for high principles. The College agreed that assistant nurses were necessary, but rejected the title, maintaining (quite correctly) that the public would not understand the difference between the two grades of nurse. It preferred 'approved invalid attendant', but this cumbersome title was not adopted. The College's decision not to contest the employment of assistant nurses broke with its traditions, but kept it in favour with government, in contrast to Mrs Bedford Fenwick and the Royal British Nurses' Association, who strongly opposed recognition of non-registered nurses, and found themselves sidelined as a result.

The press gave the Athlone report a good reception. Headlines included 'Sweeping official reform'; 'A better time coming'; 'More pay, shorter hours, fewer rules'. Only *Time and Tide* was critical, commenting 'The report contains nothing that is new, it follows very closely the lines of the *Lancet* Report on whose covers the dust of eight years now lies'. It objected that the four nurses on the committee were all members of the College, and that by taking evidence from only sixteen working nurses, compared with thirty-seven matrons, the committee reflected the matrons' conservative views. It was unreasonable to expect that Athlone's recommendations would be implemented without compulsion, and the only hope for the profession was for nursing organisations outside the College to sink their differences and make a united stand.[52] The Athlone Committee continued to meet until July 1939, but its proceedings were suspended on the outbreak of war. A draft of its final report, which was never published, indicates that it intended to address the purpose and organisation of nurse training and education.[53]

War

The Second World War laid heavy responsibilities on nurses, and gave the College more opportunity to act on their behalf. It also brought the College into contact with nurses outside its own membership. While the College continued its usual activities during the war, and indeed, made increased efforts to provide welfare services for nurses, it had to deal more routinely with government bodies, and to compromise some of its own views on nurse training in response to the national crisis. The nursing shortage was already acute, and the war created a demand that far exceeded the supply of fully trained women. The College's role in the coming struggle began early in 1938, when the Committee for Imperial Defence, which had a nursing section, consulted it over the supply of nurses. The College pressed for a civil nursing reserve ready to act in an emergency, but no action was taken until September, when the College offered its assistance directly to the Minister of Health. He requested it to prepare, as speedily as possible, a roll of state registered and certificated nurses available for civilian duties. There was grim expectation that bombing would cause many civilian casualties, and the College, like the BMA, had a major part in recruiting for the emergency services. College branches were asked to prepare local rolls of volunteers. Appeals were made on the radio and in the press, and a recruiting office opened at the College's London headquarters. The main targets were the many women with training and experience who had left the profession on marriage. But in spite of these efforts, the College reported that due to 'a complete lack of co-ordination' between the local authorities and the nursing and medical services, the number of volunteers was completely inadequate. As an alternative, the College preferred a centrally organised civil nursing reserve under a government department or central council.[54]

By the end of the year a Central Emergency Committee for Nurses was appointed, and it included a College representative. One of its key tasks was to set up the Civil Nursing Reserve (CNR). In November 1938 the Ministry asked the College if it would begin registration of both qualified and assistant nurses. It was a major departure from normal College policy to recognise assistant nurses, since the College had been arguing since its foundation that all nurses should be fully trained, but the Minister insisted that they be included, and the College's views were already beginning to change. The College accepted this duty, hoping that it would be temporary, and asked that the term 'assistant nurse' be interpreted in official statements as 'women who are, or have been, earning their living by nursing but who are only partially trained or who have had a satisfactory period of nursing experience'.[55] The Scottish Board of the College undertook the same task, and by February 1939, when the government assumed responsibility for the task, over 3,000 applications had been processed. By this period the College had dropped its opposition to refugee nurses, not only because it had more understanding of their plight, but because they offered a welcome alleviation of the nursing shortage. In this it was somewhat ahead of the popular press. The *Daily Express* ran an unedifying campaign to keep refugee nurses out of the hospitals, and appealed for English girls to serve instead. It paid for two British nurses to travel to Lenham TB Hospital to replace two 'cultivated' Jewish women from Vienna, whom the hospital employed as nursing auxiliaries when it could find no other recruits.[56]

At this time there were over 80,000 nurses on the general register. Some were retired or in private practice and so, theoretically, available for service in the Civil Nursing Reserve. But enlistment was very slow. In August 1939 only 14 per cent of those contacted directly by the Central Emergency Committee responded. A few weeks before the declaration of war, a disappointingly low total of 9,000–10,000 nurses in England and Wales had enrolled, although a further 45,000 women applied for training as nursing auxiliaries.[57] The College believed that reluctance to enrol was partly owing to uncertainty over the salaries offered by the CNR. Before the war, salaries of hospital sisters varied from £70 to £150 per annum and those of staff nurses from £60 to £90; but it was not clear whether these differentials would be maintained in the CNR. In August 1939 the Minister of Health announced guaranteed salary scales for nurses in military service or the CNR, but while this encouraged many more nurses to join, it produced inequities. Salaries for sisters and staff nurses in the Queen Alexandra's Imperial Military Nursing Service Reserve and the Territorial Army Nursing Service were set at £85 and £80 per annum respectively, which could mean less than a salary in civilian employment. Those in the CNR were to receive £90 per annum regardless of experience, and £110 if in charge of a ward. Hence an experienced sister earning £85 a year might find herself working alongside an inexperienced CNR nurse earning £90 a year. While the College highlighted these disparities, it also appealed to nurses to 'do the work that comes our way . . . without grumbling, bitterness and useless friction'.[58]

The College assisted the CNR wholeheartedly, and Cowdray Hall became a temporary enquiry bureau. From July 1939 to June 1940, during the brief lull of the 'phoney war', the College administered the London register of the

CNR. This involved allocating nurses to the sector matrons responsible for nursing in the emergency medical divisions of London. Every week, between 700 and 800 persons were interviewed and an average of 1,400 postal inquiries answered. The College continued to express its concerns about various aspects of the CNR, and was relieved when, at the end of 1939, the Ministry replaced the Central Emergency Committee with a Central Advisory Board, chaired by Florence Horsbrugh, MP. Regional nursing officers were appointed to each of the eleven civil defence regions for the hospitals of England and Wales.[59] These changes met most of the College's objections to CNR arrangements, but anxiety about working conditions continued. Nurses on the supplementary state registers, who had specialised rather than general training, were paid at the level of an untrained assistant nurse in the CNR unless they were engaged in their own specialty; pension contributions were not paid; and they had only twelve days annual leave, the same as air raid precaution staff.[60] The College argued that the CNR should have the same entitlements as the regular nursing services.

In June 1939 the College formed its own Emergency War Committee to act for the council if necessary and to assess the financial position of the College. Harsh economies were called for. If war broke out, the College could expect decreasing returns from its investments, and its members were likely to be deployed around the country, interrupting the flow of subscriptions. The College had always rented out part of its building, but since central London was a prime bombing target, tenants might evacuate and rental income fall. When war came, it did indeed put pressure on the administrative capabilities of the College, at a time when its services were in heavy demand. Its clerical staff were reduced considerably. Owing to the withdrawal of students and lecturers evacuated or enlisted, courses were cancelled and education officers released to serve in the CNR. Some administrative staff were evacuated to Edinburgh and worked from the Scottish Board for several years.[61] Those remaining in London faced much personal danger, and two were killed in air raids.

Once the blitz began, the poorer citizens of London, having no other shelter, took to the Underground stations reluctantly opened by the government. Conditions were intolerable, as the College's Public Health Section reported: 'a tube shelter a mile and a quarter long accommodates 7000 people, and the sanitary arrangements consist of four Elsan closets at each end of the tunnel'.[62] The medical peer Lord Horder urged the government to provide proper sanitation and medical services in the public shelters, but the response was very slow, and volunteers had to step in.[63] Frustrated by the lack of official action, members of the Public Health Section turned out every night to offer nursing services in the tube stations, and to publicise their demand that a doctor and a nurse should be available in all large shelters. The section formed two units taking turns to work underground, helping the volunteer nurses and the St John's Ambulance Brigade. The duty nurse reported to the first aid post, checked the logbooks of the day's activities, and then toured the platforms, the lavatories and the makeshift canteens before the arrival of the night doctor. The larger of the two stations regularly sheltered up to 2,000 people. Illnesses were often diagnosed in the shelters, and some patients were sent directly to hospital. The nurse administered medicines, and gave advice on immunisation and other health measures. A final morning round and writing up the nightly log saw the end of the nurse's shift.[64] The College wanted nurses with public health training in every shelter, but there were not enough of them; and so the College ran three-day crash courses for nurses taking on this work. The action of the Public Health Section was widely and favourably reported in the press, and probably did not endear the College to the Ministry of Health.[65]

In the decade leading up to the war, the Public Health Section had gained an influential voice on all nursing matters. Although section meetings were drastically curtailed during the war, the work of health visitors and district nurses was encouraged through articles in the *Nursing Times*. Irene Charley and her staff at the Public Health Section took a particular interest in homeless victims of the blitz. They visited the centres for the homeless, and asked the government to provide a twenty-four-hour nursing service in all large dispersal and rest centres. The council urged the Ministry of Health to set up its own Department of Nursing at the earliest opportunity, and to include public health nurses on its staff, but it was becoming apparent that the section of government most likely to co-operate with the College was the Ministry of Labour.

The reasons for this new collaboration lay in the College's role in training industrial nurses. The industrial nursing branch of the Public Health Section expanded rapidly as a direct result of the war. To emphasise the importance of properly trained nurses in maintaining a healthy workforce, the College sent a deputation to the Factory Department of the Home Office in 1939, offering its services in the recruitment, training and placing of industrial nurses. This offer was enthusiastically received. The chief medical officer of the Factory Department asked the College to continue teaching its industrial nursing courses, and also to increase the flow of students by shortening courses to three months. Later, this was cut further to six weeks, and a correspondence course was also offered for the duration of the war. In 1940 the Factories (Medical and Welfare) Order obliged factories with government contracts to employ medical personnel, including nurses. An important consequence of this was that the College, now in a position of some authority, permitted several groups of nurses who were not on the general register to affiliate to the College. These nurses, mainly from the supplementary registers, did not have voting rights, but they had access to College facilities and were encouraged to attend College training courses. They included mental nurses, and so, for the first time, male nurses came under the purview of the College, although they were not eligible for membership.[66] A number of male nurses were demanding training in industrial nursing, but since these courses were available only through the College, there were no certificated male industrial nurses. The College training courses were opened to men, and in February 1942 John Williams, an industrial nurse, became the first man to hold a College certificate.[67] Public health nursing demonstrated its importance to the war effort and contributed greatly to the friendly relationship between the College and the new Minister of Labour, Ernest Bevin.

Churchill gave Bevin great powers to organise the labour force for the needs of war. Unlike the First World War, all males of military age were immediately conscripted when war was declared, either for military service or a designated occupation. From December 1941, women between twenty and thirty were also conscripted. Bevin, whom the College viewed with much trepidation before the war, was now in control of civilian nursing recruits as part of the conscription of women, but relations between the College and the burly Minister of Labour were surprisingly cordial. He had powers to coerce the civilian population, but preferred voluntary co-operation. The support of the trade unions was essential in this, and Bevin used the emergency to force previously recalcitrant employers to accept trade unionism in their workforce. He wanted to protect workers' health, both for their own sakes and to maximise productivity, and the College, the main training body for industrial and public health nurses, was important in this. In 1943 Bevin issued regulations for the training of industrial nurses, and gave due weight to the College's views. All industrial nurses had to be on the general or supplementary registers. General nurses were offered generous government grants to cover the cost of training in industrial nursing, and a number of prominent companies such as Gillette and Pilkington provided bursaries or scholarships. The Nuffield Provincial Hospitals Trust gave £1,885 to the College to assist in expanding its courses to institutions outside London.[68] The government now valued industrial nursing as a skilled branch of professional nursing, and the College was accepted as a partner in its development. There was some irony in this. The Ministry of Health, responsible for the Emergency Medical Services, saw nurses as a labour problem, and accepted women with minimal training. The Ministry of Labour saw industrial nurses as essential to workers' health, and insisted on an appropriate level of training.

Throughout the war, the *Nursing Times* published regular articles on the nursing and medical services. Illustrated features on hospital ships, hospital trains and casualty clearing stations showed the services coping under pressure. Strategies for managing the casualties of heavy bombing and preparations for gas attacks were regular features, as were articles on general health, like 'keeping fit in the blackout'. Some of the less obvious aspects of nursing, such as help for nursing mothers whose milk had dried up due to the trauma of air raids, showed the importance of trained nurses in the community. The College used its editorial control of the *Nursing Times*, frequent contributions to the press and occasional radio broadcasts to become part of the national propaganda machine, and urged nurses to be positive in the face of often difficult and distressing work. It received funds from Commonwealth nurses to assist British nurses made homeless in the bombing, and appealed to householders outside the cities to welcome tired nurses into their homes for a weekend break. Although not directly stated, this appeal was obviously aimed at the middle classes. The College also distributed gifts from abroad, including white wedding dresses (in three sizes) from the American Federation of Women's Clubs, to be lent to hospital nurses whose hopes of a white wedding were threatened by clothes rationing. Eleanor Roosevelt personally donated a glamorous white taffeta gown.[69] As in the 1914–18 war, the government could use the image of the nurse to increase morale, by reassuring beleaguered civilians that trained and capable nurses were at hand. The College was at the centre of a shifting population of nurses in the forces and the CNR, and its facilities were welcomed by many members as they travelled between nursing stations. It tried to keep in contact with beleaguered nurses in Britain and in many theatres of war.

The College regretted the adjournment of the Athlone Committee in October 1939. The *Nursing Times* put it rather dramatically: 'It is a thousand pities that the tragedy of war has befallen the nursing profession at this critical stage in its development'.[70] There was no hope of a final report until after the war, by which time circumstances would have altered so much that the information collected would be out of date. The profession entered the war with all its old problems unresolved, particularly the question of nurses' pay.

Wartime politics and reconstruction

The College's evidence to the Athlone Committee included a memorandum on National and Regional Councils for the Nursing Profession as a desirable means of negotiation between nurses and their employers. The then Minister of Labour, Ernest Brown, had advised the College in drawing up their proposals, and it was through his Ministry, rather than the Ministry of Health, that the first negotiating machinery for nurses' salaries and conditions was set up. In 1940, when Brown was Minister of Health, a Local Authorities' Nursing Services Joint Committee was appointed to negotiate salary scales and conditions.[71] Consisting of representatives from the College, the trade unions and employers' organisations, the committee made a little progress but was opposed by the British Hospitals Association on behalf of the voluntary hospitals. The association was anxious about loss of autonomy and increased trade unionism among nurses.

In April 1941 the government announced that a Nurses' Salaries Committee would be established, on the lines of the Burnham Committee for teachers, as recommended by the Athlone report. The College and other nursing associations were disappointed. They wanted the committee to concern itself with wider issues than salaries, and to cover all aspects of work and training. Frances Goodall wrote to Brown, reminding him that as Minister of Labour he had advised the College to draw up a national and regional negotiating structure for the profession, and that this scheme was now in operation through the Local Authorities' Nursing Services Joint Committee.[72] Goodall hoped to persuade the Ministry of Health to change its plans, and had discussions with the secretary of the British Hospitals Association, J. P. Wetenhall, about how to proceed. But in July she was invited to meet the Minister informally to hear his plans for the proposed negotiating committee. When the College deputation met the Minister, he made a long statement outlining his position and confirming that the committee would be concerned only with settling minimum salaries for nurses. Frances Goodall was very discouraged, feeling that despite all their efforts they had made no impression: 'The Minister himself talked most of the time and seemed very disinclined to listen, let alone consider, any of the views which the College put forward.'[73] Goodall hoped that Bevin might stand by them in their attempt to set up a more representative body to negotiate nurses' salaries and conditions, but the College had no alternative but to accept Brown's invitation to join his committee. In doing so they formally recorded their disappointment at the committee's limited remit.

The government had examined other possible models for negotiation, including the Whitley Councils, and the national joint council structure that the College advocated. The Ministry of Health favoured a Whitley Council, but it needed to deal rapidly with the problem of nurses' salaries, and the Whitley Councils, given to lengthy negotiation between the staff and management sides, tended to be slow.[74] Meanwhile, the College co-operated with the Local Authorities' Nursing Services Joint Committee, hoping that local solutions could be reached without encouraging trade unionism among nurses. This committee had no influence on national decisions, and the government acted on its own initiative. In October 1941 Lord Rushcliffe, a former Minister of Labour, was appointed to chair a Nurses' Salaries Committee. It consisted of two panels, each with twenty members, nominated by organisations representing employers and nurses. Although the College had nine seats and the Association of Hospital Matrons one, giving them half the seats on the employees' panel, they were not happy at the number of seats allocated to the trade unions. Representation was based on membership figures supplied by the unions, and the College doubted the TUC's claim to have over 16,000 nurses in membership, for many of these were not state registered and, if non-registered members were to be taken into account, the College could claim an additional 8,000 members through its Student Nurses' Association. NALGO was also discontented, for it had only three seats based on a membership of over 7,000 nurses, and feared loss of influence. It did not wish to jeopardise the existing Whitley machinery for local government employees. Under pressure it finally agreed to join the committee, on condition that it dealt with salaries alone.[75] To the embarrassment of the Nursing Services Joint Committee, the remit of the Rushcliffe Committee was soon extended to include conditions of service, making the Joint Committee redundant.

The Rushcliffe Committee was the first official body appointed to fix salary scales and conditions for nursing. A similar committee was appointed for Scotland, and the two chairs exchanged minutes and correspondence.[76] Both committees presented their first reports at the end of January 1943, and Rushcliffe followed some of the Athlone Committee's recommendations by trying to bring nursing into line with other professions open to women. A ninety-six-hour fortnight was accepted, with the government agreeing to cover up to 50 per cent of any extra expenditure. The needs of war finally brought nursing to the forefront of national planning. In 1941, the year of the College's silver jubilee, a Division of Nursing was established at the Ministry of Health with the principal of the Civil Nursing Reserve, Katherine Watt, as the first chief nursing officer. The College welcomed this, having long advocated such a department. The day after announcing the new division, the Minister of Health appealed to the young women of the country 'to enrol for nursing service and particularly to take up nursing as a life career'.[77]

The College's reactions to the Rushcliffe Committee were mixed. Salaries were to rise, as recommended by the College. The government intended to increase salaries for probationers, to encourage recruitment. The College would not alter its view that qualified nurses should be the main beneficiaries of salary increases, since probationers were receiving expensive training, and their incentive would be the salaries they expected after qualifying, as in most other professions. Nursing, the College argued, was 'the only profession in which the principle that the maximum salary is more important than the minimum is ignored'.[78] The government was now giving a direct subsidy for nurses' salaries, but this was not expected to solve the problem of recruitment, even though the Ministry of Labour agreed to inform women conscripted for National Service that it was in their interests to begin a full training as probationers, rather than sign up as auxiliary nurses. In 1943 *The Economist* neatly described the situation, summoning up two nursing heroines of war, Florence Nightingale and Edith Cavell:

emphasis is too often laid on the sacrifices demanded, instead of on the fact that nursing is an interesting and, in the future at least, a well paid and well regulated profession. The shadow of Florence Nightingale has lain too long upon it . . . Patriotism is not enough; if nursing is made an attractive profession, as now seems likely, the recruiting campaign should concentrate on pointing it out.[79]

The College failed to win over the Ministry of Health on significant policy issues during the war, and feared that the problems of the profession would not be addressed in peacetime. With the Athlone Committee suspended, its resumption unlikely, and no guarantee that its interim report would be heeded, the College decided to act on its own account. The TUC, with similar concern for its nursing members, had already set up a National Advisory Committee for the Nursing Profession. The College followed, appointing its own reconstruction committee in 1941, and Lord Horder agreed to act as chairman. Thomas Jeeves Horder was physician to the King, and very active in medical politics and nursing issues. His committee, half from the College and half from 'kindred organisations' such as the BMA, planned for the post-war reconstruction of the nursing profession, including its regulation, education and remuneration. The appointment of the Horder Committee, the first of many high-powered investigative bodies, was a new departure for the College. In its early years it had intervened in nursing affairs in a piecemeal fashion. From this period, it attempted a more active role in the formulation of nursing policy.

Over the next eight years the Horder Committee produced four major reports. The first appeared in 1942, and was concerned with assistant nurses. It was predictable that an inquiry led by the College should make this a priority. Many untrained nursing assistants were employed during the emergency – the same situation that motivated Swift and Stanley to form the College of Nursing. There was no quick solution to the nursing shortage and the College reluctantly accepted the necessity for assistant nurses during the war. But the prospect of large numbers of untrained nurses seeking nursing posts after the war was alarming. To the government, the untrained nurse was an immediate solution to shortages; to the College, she was a threat to professional standards. Nevertheless, the first Horder report conceded that this new grade was 'pivotal to the reconstruction of nursing' and would have to be appropriately placed in a recognised hierarchy of nursing personnel.[80] The College, from necessity, finally accepted the assistant nurse and was anxious to ensure that her training, salary, status and even uniform and badges, would be clearly differentiated from state registered nurses. The College believed that, by giving assistant nurses the more basic nursing duties, student nurses would be freed from much of their heavy labour, and that assistant nurses would also be acceptable in institutions with longstanding nursing shortages, such as TB sanatoria and institutions for the chronic sick, where a high level of technical expertise was not required.[81]

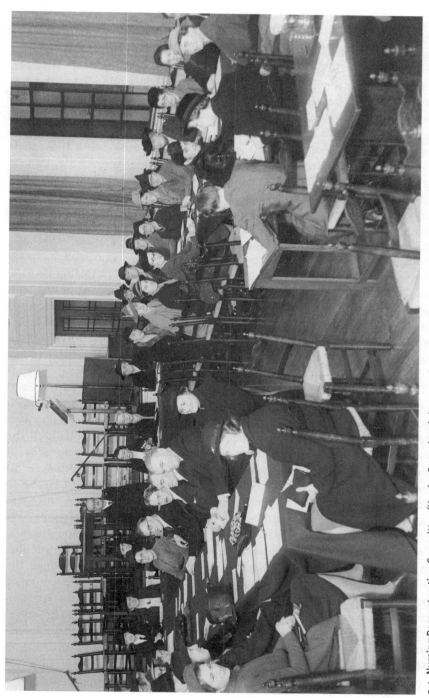

3·4 Nursing Reconstruction Committee (Horder Committee), inaugural meeting in the Cowdray Hall, College of Nursing, London, Lord Horder presiding, November 1941.

Many of Horder's policies were incorporated in the Nurses Act of 1943, for the government was anxious to increase the supply of nurses by lowering training standards, and a second tier of nurses might achieve this. The Act did not fulfil the College's desire that no one except a professionally qualified person could use the title of 'nurse', but it did meet the College's demand that nursing agencies be regulated. The Act compelled agencies to hold a licence, and to employ a doctor or qualified nurse to select their nursing staff. Clients had to be informed of the qualifications of the nurse supplied to them, and it was an offence for agencies or individuals to make false claims about their qualifications. The most significant section of the Act legitimised the assistant nurse and required the GNC to maintain a roll of assistant nurses who had fulfilled minimum conditions of training.[82] The profession was then officially divided into state registered nurses and state enrolled nurses, and the nurse training schools could offer training for either qualification. This division was contentious, and threatened to cause strife within the College. The main opposition came from the College's Scottish Board. Florence Udell, its secretary, wrote an agitated personal letter to Frances Goodall, revealing that she was having the greatest difficulty in keeping the Scottish Board in line with the College council's policy on assistant nurses. The GNC in Scotland required a higher level of entry qualifications from probationers than its English counterpart, and resistance to 'dilution' of the profession was stronger north of the border. Udell reported that the Scottish Matrons' Association, the GNC in Scotland, and other influential groups, were opposed to the Nurses (Scotland) Bill, which would extend the training and recognition of assistant nurses to Scotland. Since these organisations were well represented on the Scottish Board, Udell was greatly alarmed that the College would lose credibility with the Secretary of State and the Department of Health for Scotland if the Scottish Board resisted legislation.[83] In the smaller political community of Edinburgh, with its strong respect for medical traditions, the Scottish Board enjoyed a more harmonious relationship with the Department of Health in Scotland than its English counterpart with the Ministry of Health, and Udell was very reluctant to disrupt this. In the end there was compromise: the SEN grade was introduced in Scotland, but for only five years in the first instance. The grade was not made permanent until 1948. For this reason, Scottish hospitals did not apply for approval to train assistant nurses. Although the College's attitude towards assistant nurses was ambivalent, it encouraged them to set up their own association, and in 1944 the National Association of Assistant Nurses was formed in England.[84] It looked to the College for representation, and there was some anxiety among College members that enrolled nurses might be recruited into other organisations. At this point, affiliation to the College was offered only to associations of nurses whose names appeared on the GNC's supplementary registers. The College resisted affiliation with assistant nurses, but made no public statement 'lest it should stimulate trade union activity' among them.[85]

The College pressed on with the second and third reports from the Horder Committee, on education and training, and on recruitment. They appeared in one volume in December 1943, taking into account the recent Education Bill that would raise the school leaving age to fifteen, and hoping to influence government policy in anticipation of an imminent White Paper on post-war health services. The second report called for a wider basic training for general nursing, covering four years, with short periods of experience in other branches of nursing such as fever, TB and mental nursing, and an elective six months' training in a nursing specialty in the final year. It proposed that hospitals be grouped to provide a complete basic training, with probationer nurses spending blocks of time in the lecture rooms and in the wards, without attempting to cope with both in the same day, as was current practice. Controversially, Horder proposed that the student status of probationer nurses be confirmed by making them pay for their training rather than receiving wages from the hospitals, just as students in other professions paid fees. This suggestion was almost universally condemned, and the College was accused of being out of touch with economic realities.[86] Even though the school leaving age was to be fifteen, and possibly sixteen before long, there would still be a gap before school leavers could start nurse training. The College wanted to close the gap with theoretical training in further education colleges before practical training began, but the suggestion was condemned as middle-class elitism. Even the *Economist*, which sympathised with many of Horder's principles, commented on its impracticality:

> the vicious circle – that there can be no major reforms in nursing until there are enough nurses, but that there will not be enough nurses until the major reforms are carried out – still exists. It can, however, gradually be broken if every opportunity for making a reform is seized, and especially if teachers and school-girls alike are brought to regard nursing as a useful, well-paid and interesting career, and not merely as a means of inculcating selflessness and self-sacrifice or as a step towards the highest life.[87]

The Ministry of Health was irritated because the report appeared just before its own White Paper.[88] Katherine Watt, although a member of the College, did not approve of its ambitions, and wrote in an internal note, 'my first reading of the . . . Report gives the idea of hotch potch'.[89] The College's position was also undermined by the College of Midwives, which suspected that its recommendations for a single Central Nursing Board would undermine its own position.[90] Katherine Watt agreed to a meeting with the College to maintain the peace, and Ministry officials prepared for this, doubting whether the College was really representative of nurses:

> It is a pity that the membership of the College is still too small to make it a body truly representative of the nursing profession but I believe that the numbers have recently increased from only about ⅓ of the nurses on the register to something nearer ½ and it is, of course, the only body making anything like a 'collective voice' for nurses.[91]

In preparation for the meeting, the Ministry's officials gave Henry Willink, Brown's successor, a thumbnail sketch of all organisations that claimed to speak for nurses. The College of Midwives received approval ('they have far less of a Trade Union complex than the Royal College of Nursing'), and its secretary was praised for her co-operative approach, but the College was less favourably reviewed:

> For some considerable time the Royal College of Nursing has been devoting a great deal of its time to Trade Union activities and co-operating closely with the T.U.C. in matters relating to salaries and conditions. The Council of the Royal College have to leave a great deal to their General Secretary, Miss Goodall, who is often the only person able to represent the Royal College.[92]

The Ministry's suspicions of latent trade unionism in the College were possibly confirmed by Frances Goodall's change of title: from 1942 she was referred to as the 'General Secretary'. This reflected changing perceptions of her office, because she had to make decisions more rapidly and independently than Mary Rundle, but the new title had trade union associations.

Although the Horder Committee and the Ministry of Health were largely in agreement over assistant nurses in 1942, once the committee began to address nurses' training and conditions of service, the Ministry became hostile, even claiming that it had never been informed about the committee's appointment. In fact, Ernest Brown had received a letter from Frances Goodall on 29 May 1941. She sent a revised scale of recommended salaries for hospital nurses and added:

> [I] take this opportunity of informing you that [the Council of the College] have recently set up a special committee, composed of members of the nursing profession and kindred associations, whose function will be to make recommendations for the reconstruction of the nursing profession, specially with regard to its regulation, education and economic conditions. It has begun work on the problem of the assistant nurse.[93]

Yet in 1944 the Ministry's officials believed they had never been informed about the Horder Committee, 'either before or after they made their announcement in the press'.[94] Lord Horder exacerbated the situation, by emphasising during a meeting at the Ministry that his committee was set up with the Ministry's approval.[95]

The Ministry of Health was also concerned that the College was working too closely with the Ministry of Labour. The Ministry of Health's officials

commented sourly, 'the College is always ready to take up any new development and they have entered into all the activities of the Ministry of Labour
and National Service, working closely with the Trade Unions'. It continued,
'as you know, the Minister wishes to do everything possible to waken in the
Royal College of Nursing the sense of nursing as a profession rather than a
trade union – that is, to put it crudely, to woo them back from the Ministry
of Labour'.[96] Some key organisations feared that if they co-operated in the
Horder inquiry they would antagonise the Ministry of Health. The County
Councils' Association refused an invitation to serve on it, stating that the
Ministry of Health was 'the most appropriate body to take the lead in such
matters'. Both the principal matron in the Ministry of Labour and Harold
Balme, now regional medical officer of the Emergency Medical Service,
refused invitations to serve, on instructions from the chief medical officer at
the Ministry of Health, which found the GNC and the Association of Hospital
Matrons more congenial to work with than the College.[97] In their private
discussions, the Ministry's officials treated the College as an irritant, but it
was sufficiently important to be worth wooing. The College council and
Frances Goodall, always anxious to avoid any association with trade unionism,
would have been dismayed at the Ministry's interpretation of its activities.

Although the leaders of the Royal College of Nursing could hardly be
described as socialists, their desire for nursing reform was pushing them
towards another plan of action formulated without government approval.
William Beveridge, one of the founders of national insurance in Britain, and
director of the London School of Economics, had volunteered his services to
government during the war and been shunted off to run an obscure committee. It reported in 1942, to a lukewarm response from the government, but an
exceptionally favourable reception from the press and public. Of all the committees, sub-committees, working parties, inquiries and negotiating bodies
appointed during the war to address nursing issues, the report from the unap-
pealingly titled Committee on Social Insurance and Allied Services had the
most radical implications for the future of nursing. Beveridge's proposals for
a National Health Service were part of an ambitious strategy for a welfare
state.

Beveridge described 'five giants' – social evils from which his welfare state
would set the people free – and 'Disease' was one of them; but the precise
method of killing this giant was open to negotiation.[98] Beveridge aimed for
national insurance to cover the population's needs in times of sickness, but
did not dictate whether the organisation of health care should be local or
central, public or voluntary. The wartime government's approach to post-war
health policy was tentative, with Churchill being particularly unwilling to
make any commitments that would place further burdens on a Treasury
already heavily in debt. Rather, discussions centred around an improved

version of Chamberlain's 'regional' programme in the 1930s. In 1942, Ernest Brown made a speech on 'Regionalisation, or the Co-ordination of Hospital Services' at a College conference. He stressed that the government's future plans for health lay in regional co-operation between voluntary and municipal hospitals, but the main responsibility for health would remain with local government.[99]

Henry Willink produced his White Paper for a National Health Service in February 1944, aiming to extend free medical care to a wider section of the population, but leaving much to local authorities. Willink's plan dealt at length with the medical profession, but virtually ignored nurses, except for one short comment on domiciliary nursing. This pattern was repeated at policy meetings, where doctors were given plenty of opportunity to express their opinions, and nurses were scarcely represented. The problem was compounded by lack of communication between the nursing organisations and the nurses at the Ministry of Health. Katharine Watt had built her career in the armed services rather than civilian nursing, and during the war she was inevitably preoccupied with providing nurses for the military and the Civil Nursing Reserve.[100] When the College deputation led by Lord Horder finally met with Willink in May 1944, the Minister began in a conciliatory way, assuring them that the place of nursing in the post-war health service was of primary importance.[101] This was an ideal opportunity for Goodall, as principal speaker for the College, to discuss its anxieties on this subject, but Horder's lengthy comments soon dominated the meeting. He quickly moved on from the health service and focused on the reform of nurse education. The areas of contention between the College and the Ministry were not addressed.

In November the College published its response to the White Paper. Entitled *The Place of Nursing in a National Health Service*, the College's manifesto started by expressing disappointment that nursing was not given the same emphasis as medical treatment, except for the brief comment on domiciliary nursing.[102] In the College's view, no system would succeed without addressing the primary issues of supply of nurses and their training:

> The whole conception of a national service for health will fail unless an adequate supply of well-trained nurses can be assured. Immense numbers of nurses and midwives are involved, yet no preliminary discussions were held with them such as took place with the doctors . . . there still seems to be little public recognition of the fact that nursing is a profession parallel to that of medicine, and that it occupies an appointed and increasingly important place in the national plan for health.[103]

The College was prepared to support the plan, with certain provisos. It criticised the lack of attention to health centres and to social and preventive medicine. The College saw health centres as the focal point for all health activities, each centre having its own nurse administrator to co-ordinate the nursing work. The College had been struggling for some years for nurses to have a voice in health policy. They welcomed nurses' participation on the proposed Central Health Services Council, the main advisory body on health, but since the council would be dominated by the medical profession, it would have neither time nor knowledge to decide nursing and midwifery issues. The College wanted a separate council to advise the Minister on nursing and midwifery, to complement the work of the Division of Nursing in the Ministry of Health.

For the hospital service, the College made suggestions on better patient care, but it was particularly concerned about improving the basic training of the future nurse. Quoting from the Goodenough report on medical schools, it commented that 'the spirit of education must permeate the whole of the health service'. The College commented in detail on domiciliary nursing, believing that this should be a fully funded public service.[104] Apart from district nurses and health visitors, the College predicted that full-time domiciliary nursing would be needed because the creaking hospital system might not be adequate for the population's needs, and few would be able to afford a private nurse. The Scottish Board submitted separate comments. They believed that unless nurses and midwives had a place in the co-ordination of regional hospital planning, the proposed changes would so undermine the basic training of nurses that supplies of adequately trained staff would be perilously low. The Scottish Board reminded the Minister that in a parliamentary debate he had acknowledged that 'the success or failure of this scheme will depend in large measure on the nurse, not only in hospital and clinic, but in the home'.[105]

In the spring of 1945 representatives of the College met twice with officials of the Ministry of Health to discuss the place of nursing in the new health service. The Ministry pointed out that legislation would deal primarily with the administrative structure and not with such questions as nurses' training. The College's representatives expressed serious concerns about local government control of the health services, believing that local councils did not appreciate the importance of preventive medicine, and that their political views affected both their policies and their appointments. For the Ministry, Sir Arthur Rucker was defensive, arguing that the White Paper's lack of detail in preventive services was because it addressed personal health services only, and the new health centres would be experimental at first. He refused to discuss the training of nurses, although any reform of the hospital system was bound to affect the training schools.

The College engaged in discussions with other interested professional groups. The Ministry of Health made some concessions, allowing more professional input into the Central Health Services Council, including nursing and midwifery committees, but the members of these would be decided by the Minister, not nominated by the professions. At a local level there would be Area Planning Councils, responsible for all the health services in the area, with 60 per cent membership from local government and 40 per cent from the professions. The professional group would include one nurse and one midwife, but most of its members would be doctors. The College objected strongly to this limited recognition for nurses, but discovered that none of the other nursing organisations had been in discussion with the Ministry, or produced their own plans for nurses in the new system. Goodall's fallback position was that if the Ministry persisted in its plans, the College would accept them, as long as there was adequate nursing representation on the new local councils.[106] The College was not well disposed towards Willink's plans to leave health care in the hands of restructured local authorities. Many doctors and nurses, particularly those with experience of poor law hospitals, regarded work for local authorities as constrained by parochial penny-pinching. In the 1930s, some local authorities proved to be innovatory and generous in their approach to health, but many were held back by financial problems or ineffective management. When the Labour Party began to reveal Aneurin Bevan's plans for a more centralised National Health Service, the College raised no objections.

Conclusion

During the 1930s the College struggled to influence nursing policy, but most of its achievement was at the local level. Although it pressed for consistent standards of pay and working conditions for nurses, it had to deal with multiple employers and a variety of local conditions. It excluded many nurses by refusing to accept into membership those with lesser training, and this left the field open for other organisations. The TUC began to interest itself in nurses' welfare, arguing that only trade unionism could guarantee their interests. In its early days, the College relied on prestigious social contacts to catch the attention of government, but when it tried to intervene in nurses' working conditions, it antagonised the Ministry of Health, which suspected it of quasi-trade union activity. Ironically, although the College saw itself as a professional association, and feared 'contamination' from trade unionism, the Ministry's officials viewed it as too close to the unions. But although it was by then the largest organisation of nurses in Britain, it still represented only a minority of them, and its membership figures remained fairly stagnant.

War presented an opportunity for the College to work more closely with government and to influence nursing policy. But its influence was stronger in the Ministry of Labour, which needed its help in maintaining the health of the civilian workforce, than in the Ministry of Health, which saw it as an impediment to the constant and cheap supply of semi-trained nurses needed for the war effort. Hence, although the College could draw on a large fund of public goodwill for its welfare work, this did not translate into political capital, and schemes for post-war health reform took little note of nursing interests. The College began to take a more active role in formulating policy by appointing its own investigative committee under Lord Horder, but its priorities, particularly for enhanced nurse training, did not impress the Ministry of Health. In the event, the Churchill government's cautious regional and voluntary policies were swept away in the landslide election of 1945, and the College had to negotiate its position under a new Labour administration. Having made little headway with Conservative ministers during the war, the College was receptive to Aneurin Bevan's plans for a National Health Service, for nurses had little to lose and much to gain.

Notes

1 For a succinct history of these plans, see Charles Webster, *The National Health Service: a Political History* (Oxford and New York: Oxford University Press, 1998), pp. 1–15. For a case study of inter-war regional co-operation, see John Pickstone, *Medicine and Industrial Society: a History of Hospital Development in Manchester and its Region 1752–1946* (Manchester: Manchester University Press, 1985), ch. 12.

2 Monica E. Baly, 'Famous nursing leaders: the life and times of Frances Goodall, CBE, General Secretary of the RCN, 1935–1957', *History of Nursing Journal* 4: 5 (1992–93), 273; Monica E. Baly, 'Goodall, Frances Gowland (1893–1976)', *Oxford Dictionary of National Biography*, online edn, Oxford University Press, www.oxforddnb.com/view/article/55672, accessed 19 Feb. 2006.

3 RCN/3/1/2, Establishment and General Purposes Committee minutes, 7 June 1928.

4 Baly, 'Famous nursing leaders', p. 273.

5 See, e.g. RCN/17/4/36, press cuttings, pp. 14–15, *Northern Echo*, 21 Jan. 1941 and 5 Feb. 1941.

6 Martin Gorsky and Sally Sheard (eds), *Financing Medicine: the British Experience Since 1750* (London and New York: Routledge, 2006), especially chapters by Steven Cherry and John Mohan, pp. 72, 83.

7 M. A. Crowther, *The Workhouse System 1834–1929* (London: Methuen, 1983), pp. 187–90.

8 'The Essex scheme', *NT* 11 May 1935, pp. 471–2.

9 Dingwall et al., *Introduction to the Social History of Nursing*, pp. 196–7.

10 For the history of midwifery legislation, see Irvine Loudon, *Death in Childbirth: an International Study of Maternal Care and Maternal Mortality 1800–1950* (Oxford: Clarendon Press, 1992), pp. 206–18.

11 The history of these discussions is in RCN/4/1937/1.

12 CRC 20/NAL/4/1/6, NALGO Service Conditions and Organisation Committee, Minute Book 6, 10 July 1937, pp. 91–100.

13 RCN/13/J/4, correspondence between F. Goodall and J. Greenwood Wilson, MOH for Cardiff, 30 March to 22 May 1935.

14 RCN/13/J/2, TUC papers and correspondence.

15 Bevin was also chairman of the council of the TUC at this time.

16 Whitley Councils, named after the civil servant who devised them, were intro-
    duced in the public services after the First World War to negotiate salaries and
    conditions. They included employers' and workers' representatives.

17 RCN/17/4/34, *Eastern Daily Press*, Norwich, 8 Sept. 1937.

18 RCN/13/J/2, TUC papers.

19 RCN/17/4/34, press cuttings, *NT* 13 Nov. 1937; *Oxford Mail* 3 Nov. 1937. See also
    Tom Buchanan, *The Impact of the Spanish Civil War on Britain: War, Loss and
    Memory* (Brighton: Sussex Academic Press, 2007), pp. 45–50.

20 It was later reported that the Association of Nurses had about 1,000 members.
    RCN/17/4/34, press cuttings, *Scotsman* 18 March 1938, p. 10. For a fictionalised
    account of the formation of the Association of Nurses see Cynthia Nolan, *A Bride
    for St Thomas* (London: Constable, 1970), pp. 125–50.

21 RCN/17/4/34, press cuttings, *Reynolds News* 24 Oct. 1937; *Oxford Mail* 3 Nov. 1937;
    Nottingham Evening News 17 Dec. 1937.

22 RCN/13/J/3, TUC campaign 1937.

23 RCN/4/1938/6, 'College and TUC policy', *NT* Supplement 25 Sept. 1937.

24 RCN/4/1938/3, Notes for Miss Musson regarding the government enquiry into
    nursing conditions, 6 July 1938.

25 RCN/17/4/34, *Daily Express* 18 Nov. 1937.

26 There is some confusion over the dates of this protest march. Some sources con-
    flate the inaugural meeting of the Guild of Nurses in November 1937 with the
    march in April 1938. See Abel-Smith, *Nursing Profession*, p. 145; Rafferty, *Politics
    of Nursing Knowledge*, pp. 158–9; Hart, *Behind the Mask*, pp. 62–3; Carpenter,
    Working for Health, pp. 207–8, 214; and press cuttings in RCN/17/4/34, which cover
    the first meeting of the Guild.

27 For a fuller analysis, see Gorsky, Mohan and Powell, 'Financial health of voluntary
    hospitals', pp. 533–57, and Abel-Smith, *Nursing Profession*, p. 121.

28 'Hours and conditions of nurses, recommendations to committee', *The Times* 22
    Feb. 1938, p. 17. These movements make it hard to compare the proportion of
    single and married women in the profession (as attempted by Abel-Smith, *Nursing
    Profession*, pp. 259–60), because the population censuses on which assumptions
    rely give only the marital status of nurses on the census day, and cannot chart the
    presumed high turnover of unmarried nurses.

29 RCN/4/1938/6, Report from Financial Secretary on comparison of terms of service
    in certain professions.

30 CM 1937, pp. 183–4.

31 John Stewart, 'Angels or aliens? Refugee nurses in Britain, 1938 to 1942', *Medical
    History* 47: 2 (2003), pp. 153, 158. Stewart comments that the College's record on
    Jewish refugees stands up to hindsight better than that of the BMA.

32 'Finding jobs for girls', *The Times* 4 May 1934, p. 16; 'More girls put into work',
    The Times 17 June 1935, p. 11.

33 Abel-Smith, *Nursing Profession*, p. 153.

34 Rafferty, *Politics of Nursing Knowledge*, pp. 160–1, and footnote 33, p. 244; *Scotsman*
    17 Jan. 1938, p. 14.

35 McGann, *Battle of the Nurses*, pp. 190–216.
36 RCNA T197, transcript of interview with Frances Wakeford, 2000.
37 *BJN* Feb. 1938, p. 45.
38 RCN/17/4/34, press cuttings, *Tit-Bits* 18 Sept. 1937; *London* 3 Oct. 1937.
39 *Daily Mirror* 3 Nov. 1937.
40 RCN/4/1938/2/5, F. Goodall to A. J. Cronin, 11 Nov. 1937.
41 RCN/13/J/3, R. Pecker to F. Goodall, 12 Nov. 1937.
42 RCN/17/4/34, press cuttings, *Tribune* 31 Dec. 1937.
43 Harold Balme, *A Criticism of Nursing Education* (London: Oxford University Press, 1937).
44 Harold Balme, 'Do nurses get a square deal? 3. Grievances and remedies', *Time and Tide* 29 Jan. 1938.
45 RCN/17/4/34, *Cambridge Daily News* 26 March 1938.
46 Editorial, 'Do nurses get a square deal? No', *Time and Tide* 5 Feb. 1938.
47 The Scottish Board of the College prepared a separate memorandum for the Scottish Departmental Committee, appointed by the Secretary of State for Scotland, RCN/4/1938/2/17.
48 The General Nursing Council statistics showed no decline in the numbers entering for training. The College of Nursing, 'Memorandum relating to conditions in the nursing profession for submission to the Inter-Departmental Committee on the Nursing Services', Jan. 1938, p. 3, RCN/4/1938/2/16.
49 RCN/4/1938/2/14, The College of Nursing, Student Nurses' Association, memorandum relating to conditions in the nursing profession for submission to the Inter-Departmental Committee on the nursing services, May 1938, p. 6.
50 Ministry of Health and Board of Education, *Inter-departmental Committee on Nursing Services. Interim Report* [Athlone report] (London: HMSO, 1939).
51 *NT* 22 April 1939, pp. 498–500, and 29 April 1939, pp. 529–31.
52 RCN/17/4/35, press cuttings, 'The nurse and the nation', *Time and Tide* 4 Feb. 1939.
53 Elizabeth J.C. Scott, 'The influence of the staff of the Ministry of Health on policies for nursing 1919–1968', PhD thesis, London School of Economics (1994), p. 121.
54 CM 1938 pp. 288–9, F. Goodall to Ministry of Health, 21 Oct. 1938.
55 CM Nov. 1938, pp. 316–17.
56 RCN/17/4/35, press cuttings, *Daily Express* 17 Feb. 1939.
57 Editorial, 'The Civil Nursing Reserve' and 'Auxiliary nurses', *NT* 5 Aug. 1939, p. 978.
58 Editorial, 'Our war-time problems', *NT* 14 Oct. 1939.
59 Five of the fourteen members of the new CNR Advisory Council were nurses, whereas on the original committee, only five out of twenty members were nurses. *NT* 13 April 1940, p. 390. The names of the eleven nurse regional officers and their qualifications are in *NT* 2 March 1940, p. 222.
60 *NT* 23 Dec. 1939, p. 1536.
61 College of Nursing Scottish Board minutes, Oct. 1944.
62 RCN/17/1941, press cuttings, *Scotsman* 3 Jan. 1941, p. 7.
63 Angus Calder, *The People's War: Britain 1939–45* (London: Granada, 1982), p. 215.

64 *Local Government Service* 21: 2 (Feb. 1941), 28–30.
65 RCN/17/1941, press cuttings, *Evening Standard* 12 Dec. 1940.
66 RCN/17/4/36, press cuttings, *Public Assistance Journal* 19 Sept. 1941.
67 RCN/17/4/36, press cuttings, *News Chronicle* 20 Feb. 1942.
68 Charley, *Birth of Industrial Nursing*, p. 119.
69 RCN/17/4/37, press cuttings, *Evening Standard* 27 April 1944.
70 *NT* editorial, 14 Oct. 1939.
71 Scott, 'Influence of the staff of the Ministry of Health', p. 123.
72 RCN/13/A/6, F. Goodall to E. Brown, 1 May 1941.
73 RCN/13/A/6, F. Goodall to F. Udell, 6 Sept. 1941.
74 Scott, 'Influence of the staff of the Ministry of Health', p. 126.
75 CRC 020/NAL/4/1a, *Local Government Service* 21: 10, 10 Oct. 1941, p. 234.
76 *Report of the Scottish Departmental Committee on Nursing*, Cmd 5866, H. M. Stationery Office, 1938.
77 *AR* 1941, p. 6.
78 Athlone report, p. 10.
79 RCN/17/1/37, press cuttings, *Economist* 20 Feb. 1943.
80 Nursing Reconstruction Committee, *Report, Section I, The Assistant Nurse* [Horder report] (London: Royal College of Nursing, 1942). See also Rosemary White, *The Effects of the NHS on the Nursing Profession, 1948–1961* (London: King Edward's Hospital Fund for London, 1985), p. 15.
81 Abel-Smith, *Nursing Profession*, pp. 170–1.
82 As with the original general nursing register, women with nursing experience were placed on the first roll, even if they had no training.
83 RCN/13/A/11, F. Udell to F. Goodall, 4 May 1943.
84 CM 19 March 1943, p. 44 and 15 June 1944, p. 137. Initially the association was known as the National Association of Assistant Nurses, then the National Association of State Enrolled Assistant Nurses, and after 1961, as the National Association of State Enrolled Nurses.
85 CM 19 March 1943.
86 White, *Effects of the NHS on the Nursing Profession*, p. 18, argues that Horder was ignored, or less favourably received, compared with the Athlone report. In fact, the press gave Horder a generally good reception, though objecting to some of the details of his report. See RCN/17/4/38, press cuttings for 1943–44.
87 RCN/17/4/38, press cuttings, *Economist* 1 Jan. 1944.
88 Nursing Reconstruction Committee, *Report, Section II, Education and Training; Section III, Recruitment* [Horder report] (London: Royal College of Nursing, 1943); and, *Report, Section IV, The Social and Economic Conditions of the Nurse* [Horder report] (London: Royal College of Nursing, 1949).
89 TNA MH 55/2156, K. Watt to de Montmorency, 21 Feb. 1944.
90 TNA MH 55/1256, Central Midwives' Board to Minister of Health, 18 Jan. 1944.
91 TNA MH 55/2156, memo by BLP, 24 April 1944.
92 TNA MH 55/2156, 'Notes for Minister on some nursing and midwifery organisations', n.d. [1944].
93 RCN/13/A/6, for the public announcement of Horder's appointment, see *The Times* 23 Sept. 1941, p. 6.

94 TNA, MH55/2156, Ministry of Health memorandum re the College of Nursing formation of the Horder Committee, 19 March 1944.
95 TNA MH 55/2156, 'Note of a discussion with Royal College of Nursing', 2 May 1944, p. 3.
96 TNA MH 55/2156, 'Notes for Minister on some Nursing and Midwifery Organisations', n.d. [1944], and memo from Sir John Wrigley re the forthcoming deputation from the Royal College of Nursing, 12 April 1944.
97 TNA, MH55/2156, Ministry of Health memorandum re the College of Nursing formation of the Horder Committee, 19 March 1944, and F. R. Fraser to H. Balme, 11 Nov. 1941, and 'Notes for Minister on some nursing and midwifery organisations' n.d. [1944]; Scott, 'Influence of the staff of the Ministry of Health', pp. 185, 192.
98 William Beveridge, *Social Insurance and Allied Services* (London: HMSO, 1942), pp. 158–9.
99 RCN/17/4/38, press cuttings, *Local Government Chronicle* 20 June 1942.
100 For the lack of communication between the Division of Nursing and the nurses' organisations, see Scott, 'Influence of the staff of the Ministry of Health', pp. 196–9. Scott also argues that nurses in the Ministry were reluctant to become involved in policy-making.
101 Notes of the meeting are in TNA MH55/2156.
102 The term 'domiciliary nursing' referred to district nurses, midwives and health visitors.
103 *NT* 11 Nov. 1944, editorial, p. 769.
104 As indicated in the College's memorandum to the Athlone Committee in 1938.
105 RCN/5/7/26.
106 RCN/5/7/26.

4

Nursing and the National Health Service, 1945–50

The arrival of the Labour government in 1945, with Aneurin Bevan as a dynamic Minister of Health, profoundly changed the health services in Britain. Under the new National Health Service, which came into operation in 1948, many nurses became employees of state-funded regional health authorities. The poor law was abolished, and its hospitals, if fit for the purpose, were incorporated into the NHS, as were the voluntary hospitals, the most prestigious centres of nurse training. The Labour government's programme for state control of vital industries also stimulated the growth of larger trade unions, for they could now negotiate directly with government rather than a multitude of local employers. As public employees, nurses would have national pay scales and, it was assumed, less variable conditions of service. This new world offered considerable opportunities to the Royal College of Nursing, for its wartime activities gave it increased credibility as the voice of the nursing profession. Nevertheless, its position in the post-war years was difficult, as its interests were hard to reconcile with those of government, employers and the trade unions.

Bevan's National Health Service Act was passed in November 1946. His plans were far more radical than Willink's, and the College council received them more enthusiastically. He retained a Central Health Services Council as the advisory body for the NHS, and it was still to be a forum mainly for doctors. There would also be a new Standing Nursing Advisory Committee (SNAC), which promised a more prominent role for nurses. The midwifery and maternity services had their own advisory committee. While the College welcomed the grouping of hospitals under regional boards rather than local government, it also called for an overhaul of local government provision, for the NHS was notoriously skewed towards curative rather than preventive services. The College wanted nurses on these official committees to be nominated by their professional bodies, but Bevan, like Willink, insisted that nurses be appointed as individuals, not as delegates of the nursing organisations. Bevan wished to appear even-handed in his dealings with the professions, but it is likely that his increasingly difficult relations with the BMA made him suspicious of 'interest groups' like the College. The College was invited to submit nominations for the two nurse members of the Central Health Services Council, but neither of its nominees was selected. Again, when the constitution of the Standing Nursing Advisory Committee was drawn up in 1948, the College council was dismayed at the number of members from outside the profession. Twelve members of the SNAC were to come from the Central Health Services Council, but since the SNAC's membership included only two nurses and one midwife, this could hardly guarantee a voice for nurses. Perhaps as a gesture of appeasement, Bevan invited Frances Goodall to join the committee, and its nursing component was increased. The other members came from bodies such as the BMA and the Society of Medical Officers of Health, who also had their own advisory committees. The SNAC's counterpart in Scotland, which included midwives as well as nurses, successfully insisted that its members be drawn only from the relevant professions. Webster comments that the SNAC, although very active, was on several occasions thwarted by opposing interests in the medical committees, and that it was treated with 'contempt' by professional bodies.[1]

The College has been criticised for employing 'little external pressure' in its negotiations with government over nursing representation, in contrast with the recalcitrance and assertiveness of the BMA leadership.[2] It is expecting too much of the leaders of the College at this time to compare their position to that of the leaders of the medical profession. Nurses did not have the same status as doctors, and while the College leaders were confident that they represented its 41,500 members, there were as many nurses outside its membership, for whom they could not speak.[3] Most doctors joined a single professional association, the BMA, but nurses were divided between several organisations. None of these, apart from the College, had prepared a case for nursing policy, in anticipation of the new structure, and the College was the most coherent advocate for nurses, in spite of its own divisions over certain aspects of policy, as will be seen. Delegates at the BMA annual conference were not helpful to the nurses' cause, grumbling that nursing leaders made the shortage worse by putting too much emphasis on examinations and not enough on practical work in the wards.[4] Somewhat inconsistently, the doctors also objected to employing part-time (usually married) nurses, because they preferred a full-time nurse on call when the doctor required her.

In contrast to the hostile BMA, wresting concessions over private practice from a reluctant Bevan, the College may have weakened its negotiating position by its enthusiasm for the new health service. Unlike the affluent consultants who influenced the BMA's opposition to the NHS, nurses did not have

lucrative private practices to protect. Nurses approached the NHS optimisti-
cally, since they did not think their patients or themselves well served by the
existing system. The College held a conference in June 1946 to welcome the
new Minister of Health, and Hilary Blair-Fish spoke for the College, praising
his 'great Bill', which was framed for the good of the community. The conference, she said, might have been called 'Putting the Patient First'.[5] Bevan replied
that he was anxious to avoid warring factions on the regional hospital boards,
and so no professional body would be represented on them.[6] Despite its disappointment at the limited nurse representation in the new structures, and the
modest provisions for health education and preventive medicine, the College
approved his proposals for the hospital service, and hoped, perhaps naively,
that the Minister would in time pay more attention to nurses.

The nursing shortage

The war aggravated the nursing shortage, not only because of the needs of
the armed forces, but by increasing the numbers of hospital beds in Britain,
opening new fields of nursing activity, and stimulating competition for female
labour. War also encouraged medical research and new medical procedures,
requiring a greater degree of technical competence from nurses. The NHS
would also need more nurses, because the whole population would have
access to free medical care.

During the war, the College accepted that 'dilution' of the nursing service
with assistant nurses (the SEN grade) was inevitable. In fact, most assistant
nurses in civilian hospitals preferred to sign up as probationers, to keep open
the possibility of becoming state registered nurses.[7] The employment of
married women was also necessary to meet the emergency, and from 1943 the
government encouraged employers to take on married women with family
responsibilities as part-time workers. But when the war ended, the nursing
shortage was not eased. Many nurses in the armed forces and civilian conscripts were leaving the service just as demand for nurses was growing. Under
these circumstances, government, hospitals and other employers looked for
ways to attract recruits and train them as rapidly as possible. The SEN grade,
although imposing a shorter period of training than for registered nurses,
failed to attract enough recruits. Student nurses, usually seen by the hospitals
as cheap labour, were the most obvious solution. The government considered
ways of speeding up nurse training for the register to reduce the high dropout rate among probationers, but the College, firmly attached to the concept
of rigorous training over three, or even four, years, appeared as an obstacle
rather than an ally. Nor could the College expect support from the medical
profession, also undergoing major changes. Whenever the future of nursing
was discussed, doctors were divided over the nurse's role. Some thought the

shortage would rapidly resolve itself if nurse training were kept short and simple. A *Lancet* editorial of 1946 stated:

> For most patients most of the time, nursing does not mean the more technical feats of the sister – the skilled dressing, the saline-drip, or even the regular careful dosage with medicines. It means having his bed properly made, having his pillows well placed, hearing simple reassuring words at the right moment, getting a hot-water bottle as soon as he wants it, being prepared deftly for operation, being amused and stimulated at one moment, soothed and settled at another. The 'born nurse' – the girl who does these things well – is extremely common, just as the maternal instinct is extremely common; and she may not necessarily be good at her books, though she often is.[8]

In this scenario, the College seemed to speak only for the 'sister' with her saline drip, not for the good-natured handmaid who seemed so desirable in a time of shortage. *The Lancet* stood its ground after an angry rejoinder from the *Nursing Times* accused it of advocating semi-literate nurses who might well poison their patients. *The Lancet* kept up this line of argument for some time, being convinced that the nursing shortage could be solved by employing assistant nurses with a two-year basic training, much of which would be done in the wards. Its view of the ideal assistant nurse was distinctly domestic:

> She will learn bed-making – especially how to make a bed comfortable though neat – how to give an enema, how to turn and lift a patient, how to prevent bedsores and dropped feet, how to cleanse and sterilise the bedpan, how to avoid infection when nursing the tuberculous, and how to dispose safely of their sputum, how to lay infected dust and sweep it up, how to give an injection and put drops in an eye or ear, how to barrier-nurse an infectious disease, how to assist at a minor operation, for all these are things she might sometime have to do for her family . . . If at the end of two years of this kind of training a girl of average intelligence is not a competent and handy nurse the fault must be with her teachers.[9]

The Lancet was soon deploring the rift between the medical and nursing professions, which should be a support to each another.[10] But divergent views over the amount of training required to produce a competent nurse made consensus difficult, and began to sour the College's relations with government.

In August 1945 the Ministry of Labour's National Advisory Council on Nurses and Midwives produced a memorandum entitled 'Recruitment of nurses and midwives to training institutions'. The council monitored nursing recruitment in relation to the demand for nurses, and reported that the situation was dire. In March 1945 there were approximately 190,000 nurses, midwives and probationers employed in hospitals, nursing services and other institutions in Britain. About 11,000 vacancies needed to be filled urgently.

The number of state registered nurses qualifying in the UK, for all parts of the register, averaged fewer than 9,000 per year in 1943 and 1944. There was already a shortfall of some 2,000 between the nation's urgent requirements for nurses, and the number recruited that year, and the situation would inevitably worsen as conscripted women and older nurses who had postponed retirement left the workforce. Apart from Britain's need for nurses, there were additional demands from the Commonwealth and liberated Europe. The National Advisory Council was convinced that the 11,000 vacancies greatly underestimated the real needs of the country. Nine hundred sister tutors were required immediately, and this was only for training student nurses in general hospitals, without taking account of the training needs of mental nurses or assistant nurses. The real number of vacancies might be as much as 34,000, and, with a high turnover in the profession, supply of nurses was far short of demand.[11]

The National Advisory Council stressed the wastage rate among student nurses. Annual student intake was estimated at 19,000–20,000, with less than half that number becoming state registered nurses. Between 25 and 30 per cent left during their first year, about one third of the entrants for the preliminary state examination failed, and in the final examination 20 per cent failed. The council estimated that, allowing for such wastage, 22,000 students were needed each year to meet demand. They wanted hospital authorities to reduce wastage by improving conditions for student nurses and by relaxing traditional hospital discipline. They recommended setting up nurses' councils, on the lines advocated by the College, retaining married students, and employing more ancillary staff to release nurses from unskilled tasks. The council believed that recruiting more assistant nurses could reduce the nursing shortage, and was concerned that very few hospitals seemed keen to train them. The College had pragmatically, but reluctantly, accepted the need for a 'second tier' of SENs during the war, but in the post-war shortage, the enrolled nurse seemed far more desirable than the alternative of virtually untrained staff. Since SEN training was introduced in 1943, only thirty-one applications for approval to set up a training school had been received in England and Wales, and only seventeen approved. In Scotland none were approved, since the assistant nurse grade was at that stage only temporary. Unless arrangements were made quickly, many suitable recruits from the Forces would be lost to the profession.

The General Nursing Councils reconsidered a previous decision and permitted members of the Civil Nursing Reserve, VADs and nursing orderlies to enrol as assistant nurses on the basis of their wartime experience. The College had to accept that for some time to come, nurses could be recruited from girls with no education past the age of fourteen, and that the profession would include men and women with wartime experience but little formal training.

The profession could expect even more competition in trying to attract recruits from school leavers after the war. The 1944 Education Act expanded secondary education. The school leaving age would be raised, so that more schoolteachers would be needed; and teaching always competed with nursing as a profession for women. The Act also abolished university fees, encouraging middle-class girls to aim for higher education. Nursing was caught in the class divide. For middle-class women, other opportunities were opening up; while for girls from poorer homes, the gap between leaving school, even at fifteen or sixteen, and beginning nurse training at the GNC's minimum age, was still a barrier to nursing.

In September 1945 the Ministry of Health launched a major recruitment campaign. It contacted nursing organisations and hospitals and held several meetings on how to improve the image of nursing. The post-war labour shortage meant that hospitals had trouble recruiting any type of worker, let alone nurses, and the absence of cleaners and other domestic staff made it difficult to reduce nurses' working hours. In many wards the students did much of the cleaning, carried messages and moved equipment, and nurses made the patients' tea and light meals. Over several meetings a New Deal was negotiated for nurses and domestic staff in hospitals, and a document referred to by the Ministry's staff as the 'Hospital Nurses' Charter' was prepared. It urged immediate changes in working conditions, or, if this proved impossible, that hospital authorities should introduce them by a given date.[12] The government launched its publicity campaign with a broadcast by the Minister of Health and a booklet based on the charter, entitled *Staffing the Hospitals: An Urgent National Need*. It opened with 'An appeal to all men and women . . . to come and play their part in this great field of service . . . The country stands in urgent need of nurses and midwives . . . the situation is extremely serious'. The campaign targeted nurses and VADs leaving the Forces, and all types of hospital were encouraged to recruit ex-servicemen for training as male nurses. In his broadcast Bevan announced a new scheme of special allowances for men and women leaving the Forces who took up nurse training. Those with relevant experience would be excused six months of the training period. Nurses would be released from the Civil Nursing Reserve by stages, and the Ministry hoped that many would stay on and serve in the difficult period ahead. Hospitals should offer part-time employment to married nurses. The Ministry hoped that opening the roll of assistant nurses to those with wartime experience would reduce the shortage. Eventually admission to the roll would be conditional on training and an examination, but for the present this was not enforced.

The Code of Conditions of Service for Hospital Nurses and Midwives, the 'New Deal for Nurses', gave detailed instructions on every aspect of nurses' work and training – salaries, superannuation, hours of work, off-duty periods, health, food, accommodation, recreation, social life, living out and discipline. The government intended that these instructions, agreed with the professional organisations and trade unions, would become the accepted standard 'as soon as circumstances permitted'. The objective for all hospitals was a ninety-six-hour working fortnight, and it was intended to fix a date on which this condition would come into universal operation. Hospitals were also urged to provide better accommodation for nurses, with more privacy and greater freedom in their off-duty periods. To encourage recruitment there would be an immediate salary increase, as recommended by the Nurses' Salaries Committee. Bevan admitted that the whole question of nurses' training and prevention of wastage required more detailed study, and promised that the government would investigate it without delay.[13]

The day after the Minister's broadcast the College held a press conference. Frances Goodall was pleased with the government's position, for the Minister had accepted many College policies, including Nurses' Representative Councils for every hospital (though in the event, these were left to the discretion of individual hospitals). The government's booklet on the new arrangements made several references to the Horder reports, indicating that these had influenced the New Deal. The government received monthly reports from the nursing sections of the regional appointments offices. In the week before the campaign began, enquiries numbered only 700, but within a fortnight of the launch this rose to 3,000. A newspaper report four weeks into the campaign claimed: 'Thousands of young people are answering the nation's call for more nurses'.[14] Nevertheless, the campaign was not universally supported. The British Hospitals Association feared that many of the Ministry's promises would require expensive new building programmes and it would be several years before these could begin. When the Department of Health for Scotland received a draft of the New Deal, the Secretary of State reportedly dismissed some of its recommendations as 'fairy tales'. He commented that it would be counter-productive to say 'this is what you should have but you won't find anything like it in many or indeed in most hospitals, and you won't get it for five years or longer'.[15] The New Deal promised better accommodation for nurses, but all building programmes had to compete for scarce resources in the building trade, since the government also planned a major housing programme to replace the slums and repair the ravages of war. Civil servants in Northern Ireland had no warning of the New Deal, and complained that they had no official confirmation from London.

Among all these debates on how to solve the nursing shortage, retention of married women was not at first a major issue, even though they were an important part of the workforce during the war. The formal or informal 'marriage bar' applied by public bodies and many private firms before 1939 had to be relaxed during the war, and in most cases was not reintroduced because of the post-war labour shortage. The 1944 Education Act released married teachers from this restriction. The government certainly encouraged employers to offer part-time positions to married nurses, but these did not accommodate well to traditional hospital routines, or to hospitals where nurses were expected to live in. It was assumed that married women, if they wished to continue in the profession, would be better employed in community or industrial nursing. High marriage rates and the post-war bulge in the birth rate also removed younger married women from the labour force, though this proved to be temporary. Between the censuses of 1931 and 1951 there was a major shift in the composition of the profession, with the numbers of married women rising from 4.8 per cent to 21.6 per cent.[16] But in the immediate post-war period, the importance of married women's work was not anticipated. The tone of the *Lancet*'s comments on the nursing shortage indicated that many doctors still assumed that nursing was usually a short-term career, or a kind of special training for family duties. There is little indication that College leaders, drawn from the much larger pool of unmarried women who began their careers before 1939, saw things differently. The problems of married nurses were not high on their agenda.

Although the College welcomed the NHS enthusiastically, it soon parted company from the government over dilution of the profession and how to overcome the nursing shortage. The College held to the views of its founders, that if the status of nursing were raised, a more 'suitable' kind of recruit would be attracted, and nursing would be able to compete with other professions for women. The government, faced with the immediate problem of staffing the NHS, could not afford to take this long-term view.

The College advisory service

Although the College did not always achieve its ends in negotiations with government, it was more effective in assisting individual nurses, particularly those leaving the Forces. By the end of 1945 the Ministry of Labour had appointed nursing officers to each of its thirty-one appointments offices to help demobbed nurses. When a trained nurse left the Forces she had eight weeks' leave to decide her future. After that, if a nurse under the age of forty-one had not found work, she had to obtain permission from the nursing appointments office before taking up a new post. The College started an advisory service providing nurses with information about adjusting to civilian life. Its literature supported the government's recruitment campaign: 'While you have been away those at home have had to carry on as best they could . . . the civilian nursing service desperately needs your help. Many older nurses have held on waiting for your return'.[17] The advisory service issued information on training and refresher courses, grants and scholarships, and about future prospects in the different fields of nursing: 'while at present the demand for private nurses far exceeds the supply, prospects in this field are likely to be profoundly modified when the National Health service comes into force'.[18] They anticipated major demand from overseas nursing, especially in the Colonial Nursing Service, and set up a central register of nurses wishing to volunteer for relief work abroad. Florence Udell led the way in 1944, when she was released by the Scottish Board of the College to work for the United Nations Relief and Rehabilitation Administration, recruiting nurses for emergency work in the liberated countries of Europe. The *Evening Standard* reported this under the headline 'Europe's no. 1 nurse looks for tactful women'.[19]

After the College received many enquiries from nurses in the Forces, the War Office invited Frances Goodall to make an official visit to nurses serving in the British Army of Occupation on the Rhine in February 1946. The government wanted nurses in the Forces to be given every encouragement to go into civilian nursing when they returned to Britain. Goodall's mission received much favourable press coverage, and a photograph of the general secretary, soigné in fur coat, waving regally from the steps of the aircraft, was published in several papers.[20] Goodall visited fifteen groups of nursing sisters along the Rhine and in Belgium. She found them anxious and undecided about their futures. All wanted to know about the effect of the National Health Service on nurses and nursing. While some were concerned mainly about future salaries, others were interested in professional and educational matters. Goodall told them that civilian nurses were looking forward to their return, so that some of the long awaited reforms could be implemented. Many army nurses expressed reluctance to return to the petty restrictions and discipline of hospital life after the informal atmosphere of the sisters' mess, and they were unanimous in their intention to live out. Many said they would rather give up nursing than return to the rigid hospital regimes they remembered. They worried about being out of touch with civilian nursing and felt they needed short refresher courses. Older nurses wanted help to take courses at the College so that they could apply for matrons' and administrative posts. Goodall recommended that this help should be given, because many potential leaders of the profession had volunteered for the armed services during the war. The government was more generous to doctors leaving the forces than to nurses, and would not pay for nurses to attend post-qualification courses. In her report Goodall wrote:

> Many expressed their great disappointment that the government had not found it possible to extend to the nursing profession the same financial help which was given to the medical profession. In my opinion this has had a very bad psychological effect, giving rise to discouragement and a feeling that the status of the profession was being overlooked.[21]

The need for reconstruction

Despite the government's recruitment campaign of late 1945 and the promise of a New Deal, the nursing shortage continued. In an article in the *Sunday Times*, the secretary of the BMA described the situation as desperate, while the Socialist Medical Association, a small group whose ideas were influential in the establishment of the NHS, published a pamphlet entitled *Nursing in the Post-War World, a Memorandum on the Shortage of Nurses, with Constructive Proposals.*[22] These doctors believed that the exploitation of nurses was now affecting patients, and that the only way forward was an improvement in the conditions and prospects of nurses and hospital workers. They objected to Willink's White Paper, which described nurses and midwives as an 'ancillary service' to the medical profession. Unlike the editor of *The Lancet*, still hankering after docile and motherly nurses, the SMA believed that nurses were professional colleagues, and that no permanent solution for the nursing shortage was possible without a public enquiry into the standards of care in every type of institution. They too proposed a job analysis to show which of a nurse's duties could properly be described as nursing, and which could be left to domestic staff. The SMA believed that once nurses' duties were amended, it would be possible to find enough recruits. They reached the same conclusion as the more conservative *Lancet* in their suggestions for 'modernising' nurse training. The SMA believed there would never be enough recruits for assistant nurse posts, and that this grade should be abolished. Instead, the government should fund the training schools to provide an intensive two-year nursing course for all nurses, after which, the ambitious or specialised should have free and compulsory post-certificate training. If nurses were relieved of domestic and cleaning duties, a thorough basic training could be given in two years, and local authorities and voluntary hospitals should be permitted to conduct experiments in shortened training. Nurses, both inside and outside the hospitals, were essential in health education, and the quality of the NHS would depend on the quality and quantity of nurses.[23]

All these suggestions for a shorter training ran counter to the view of the College leaders that four years was the ideal period, and their position seemed reactionary to reformers. At the beginning of 1946 a series of articles appeared in the *Nursing Mirror* written by Evelyn Pearce, a well-known author of nursing textbooks, and Gladys Carter, a nurse with a degree in economics, author of textbooks on midwifery, and a perceptive critic of the state of nursing.[24] Their views are given here, since they show that in the nursing profession, alternative theories of nurse training were emerging that challenged the College's adherence to the old apprenticeship system. Pearce and Carter referred to the imminent publication of the NHS Bill: 'we do not know if it will contain explicit references to the nurses calculated to raise the prestige of the profession or will just take them and all the other members of the health team, except the doctors, for granted'. Carter was critical of the nursing organisations and blamed nurses themselves for their lack of influence in the Ministry of Health. Like the SMA, she made the case for an independent job analysis of nursing, to determine what needed to be done by nurses, and what could be done by other staff. She attacked the GNCs, which were still dominated by matrons from the voluntary hospitals, considering them out of touch with reality. Municipal hospitals were now responsible for about five times the number of beds provided by the voluntary hospitals and yet, in the decades since the GNCs were established, there had been years when none of the GNCs' members was from the municipal hospitals. Because the GNCs and the College council usually had overlapping membership, the College could not view the GNCs objectively. Carter was reiterating views expressed in her 1939 book, *A New Deal for Nurses*.[25] Although she was one of a handful of British nurses with a university degree, and her experience of working in Canada made her an advocate of nursing as a university discipline, she took an inclusive view of the nature of the profession. She believed that British nurses needed a new professional structure, a federation for all nurses, not only those on the state register.

> Sooner or later at every public meeting discussing nursing, there crops up the question of an organisation to take in all nurses and the answer that State Registered Nurses already have a powerful organisation in the Royal College of Nursing does not give satisfaction.[26]

Although the College leaders did not then heed such views, and remained very anxious about 'dilution' of the profession, Carter's views represented a new current of opinion in nursing, and indicated the matron-dominated College council did not necessarily speak for the new generation of nurses. At this point, the matrons also found themselves under attack from a more official source.

The Wood report

At the same time as these articles were appearing in the *Nursing Mirror*, the government indicated that it was setting up another study of the recruitment and training of nurses. In a letter to the nursing organisations announcing this initiative, Bevan indicated that he did not think another formal inquiry into nursing was needed, but he proposed a small working party to examine the reviews already made, and to collect further evidence. The College welcomed this, hoping that nurses would be involved, but the Ministry appointed the working party without reference to the nursing organisations. Its chairman was Sir Robert Wood, recently retired from the Ministry of Education, and now principal of Southampton University College. Other members were Dr John Cohen, a psychologist from the Cabinet Office, Dr Thomas Inch of the Department of Health for Scotland, and two nurses, Elizabeth Cockayne and Daisy Bridges. Cockayne, matron of the Royal Free Hospital, was a former member of the College council and had chaired an investigation into recruitment under the Horder Committee. She was also honorary secretary of the Association of Hospital Matrons, and had worked closely with the Ministry of Supply as an advisor during the war. Bridges was a public health nurse with experience of nursing education at home and abroad. Wood wanted his report to be based on solid evidence rather than 'hunches' and employed field workers to carry out 'scientific enquiries' into different aspects of nursing.[27] The working party deliberated for twelve months and, in Abel-Smith's words, collected enough evidence to shame many a 'leisurely Royal commission'.[28] They tried to define nurses' work and the type of training needed to support it, to determine the annual number of recruits needed for the profession, how they might be found, and what sections of the population they should be recruited from. As Wood's work progressed, the emphasis shifted to the high drop out rate among student nurses, and how to increase the number of trained nurses.

The Wood report is remembered for the hostile reaction it provoked from the leaders of the profession, largely because of its conclusion that the authoritarian discipline of the nursing hierarchy was a prime cause of student disaffection.[29] Abel-Smith described the report as 'the most outspoken and well-documented condemnation of the attitudes and behaviour of senior nurses in hospitals'.[30] It provoked a lively debate that continued for some years. It also reinforced a well-worn stereotype of the frustrated spinster matron seeking to enforce petty restrictions on the personal freedom of spirited and modern young nurses, who would not put up with interference in their off-duty lives. This, of course, echoed the long-standing criticisms from the Guild of Nurses, that 'there are too many elderly matrons and too many matrons who rule a hospital as though it were a penal reform school'.[31] Cockayne reflected ruefully many years later that many senior nurses, particularly the powerful matrons on the College council and the GNC, never forgave her for the revelations about training and discipline in the Wood report, and that she herself was shocked to hear what the nurses actually felt about their training.[32] Unfortunately, her association with the Wood report exacerbated divisions between the College and the Ministry of Health, and when Cockayne was appointed chief nursing officer in 1948, there was a legacy of distrust, even though she was far more active than her predecessor in making the Ministry include nursing interests in their policy discussions.[33]

Wood aimed to make nurse training more consistent with the trend in the health services towards social and preventive medicine. Nurse training should be reduced to two years, with a basic general education in the first eighteen months, followed by six months' specialisation in a field chosen by the student. The shortened training would be possible if nurses were relieved of domestic duties and probationers treated as students rather than cheap labour. Students should be responsible to their training schools rather than to the hospitals where they worked. They would qualify for registration after two years, and have the pay and status of a qualified nurse, but would work under supervision for a further year. The College published its response in March 1948, after a conflict of opinion between the council and its salaried staff that also revealed some splits in the College's position, though these were not made public. A small group consisting of Frances Goodall, Mary Carpenter, the Director of Education, and Hilary Blair-Fish, secretary of the Public Health Section, drafted the response. They agreed that some modification of the length and type of training was desirable. They were not in favour of the two-year training proposed by Wood, but preferred a three-year course with the state examination after two years and registration after three. When the council discussed this, Ada Woodman, the vice-chairman, said that public health nurses had for many years felt that the present general training was too long. In effect, they agreed with Wood, because they wished to spend more time studying their own subject, rather than being compelled to take additional training after qualification. Woodman believed that unless the basic training course was shortened, public health nurses might leave general nursing and demand a separate training. The council, still composed mainly of hospital matrons, reluctantly accepted that a shorter basic training might be necessary for some nurses, but were not ready to separate the training schools from the hospitals during training, since this would remove students from the authority of the matron. They replaced the term 'student status' with 'student-nurse status' in their draft comments to make this clear: 'the status of a nurse in training was really that of "student nurse apprentice" . . . no hospital employers could allow nurses over whom they had no control to work in their wards. Student nurses would be responsible to the matron as long as they were engaged in nursing patients'.[34]

The College's published response, amended after this internal argument, welcomed the sections of the Wood report that were close to its own policies, but, as expected, disagreed with Wood's proposals on nurse training. Wood proposed liberal holidays and a forty-hour week, which the College thought would actually reduce the training period to about eighteen months. The College believed that the basic course should take three years, to include both curative and preventive nursing. It offered an alternative training scheme, proposed by the Public Health Section, with a two-year training devoted to the fundamentals common to all fields of nursing, and a third year spent studying a special area of nursing. All agreed that experimental nurse training schemes were desirable to work out a comprehensive and integrated basic syllabus. The College accepted that there should be a single register for men and women, and that the supplementary registers should ultimately be closed, their fields being partly covered in the basic training and partly by the qualified nurse's subsequent study in a chosen field. Wood recommended grants for nursing students, to be paid by the training authority not the hospitals, in sharp contrast to Horder's notion that students should pay for their own training. Horder was allegedly influenced by certain matrons, such as Emily MacManus, matron of Guy's Hospital, who believed that 'during her first two years, a student nurse was more of a liability than an asset'.[35] The College clung to the principle of means-tested grants for students, arguing that financial arrangements in nurse training should be as close to other professions as possible, for if all student nurses received grants, this would imply lower status than other students.[36]

Wood's most innovative proposal was for restructured nurse training based on Regional Nurse Training Boards for each NHS region. Hospitals and public health agencies in each region would be grouped into nurse training units. Each training school would have its own director, entirely independent of the hospital administration. The Division of Nursing at the Ministry of Health and the Department of Health for Scotland would be the controlling bodies, and should be enlarged to include advisers on nurse education and inspectors of training schools. The College council rejected all this, believing that nurse education should remain in the hands of the profession and not be handed over to the Ministry. They endorsed the idea of regional committees to plan and co-ordinate nurse training, but did not want independent training schools, nor for matrons to lose their authority over nursing students. The College and Wood also fell out over the reform of the GNC. Wood shared Gladys Carter's view that the matrons from the London voluntary hospitals dominated the GNC for England and Wales, while municipal hospitals and public health were under-represented. Wood proposed to combine the two GNCs (England and Wales, and Scotland) into one, possibly to include midwifery. The College council, which included several London matrons, was very conservative on this issue, and argued that any major alteration to the GNC should wait until the NHS was at least three years old.

Wood criticised recruitment campaigns that presented nursing as an attractive and even glamorous career. This type of publicity was counter-productive, because disillusioned probationers were more likely to drop out when they encountered the harsh discipline of the training schools.[37] The main culprits, once more, were senior nurses and their old-fashioned ways:

Self-abnegation was the keynote of this tradition which the insularity of institutional life has preserved more or less unaltered by the profound changes in

social outlook which have affected the community as a whole . . . During the
inter-war years a generation has grown up nurtured on modern ideas of personal freedom and relationship between the sexes and, inevitably, a gulf has
separated the representatives of the old order from the newcomers to nursing.
Potential student nurses today . . . regard nursing as a profession with no more
justification than any other for encroaching unduly upon the personal life.[38]

Not surprisingly, the College council was much irritated by this, being largely
composed of matrons of the old school. Wood exposed the generation gap in
the nursing profession. Yet although matrons were reluctant to loosen their
hold over nurse training and discipline, their position was not based entirely
on outdated principles or snobbery. Throughout the war, they had to cope
with severe shortages of nursing and ancillary staff, and to manage reluctant
conscripts or semi-trained volunteers. Also, as Emily MacManus pointed out,
during the war even the most modern infirmaries had trouble keeping equipment in good repair. When vacuum cleaners and electric floor polishers wore
out and were not renewed, nurses were forced into the hard manual work that
many progressive matrons wished to replace with labour-saving devices.[39]
These shortages of staff and equipment persisted for some years after the war.
In the circumstances, the iron discipline of Nightingale days seemed the only
way to keep a hospital running efficiently.

One member of the Wood Committee, Dr John Cohen, embarrassed his
colleagues by producing a minority report.[40] Cohen disassociated himself
from the majority's conclusions on the numbers of nurses required by the
future health service, and wanted numbers to be proportional to the number
of beds. He criticised Wood's methodology and considered that it was foolish
to decide the method of training nurses before addressing the future demand
for health services, the changing role of hospitals and the proper function of
the nurse. If the two-year training scheme were adopted without further
research, it might be detrimental to the public interest. Anne Marie Rafferty
doubts whether Cohen's analysis was ever taken seriously by the planners of
the new health service; and nursing organisations, upset by his attack on
nursing discipline, failed to notice how useful his argument might be to them
when seeking funds for research into nursing.[41] Cohen wanted nurses to participate in life outside the hospital, 'not cloistered within four walls as in a
mediaeval nunnery'. Elaborating his views to a meeting of the Yorkshire
branch of the College, he contended that historically nursing was a segregated
profession, separated by powerful barriers from contact with the community.
Low salaries, poor working conditions and harsh discipline were evidence that
nursing was not highly valued. As a psychologist, he offered a professional
insight into this, and argued that the praise lavished on nursing by distinguished persons at prize-givings and conferences was a defence against the
unconscious guilt they felt at the shabby treatment of the profession.[42] Cohen's

report included a number of comments from former student nurses who had given up their training. Two typical examples were:

> The attitude of the sisters to the probationer was not that of an instructor to a student, but of a Victorian housewife to the scullery maid.

and,

> I know discipline is very essential, but the following is not discipline – one late pass a week, no friends allowed in the home, no smoking in our rooms, no visitors allowed when I was off sick, and I was told on one occasion to take my photographs off my table.[43]

The majority report was well received by the Ministry of Health, and it found the response of the nursing organisations disappointing. The most positive reaction came from the Ten Group of influential nurses, who prudently remained anonymous because some of them held official positions and they were out of line with the official College view. They included Gladys Carter, Evelyn Pearce, Olive Baggallay, and Bethina Bennett, principal matron at the Ministry of Labour. They believed that the profession was entirely unprepared for its key position in the NHS. Welcoming the Wood report, they wanted to see nurses leaving behind the narrow, hospital-based world of the past. More and better teachers would broaden nurses' outlook, and suitable young nurses should be selected for degree courses in science, sociology or arts, to prepare nursing for wider horizons and a new research culture.[44] The College, however, continued to see the matrons as appropriate managers of student nurses. Although the College was in fact divided over whether to separate nurse training from hospital duties, it would not officially endorse the Wood report.

Bevan had promised to present a Nurses Bill before the end of 1948, and he sent draft proposals to the nursing organisations as the basis for discussion at the Ministry. Rosemary White's study of nurses in the early years of the NHS describes the draft as 'extraordinarily ambitious', and credits Bevan with far greater goodwill towards nursing than the officials in the Ministry of Health had ever shown. He proposed to set up new regional training councils, responsible for nurse training in each NHS region. The councils would run new training schools, independent of the hospitals, and funding would be separate from the hospital budget. The College council considered this a wasteful duplication of resources, and preferred nurse education committees under the NHS Regional Hospital Boards. White argues that both the College and the GNC failed to realise that they were being offered professional independence, like that of the University Grants Committee in the training of doctors, and that they did not appreciate the far-reaching possibilities of this scheme. The matrons, as ever, prioritised hospital labour needs over the education of the profession, and 'the matrons' interests were directly antithetical to the development of the profession and professional control'.[45] Divisions among the Wood Committee, and the hostile response of nursing organisations, dampened the Ministry's brief interest in reforming nurse training, but Elizabeth Cockayne later revealed that the Ministry was disappointed in the Wood report because it proposed no radical shortening of the training period, and no quick solution to the nursing shortage.[46] Although it is debateable whether the regional training councils would have been as independent as White suggests, in the event nurses had no training body to separate nursing education from hospital labour.

Despite all the suggestions of the Athlone, Horder and Wood reports, the Nurses Act of 1949 did not reconstruct nursing. The nursing establishment had successfully prevented any sweeping reforms of nurse training, and the Act left it in the hands of the matrons and enlarged General Nursing Councils. The councils set up Area Nurse Training Committees in each NHS region. Some of these experimented with new training programmes, but their powers were limited. They had budgets for nurse training, separate from hospital finances, but the hospital, rather than the training body, determined the students' conditions of service. Students did not receive grants from an independent education authority, but a 'training allowance' from the NHS.[47] They remained low-paid employees of the hospitals and, with ancillary staff in short supply, did time-consuming unskilled work, including cleaning and general fetching and carrying.[48] Bevan left the Ministry of Health in November 1949, and his successors did not occupy a seat in the Cabinet again until the 1960s. The Ministry itself was much shrunken after economies by the Labour government in 1951, and continued to see nursing as a rather low priority. At the beginning of the NHS the vicious circle in nursing recruitment was not broken. While the shortage persisted, nurses would be overworked and given unskilled duties, the very conditions that made nursing seem unattractive, and discouraged recruits.

Public activities

War and reconstruction immersed the College's leaders in constant negotiations with bureaucracy, whose linguistic habits unfortunately began to permeate the College's own communications. It was the age of the memorandum, the sub-committee and the working party. But while the official records of the College in this period inevitably concentrate on its political activities, everyday life in Henrietta Place and in the branches focused on services to members. The College aimed to prepare nurses for the health service reform, and held a series of conferences on 'The Nation's Nurses' between 1947 and 1951. The conferences brought together prominent speakers, including Cabinet ministers, high-ranking civil servants, university staff and professionals from the private sector. The first, in March 1947, dealt with nurses' future responsibilities under the NHS. Bevan was the main speaker. He charmed a large audience of senior nurses by feigning shyness, and admitting coyly, 'You know, you rather frighten me'.[49]

The second conference, held in November 1947 after the publication of the Wood report, had Sir Robert Wood as the main speaker. Subsequent conferences focused on job analysis, modern methods of selection of recruits and in human relations, public health, the industrial nursing service and hospital management. The fifth conference, in the spring of 1949 emphasised public health in nurse training and practice. It received much publicity after a speech by Colonel E. W. Northfield, governor of Gloucester prison, who described in moving detail the long night shifts, poor food and discouraging atmosphere endured by his daughter, a student nurse. Press attention was caught by his demand that nurses be allowed to wear cosmetics on duty: 'attractive nurses cheer up the patients. Outside the hospital make-up now seems to be regarded as essential to any woman's morale. For a tired and jaded nurse it might not only be a disguise but a tonic and restorative'.[50]

The College also offered educational support for nurses in the new Library of Nursing, opened by Princess Elizabeth in July 1945. The library's Carnegie grant, which in its first ten years amounted to £1,000, was discontinued in 1931. The library was open to all nurses whether College members or not, though from 1943 it charged an annual subscription of ten shillings to non-members who wished to borrow books. In the same year, the first full-time librarian was appointed, and in 1944 the library moved into the more spacious accommodation it still occupies in Henrietta Place. More material needs were also catered for. One of the benefits of College membership, besides legal and professional aid, was the Uniform Department that provided extra clothing coupons for nurses working outside the hospital service – private nurses, industrial nurses and school matrons. Throughout the war and the years of rationing, hospital nurses complained bitterly that their allowance of clothing coupons had to be used to replace the shoes and stockings worn out during their long working hours, leaving them nothing for their off-duty clothing. A hospital nurse, it was claimed, walked 12 to 15 miles a day. The subject was raised in parliament, and the College secured some relaxation of the regulations. The College also offered convalescent care for overstrained members, in its newly acquired Barton House Hotel near Bournemouth. In 1948 it bought a second convalescent home, Drygrange, a handsome baronial mansion near Melrose. The money for this came from a thank-offering gift from South Africa to Britain. In November 1947 Sir Arthur Stanley died, leaving the College £1,000 – a modest proportion of his considerable estate. He remained a life-long supporter of the College, attending council meetings until his last years. The College benefited in other ways from a grateful nation, as both government and private donors gave grants to nurses taking College courses. These hardly met the need for specialised nurse training, but in the absence of any official system of post-qualification training, the College continued to fill the gap.

The College took part in government-sponsored recruitment campaigns, with nursing exhibitions in local hospitals, and continued its own drive in the more prestigious girls' schools by offering lectures on anatomy to science mistresses who were willing to encourage girls to enter the profession. Even publicity drives caused some friction with the Ministry of Health. Mindful of criticisms that nursing life inhibited romance, the Ministry produced recruiting leaflets in 1947 featuring 'glamour drawings' of fetching nurses alongside handsome young doctors. Several critics pointed out that the drawings showed a nurse using sterilising equipment without wearing rubber gloves. The College complained that such advertising attracted the 'wrong' type of recruit, and would exacerbate the dropout rate among student nurses.[51] Undeterred, in 1949 the Ministry produced recruiting leaflets and posters featuring the film star Patricia Neal in her role as the nursing heroine of the popular film *The Hasty Heart*. The Ministry appeared to endorse Colonel Northfield's views, as Miss Neal wore full make-up on duty. Uniformed nurses were drafted in to

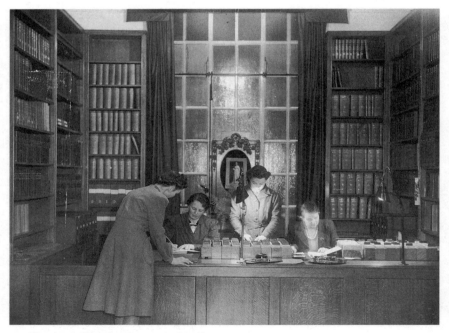

4.1 Library, College headquarters, London, 1945.

hand out the leaflet in cinema foyers. The College protested again, and also complained that hospital managements were pressurising matrons to take part in this campaign, which presented nurses in an unrealistic way. The College was not supported by a correspondent in the *Beckenham Advertiser*, who accused it of stuffiness. In Beckenham, it appeared, posters featuring Neal were balanced by others showing 'a typical, real-life nurse'. Unfortunately, no examples of these have been located.[52]

Reluctant trade unionists

Although the coming of the NHS made little difference to the professional status of nurses, partly because of the College's conservatism over nurse training, other changes were occurring that would, in time, fundamentally alter the College's role. One of the unforeseen consequences of its wartime activities was slow but inexorable pressure towards trade unionism. Trade unions were increasing in power and confidence, especially because Bevin was anxious to secure their co-operation for the war effort. After the war, the College had to sit alongside the unions in many committees discussing nurses' pay and conditions. Frances Goodall had worried about the 'contamination' of association with the TUC in the 1930s, but good relations with the Ministry of Labour during the war soothed some of these anxieties, to the point where the Ministry of Health feared that the College was developing a 'trade union complex'.

The coming of the NHS encouraged the growth of unionism in the health services. From 1948, most nurses became public employees with nationally agreed pay structures, and the College was dealing not with local hospital committees, but with a national negotiating body. Like other sections of the civil service, nurses' pay was now arbitrated by a Whitley Council, the new Nurses and Midwives Whitley Council. The staff side of the council was a mixture of professional associations and trade unions, including the College, the Association of Hospital Matrons, the Royal College of Midwives, the Association of Supervisors of Midwives, the Scottish Matrons' Association, the Women Public Health Officers' Association, NALGO, and five of the larger unions of nurses in the public sector.[53] At this point, twenty-seven organisations claimed to speak for nurses, but only thirteen were recognised by the Whitley Council.[54] It had sub-committees to deal with nurses, midwives, public health nurses (including health visitors, tuberculosis visitors, domiciliary nurses and school nurses), mental nurses and nursery staff.

In November 1945 Frances Goodall reported to the College council on trade unionism among nurses, after attending meetings at the Ministry of Health to assist Bevan in preparing his broadcast appeal for more nurses, midwives and hospital staff.[55] The unions were well represented at these meetings, and although the Minister's statement was generally acceptable to the College, Goodall feared that some of his views were bound to affect its position. Bevan wanted a national negotiating machinery for all ancillary staff in NHS hospitals. They would be represented through trade unions, which would thus gain entrance to every hospital. Goodall believed that unless the College took action the unions would use the opportunity to recruit trained nurses and students. The College must publicise its work in defending nurses' individual and collective interests, and matrons should encourage nurses' representative councils in their hospitals. Goodall wrote:

> I feel that the College is being challenged and that unless this is met by a determined stand and strong counter action the College will find its position as a professional body usurped by the trade unions. This may seem to be an overstatement but evidence from the Area Organisers and others . . . confirms this.[56]

Although the College and the unions had worked together harmoniously on the Rushcliffe Committee and the National Advisory Council for Nurses and Midwives, they differed in their approach to nursing. A few unions were still challenging the College. Thora Silverthorne's Association of Nurses, which failed to attract many members, had merged with the National Union of Public Employees. The Guild of Nurses, now part of the Hospitals and Welfare Services Union, had a history of persistent opposition to the College, especially over the College's earlier objections to the ninety-six-hour fortnight.[57] The Guild continued to act as gadfly, portraying the College as a group of high-handed matrons incapable of understanding nurses' interests. An anonymous letter to the *New Leader* stated:

> The Union recognised by most hospitals is one which is not affiliated to the T.U.C. – the Royal College of Nursing. In most hospitals it has the Matrons and Administrative Staff at its head. As you can see, this is rather like running a Union with the Manager and all the foremen on the E[xecutive] C[ommittee]! So we in the real T.U.'s have to work quietly underground, or else to be open to petty, but potent, victimisation.[58]

In 1944 the Guild advised its members to join the College for educational purposes, but maintained that nurses needed a trade union to defend them. Goodall considered this a dangerous message, and argued that the College must take the trade union 'threat' very seriously. Her first instinct was to improve College publicity, since many members of the College and the Student Nurses' Association apparently did not know of its work in defending individual members, and it was not the council's policy to publish details of successful negotiations in individual cases. She urged matrons and sister tutors to arouse the professional consciousness of nurses in their charge, and encourage them to take an active part in their professional body. The trade unions had an advantage because, she thought, some of their members were almost fanatical in pursuing their aims.

Frances Goodall persuaded the council to reorganise the Student Nurses' Association, and to appoint an extra officer to bring its recruitment literature up to date and encourage activism, for she worried about 'sleeping members'. In 1949 the council followed her advice and set up a new Ward Sisters' Section for hospital nurses, but her desire for a Nurses' Defence Union, akin to the Medical Defence Union, was not realised. Setting up an independent body of this kind would be complex and possibly costly, but the College continued to pay for insurance policies to give its members legal protection, and stressed this prominently in its recruitment literature.

The *Nursing Times* reflected some of this new mood in 1945, stating that the College 'is not simply an educational body, but is essentially a professional organisation like the British Medical Association', recognised by employers and the Ministries as a negotiating body.[59] The comparison with the BMA certainly accorded with the self-image of that body, but side-stepped the BMA's vigorous political campaigns, for the doctors were particularly vocal and fractious in their negotiations with Bevan over the introduction of the NHS. The BMA did not consider itself a medical trade union, but it certainly

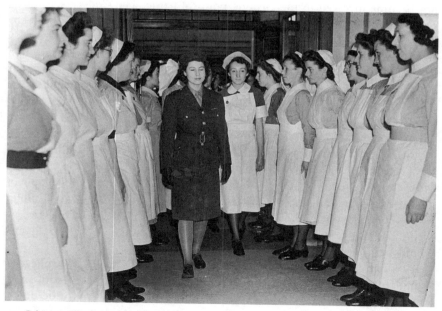

4.2 Princess Elizabeth, president of the Student Nurses' Association, with guard of honour, College headquarters, London, July 1945.

behaved like one when threatening to boycott the NHS if its terms were not met. The College's view of its own position was put to the test when in 1946 the government repealed the Trade Disputes and Trade Unions Act of 1927. Employers in the public sector could once again require their employees to be members of a trade union, but would they accept College membership instead, given the College's resolute non-union stance? Goodall wrote to all members of the College in September 1946 reassuring them that theirs was the largest association for nurses in the country, as demonstrated by its majority on the nurses' panel of the Whitley Council. It was recognised by the government, the employers and the TUC as a negotiating body, and it represented the profession on forty-three other bodies, especially the National Advisory Council on Nurses and Midwives. Goodall chose her language with care to reconcile the warring claims of professionalism and trade unionism. She stated that the College, with over 40,000 members, was 'a professional union.'[60]

Within months of the repeal of the Act, Willesden Borough Council decreed that all its staff must belong to a union. Since professional associations did not have the legal status of trade unions, the council served notices of dismissal on two doctors, two matrons and forty-eight sisters, nurses and midwives who refused to comply. Most of the nurses were members of the College and followed its advice to maintain a dignified and professional attitude and not become involved in the ensuing political battle. The College set out its policy in a letter to *The Times*, and released a press statement.[61] It took advantage of the situation to increase its membership, and a letter was sent to every state registered nurse setting out the function of the College, together with a membership application form. Durham County Council imposed a similar closed shop policy in 1950. Organisations affected by the ruling, including the BMA, the National Union of Teachers and the College of Midwives, joined the College of Nursing in advising their members to disregard Durham Council's request for proof of union membership. These organisations, joined by the British Dental Association, formed a Joint Emergency Committee of the Professions and began negotiating with Durham County Council. The professions claimed that the Durham order was contrary to the principle of voluntary association, and the matter was referred to the Minister of Labour, who found in favour of the professions.[62] Roundly condemned by the government, Durham eventually conceded that it would take no action against members of professional bodies.

Although the government pressed local authorities to accept the College as a union for purposes of negotiation, not all nurses were happy at this outcome. Some clearly felt that the College was not presenting itself as a trade union should. One nurse, a member of the Labour Party, wrote personally to Bevan after receiving the College's recruitment letter:

I have been nursing 14 years and have witnessed the attempts of a few nurses to form unions. These attempts have been quickly suppressed by the matrons or medical directors. The nurses have been labelled as 'agitators' and have been black-marked.

Matrons encourage the idea among nurses that to belong to a union will place them on the same level as factory workers. This line of thought is foolish but a number of nurses unfortunately think along these lines.

I have no intention of joining the Royal College of Nursing but would like to join a union on similar lines as other workers.

I do not know if any such union exists for nurses but would be very pleased to have any information.[63]

Keeping the unions at bay was not easy, especially if nurses began to demonstrate militant tendencies. An incident occurred immediately after the National Health Service Act came into force in 1948. When the student nurses received their first pay packet from their new employer in July 1948, many were shocked to find that they were worse off than before. They were now liable for national insurance and superannuation contributions of almost £20 a year, and this left them 10 shillings worse off every month. For seventeen student nurses at St Mary's Hospital, Plaistow, in the East End of London, this was intolerable. They wrote to Bevan, to the chair of their Regional Hospital Board, to their local MP and to the press, complaining that it was impossible to exist on a student nurse's salary of £3 3s 4d per month, and that they would have to resign. The Nurses' Salaries Committee (Rushcliffe) had recommended an additional £15 per year for student nurses, to be paid immediately, and the Ministry of Health hastily announced this. But the students were still paid less than their pre-NHS salary. Over 600 student nurses from hospitals in the East End of London attended a heated meeting at St Mary's, and telegrams and messages of support came from all over the country promising to follow the lead of the St Mary's nurses. The seventeen students agreed to meet representatives of the Royal College of Nursing, and, after discussions with members of the Hospital Board, withdrew their resignations. That evening the College held an open meeting for student nurses. The College reiterated its usual position on the status of student nurses.

The College has always maintained that if the nurse in training is to be recognised as a genuine student of nursing her remuneration during training should take the form of educational grants and adequate maintenance allowances rather than salary or wages as an employee.[64]

The threatened resignation of the student nurses was well covered by the press. Some students were members of trade unions, and the Confederation of Health Service Employees organised a public march from Trafalgar Square to Hyde Park. The *Nursing Times* reporter described this meeting as orderly

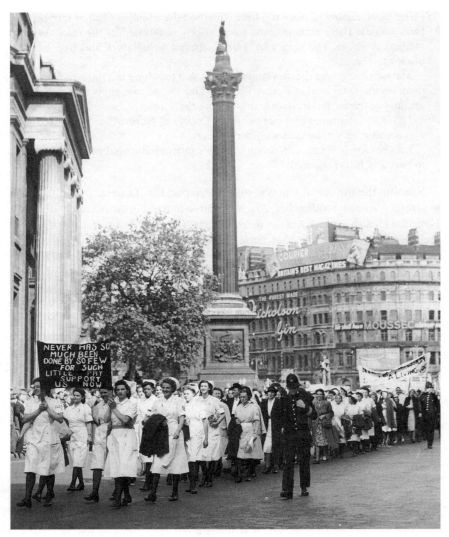

4.3 Student nurses' protest, London, August 1948.

and dull, and concluded that there was little sympathy between the union officials and their nurse members. The College sent a member of staff to the demonstration who reported that COHSE was using the dispute as an excuse to recruit student nurses. For several years the professional organisations and the trade unions had argued over the status of student nurses. The professional organisations contended that they were students and that their pay should not be regarded as a salary, while the unions regarded them as employees and were more concerned about their pay and working conditions than their professional development and education. Both sides had a vested interest in recruitment, for if probationers became 'students' they would not be eligible for union membership, but if they were 'employees' then the Student Nurses' Association of the College was not empowered to negotiate for them. The association issued a statement on student nurses in July 1948, proposing that they be paid a gross salary, out of which the student would pay the hospital for board and lodging.

The medical press took much interest in the students' plight and *The Lancet* commented that it was stimulating to find nurses – 'who usually seem too busy or too tired for polemics' – standing up for themselves. The whole affair had been so badly mismanaged that the students were threatening to strike.[65] The Rushcliffe Committee tried to resolve the problem, but the employers were not prepared to concede more than the £15 a year pay rise, and the staff side would not accept this. The staff side considered going to arbitration, but the Ministry of Labour told them that the issue could not be regarded as a trade dispute, and arbitration could not be invoked. The advice of the Ministry was to let the matter rest until the new Whitley Council met in August, and this was reluctantly agreed by the staff side. When the relevant Whitley committee met, it agreed that an increase was justified by the rising cost of living, and by the end of 1948 student nurses' pay was increased by £8 a month. One outcome of the student nurses' threatened strike was a sharp rise in membership of the Student Nurses' Association. By the end of 1948, over 10,000 new student nurses had joined, over 3,000 more than in any previous year, bringing the total membership up to 19,000. Despite their minimal salaries, the blandishments of the trade unions, and the College's ambivalent attitude to student nurses' pay, many students looked to the College to defend their interests. They settled for very little, accepting their role as trainee professionals rather than employees, in spite of their major contribution to the daily work of the hospital wards.

Male nurses and equal pay

Among the various post-war strategies to overcome the nursing shortage, the value of male nurses to the hospital service was recognised. The Ministry of Health arranged for a special one-year course of general training for men released from the Forces, to speed up their qualification for state registration. Any man with at least two years' ward experience under trained nurses and the status of a nursing orderly in the army or air force, or of a leading sick berth attendant in the navy, was eligible for this course. Other ex-servicemen were eligible for enrolment as assistant nurses if they had at least two years' wartime experience of hospital nursing under the supervision of a trained nurse. If they wished to qualify for the register, their training period was reduced by six months. Although Frances Goodall fostered cordial relations with the male nurses' organisations, there was lingering anxiety in the College over their integration into the hospital system. In 1943, the president of the College, Emily MacManus, welcomed them as district nurses, but admitted 'she did not know whether she was herself quite educated to male nurses for women patients'.[66] The possibility of more male nurses in the general hospitals also brought the question of equal pay into sharper focus.

During the war, the Rushcliffe Committee recommended higher salaries for nurses, and these were generally accepted by employers, although the committee had no official powers. Rushcliffe reluctantly agreed to recognise the practice, 'in existing economic circumstances', of paying male nurses at a higher rate than female nurses of similar grade, despite vigorous protests from the College. The principle of equal pay for equal work was far from the normal practice in Britain. In commerce and industry women were paid about 53 per cent of men's rates, though this average disguised wide and erratic variations.[67] Some male-dominated professions accepted equal pay, mainly to prevent salaries from being undercut by competition from women, but in the civil service, local government, teaching and nursing, different rates for men and women were normal. Nursing was a unique case, for although most nurses were women and, unusually, had a higher status than their male colleagues, they were paid at a lower rate than male nurses for the same work. The College had long supported the principle of equal pay for equal work and was a founder member of the Equal Pay Campaign Committee, on which Frances Goodall sat.

During the war, there was much agitation over equal pay for equal work, particularly in industry. As more women moved into work previously done by men, at lower rates of pay, some trade unions feared that employers would prefer women workers to men once the war ended, to cut costs, and supported equal pay for that reason.[68] Although professional and white-collar groups were less inclined to strike over the issue, many were strongly committed to the principle of equal pay, and the Equal Pay Campaign Committee was formed in January 1944. Its members were mainly from professional and middle-class women's organisations, including the British Federation of University Women, the Council of Women Civil Servants, NALGO, the National Council of Women, the National Union of Women Teachers, the Women Public Health Officers' Association, and others. The campaign concentrated on the public sector, believing that if government introduced equal pay then the private sector would follow. The movement came close to a major success when an amendment to the 1944 Education Act introduced equal pay for schoolteachers, and the government had to take extraordinary steps to reverse this. Churchill temporised by appointing a Royal Commission on Equal Pay. To successive governments, financial considerations were paramount. Although the principle of equal pay for equal work had a wide measure of political support, inter-war governments had refused to implement it, citing the poor state of the economy. Wartime and post-war governments resisted equal pay on financial grounds, fearing inflationary pressures and the additional burden on the public payroll.

In the 1940s Goodall was chairman of the British Federation of Business and Professional Women, which was also involved in the Equal Pay Campaign, and the federation's evidence to the Royal Commission singled out the nursing profession along with women police officers. The College gave evidence in December 1945, calling for an end to sex discrimination in pay. It described the peculiar nature of the nursing profession:

> The training is essentially the same but the status of women in the profession is higher. All the top posts are occupied by women. The revised scales of salaries, introduced by the Rushcliffe committee, for all branches of nursing, recommended improvements but women nurses' confidence in the committee was shaken by the marked discrimination in favour of the male nurse, male student nurse and male assistant nurse, particularly in contrast to the female ward sister and staff nurse in hospital.[69]

The Association of Male Nurses, which was now affiliated to the College, supported its claim for equal pay; but the College was not universally popular among male nurses, who, excluded from formal membership, not unreasonably regarded it as concerned only with women's issues. One disgruntled male nurse wrote:

> The R.C.N. represents only the female, general trained, State registered nurses. What of those on the so-called 'supplementary' registers (male nurses, mental nurses, fever and sick children's nurses) and the large number on the R[oyal] M[edico-]P[sychological] A[ssociation] and assistant nurses' registers? All these can and do join in the one representative body – the union.[70]

When the Royal Commission's report was published in November 1946, the Equal Pay Campaign Committee could only regard it as a challenge. The commission was forbidden to make policy recommendations, and concentrated on analysing the wage gap and the consequences of accepting equal pay. It produced the following figures for nursing in 1946, when there were estimated to be 154,400 women and 18,700 men in the profession, both registered and unregistered, distributed as follows:

Table 4.1 Distribution of male and female nurses in different types of institution, March 1946

	Males	Females	Total
Hospitals, including sanatoria	4,400	97,600	102,000
Mental hospitals	13,200	14,800	28,000
Nursing homes, district nursing, homes for the aged, etc.	1,100	42,000	43,100
Total	18,700	154,400	173,100

Source: *Report of the Royal Commission on Equal Pay 1944–46* Cmd 6937 (London: HMSO, 1946), p. 41. Two part-time nurses were counted as one individual in these figures, and private nurses were excluded.

The pay differentials were considerable, even when board and lodging for female hospital nurses were taken into account. Official calculations always treated nurses' accommodation as 'emoluments', although some nurses' homes were of poor quality, and many female hospital nurses were not given the choice of living out. Men's salaries were calculated purely on a monetary basis.

Table 4.2 Rates of pay for male and female nurses in selected grades, July 1946

Grade	Females			Males	
	Salary	Emoluments (estimated)	Total remuneration	Salary (London)	Salary (outside London)
State-registered student nurse	£95	£75	£170	£258.4.0	£234.0.0
Staff nurse	£120–80	£100	£220–80	£284.14.0–£336.14.0	£260–£312

Source: *Report of the Royal Commission on Equal Pay 1944–46* Cmd 6937 (London: HMSO, 1946), pp. 42–3

A majority on the Equal Pay Commission thought that the difference between men's and women's earnings in certain occupations reflected their unequal value as workers. Women, allegedly, showed less initiative, were bad time-keepers and took time off work for family reasons, thus making themselves less attractive to employers. Although differences between male and female physique certainly did not account for the wide variations in pay in many occupations, there were many jobs where women were less effective for physical reasons. Not surprisingly, three of the four women commissioners rejected several of these arguments, arguing that 'natural' differences in male and female physique were being rapidly overcome by labour-saving equipment, and that individuals should not be penalised because of (often unsubstantiated) ideas about the capacity of the 'average' female worker.[71] Rather, they contended that women had low pay because they had no bargaining power and weak trade unions. The majority report, according to its brief, noted that equal pay would be relatively costly for national and local government; while the minority resisted this stark choice between 'exact justice' and 'oiling the wheels of economic progress', claiming that equal pay would bring greater productivity.[72] The Labour Chancellor, Hugh Dalton, accepted the justice of equal pay but stated that, at an estimated £24 million, it would be inflationary. The response of the Campaign Committee to this well-worn argument was that no section of workers should be expected to forego their rights in order to spare the Chancellor financial troubles. This was a matter of fundamental justice, and they pointed out that the British delegates to the United Nations had subscribed to the UN charter proclaiming that there should be no discrimination by reason of race, sex, language or religion.

Women's groups continued to lobby the government for equal pay in the civil service, local government and other areas where it was directly involved. It aroused strong feelings, for many women were passionately against equal pay, particularly within the Conservative Party, where the subject was extremely divisive.[73] The party was officially in favour of equal pay, but its women's section was not, believing that equal pay would make employment more attractive to women and thus deter them from marriage and childbearing, or that it would encourage married women to work and leave their children in the care of the state. Rather, they considered that it was more important to improve the status of housewives. Conservative women saw equal pay as part of a feminist campaign for sex equality, and this meant loss of femininity. To most nurses, it was a clear-cut issue, and the more forceful public outburst came from nurses in Scotland. The Edinburgh branch of the College submitted a resolution to the Standing Conference of Women's Organisations, calling for an end to inequality.

In July 1947 the College council made a firm statement on equal pay for equal work in the nursing profession, stressing that salaries should be based on the rate for the job. The assumption that men had greater liabilities was no longer valid, because women who remained unmarried (and widows) needed a career for life, and women often had dependants to support. At this stage, of the forty-one members of the College council, three were men and thirty-six were unmarried women. The married senior nurse was still a rarity. If it were inequitable for a man to support his wife and family on the same salary as his spinster colleague, it was equally inequitable that a single woman should have to support aged parents on a salary less than that of her bachelor colleague. Anomalies were most marked in general training schools where increasing numbers of male students were being accepted. Male student nurses' weekly rates were more than double those of female students and often exceeded the pay of the female staff nurses and junior sisters.[74] A male assistant nurse earned a higher salary than the maximum of a female staff nurse and his starting salary was higher than the starting salary of a female ward sister. The College followed its statement with an unsuccessful request that the Minister receive a deputation from the College, the Student Nurses' Association and the Society of Registered Male Nurses. It was perturbed that the new hospital boards were beginning to advertise for staff at unequal rates, and lobbied vigorously against this.[75] In 1955, the Conservative government, at a time of economic boom and continuing labour shortage, and mindful of the female vote, finally agreed to introduce equal pay for the public service, to be introduced over six years. The principle was not applied to the rest of the workforce for another twenty years.

Conclusion

The College welcomed the NHS, but rapidly realised that the new structure gave nurses little more influence in health policy than the old. Hospital matrons certainly remained powerful within their own domain, and their leading role in the College council meant that its policy towards nurse training still favoured an apprenticeship system, under the matrons' control, rather than independent training schools outside the hospitals. In the early years of the NHS, the government's strategy for nursing staff was determined mainly by the nursing shortage, and this frustrated all efforts to raise the educational qualification of recruits, or to alter the status of nursing students, the vital source of cheap labour. Traditional gender roles exacerbated the problem, since neither the government nor the College saw the contribution of married women as a possible solution to the shortage, in spite of wartime experience of married women's work. Rather, official views, as expressed in the Wood report, tended to stress the conservatism of senior nurses, and their attachment to rigid hospital routines, as a major obstacle to recruitment. This was an implicit criticism of the College, whose leaders were senior, unmarried, career nurses.

However, the new national pay structures of the NHS gave the College more opportunity to speak for nurses in negotiations over pay and working conditions. Its leaders may have been conservative in their support of traditional management for hospital nurses, but they were in the vanguard of the contemporary struggle for equal pay for men and women. Although the College began its relationship with the NHS without official union status, and its leaders rejected unionism for nurses, the College was effectively taking on the tasks of a union in pay bargaining, and sat alongside trade unionists in many meetings. For a time, the description of 'professional union' seemed a satisfactory compromise, as long as government was prepared to accept membership of the College as 'virtual' union membership. Trade unions, however, had a legal status in industrial relations that the College did not possess, and its claims to official recognition rested on informal arrangements. As Britain entered a more contentious period in trade union history, the College faced more severe challenges to its position, and these coincided with major changes in the gender and racial mix of the profession.

Notes

1 Charles Webster, *The Health Services Since the War. Vol. 1* (London: HMSO, 1988), pp. 243–8.
2 Rafferty, *Politics of Nursing Knowledge*, p. 173.
3 The membership figure for 1945.
4 RCN/17/4/39, press cuttings, *BMJ* 2 Aug. 1947 and *The Lancet* 26 Oct. 1946.
5 RCN/5/7/28, Digest of speech by Mrs H. Blair-Fish, 21 June 1946.

6 RCN/17/4/39, press cuttings, *Daily Sketch* 22 June 1946.

7 Abel-Smith, *Nursing Profession*, pp. 176–7.

8 *The Lancet*, 1 June 1946, p. 819.

9 RCN/17/4/39, press cuttings, *The Lancet*, 26 May 1945.

10 RCN/17/4/39, press cuttings, *The Lancet* 26 Oct. 1946.

11 RCNA pamphlet collection 11a, 'Recruitment of nurses and midwives to training institutions' (HMSO, not published, 1945). The pamphlet was printed for the Ministry of Labour and National Services, the Ministry of Health and the Department of Health for Scotland by HMSO, August 1945.

12 TNA MH 55/2056, 'Nurses recruitment and distribution, Hospital Nurses' Charter'. The document was first referred to internally as a charter, but by time it was published it was referred to as a New Deal.

13 TNA MH55/20/56.

14 TNA MH55/20/56, newscutting, not identified, 8 Dec. 1945.

15 TNA MH55/20/56, letter to A. E. Neville, 22 Sept. 1945.

16 Abel-Smith, *Nursing Profession*, p. 259. The College did not keep a record of the proportion of married women among its members.

17 RCN/28/11AC, advisory service of the Royal College of Nursing, Dec. 1945.

18 Ibid.

19 RCN/17/4/37 press cuttings, n.p., *Evening Standard* 2 Dec. 1944.

20 RCN/17/4/39, press cuttings, p. 36.

21 RCN/5/9/2, visit by Frances Goodall to nurses serving in the British Army of Occupation on the Rhine, Feb. 1946, on invitation of the War Office.

22 This was issued in December 1945. The Ministry of Health received a typed copy (TNA MH55/2059) in advance of publication, and a note on the back of this indicates that the government pamphlet *Staffing the Hospitals* was issued after receiving the SMA's communication. For the history of the SMA, see John Stewart, *The Battle for Health: a Political History of the Socialist Medical Association, 1930–51* (Aldershot: Ashgate, 1999).

23 Socialist Medical Association, *Nursing in the Post-war World: a Memorandum on the Shortage of Nurses, With Constructive Proposals* (London: Socialist Medical Association, 1945), p. 10.

24 Gladys Beaumont Carter, *Reconsideration of Nursing: its Fundamentals, Purposes and Place in the Community* (London: Nursing Mirror, 1946). This pamphlet was reprinted from articles in the *NM* in January, February and March of that year. See also, Rosemary Weir, 'Gladys Carter – an advocate of higher education for nurses', *International History of Nursing Journal* 4: 2 (Winter 1998/1999), 22–7.

25 Gladys Beaumont Carter, *A New Deal for Nurses* (London: Gollancz, 1939). New Deals were part of the political language in the late 1930s, but Carter's new deal for nurses anticipated Bevan's by some years.

26 Carter, *Reconsideration of Nursing*, p. 15.

27 TNA MH55/2059.

28 Abel-Smith, *Nursing Profession*, p. 182.

29 Ministry of Health, Department of Health for Scotland, Ministry of Labour and National Service, *Report of the Working Party on the Recruitment and Training of Nurses* [Wood report] (London: HMSO, 1947).

30 Abel-Smith, *Nursing Profession*, p. 182.

31 E.g. Beatrice Drapper's earlier comments, RCN/17/4/36, press cuttings, *Daily Herald* 27 May 1941.

32 RCNA T10, interview with Dame Elizabeth Cockayne, 1984.

33 Scott, 'Influence of the staff of the Ministry of Health', pp. 54–5, 199–200.

34 CM 17 Nov. 1947, p. 288. For a discussion of responses to the Working Party Report, including the divided opinion within the College, see White, *Effects of the NHS on the Nursing Profession*, pp. 24–33.

35 TNA MH 55/2156, note of discussion with Royal College of Nursing, 2 May 1944, p. 8.

36 Royal College of Nursing, *Memorandum on the Report of the Working Party on the Recruitment and Training of Nurses* (London: Staples Press, 1948), p. 10.

37 Wood report, p. 63.

38 Ibid., p. 41.

39 RCN/17/4/38, press cuttings, *Sunday Times* 7 Oct. 1945, p. 89.

40 Ministry of Health, Department of Health for Scotland, Ministry of Labour and National Service, *Working Party on the Recruitment and Training of Nurses, Minority Report* (London: HMSO, 1948). See also Scott, 'Influence of the staff of the Ministry of Health', p. 140.

41 Rafferty, *Politics of Nursing Knowledge*, pp. 180–1.

42 *NT* 20 Nov. 1948, pp. 850–1.

43 *Working Party on the Recruitment and Training of Nurses, Minority Report*, p. 64.

44 RCN/4/1947/4, comments submitted to the Ministry of Health by the Ten Group, 1948.

45 White, *Effects of the NHS on the Nursing Profession*, pp. 34–51.

46 Scott, 'Influence of the staff of the Ministry of Health', pp. 152–4, shows how the Ministry canvassed numerous nursing and other bodies, but received little support. See also RCNA T10, interview with Dame Elizabeth Cockayne, 1984.

47 Monica Baly, *Nursing and Social Change*, 3rd edn (London: Routledge, 1995), pp. 205–6. Baly gives details of committees who did use the Act to promote new types of curriculum.

48 Baly, *Nursing and Social Change*, pp. 190–2.

49 RCN/17/4/39, press cuttings, *Daily Graphic* 3 June 1947.

50 RCN/17/4/41, press cuttings, *Manchester Guardian* 15 Dec. 1949, p. 3. Northfield later claimed to have received fan mail from all over the country on this subject.

51 RCN/17/4/1949, press cuttings, *Evening Standard* 3 Jan. 1947, p. 125 ff.

52 RCN/17/4/40, press cuttings, *Evening News* 27 Oct. 1949; *Beckenham Advertiser* 17 Nov. 1949.

53 These were: the National Union of Public Employees, National Union of General and Municipal Workers, the Guild of Nurses and National Union of County Officers, the Mental Hospital and Institutional Workers' Union, and the Women Public Health Officers' Association.

54 As stated by Stanley Mayne of the Ministry of Health in a public speech. RCN/17/4/39, press cuttings, *Lincolnshire Echo* 24 April 1948.

55 CM 15 Nov. 1945, pp. 278–80.

56 CM 18 Oct. 1945, p. 245.

57 College had opposed the TUC-sponsored Limitation of Hours Bill in 1937.

58 RCN/17/4/37, press cuttings, *New Leader* 26 Feb. 1944.

59 Editorial, 'A negotiating body', *NT* 29 Dec. 1945.

60 RCN/3/12/6, Professional Association Committee minutes, Sept. 1946.

61 RCN/13/EE/2, papers relating to the Willesden dispute, 1946–48.

62 These were not the only councils to attempt the closed shop. A similar situation occurred in Motherwell. RCN/17/4/39, press cuttings, *Evening Dispatch* 17 Jan. 1948.

63 TNA MH55/1986, F. Fieldhouse to A. Bevan, 29 Dec. 1946.

64 RCN/17/2/41, papers relating to the student nurses' dispute. See also, S. McGann, 'No wonder nurses quit! What the new health service meant for nurses in 1948', in C. Nottingham (ed.), *The NHS in Scotland, the Legacy of the Past and the Prospect of the Future* (Aldershot: Ashgate, 2000), pp. 34–48.

65 RCN/17/2/41, press cuttings, *The Lancet* 7 Aug. 1948.

66 RCN/17/4/37, press cuttings, *Public Assistance Journal*, 11 Feb. 1943.

67 Pat Thane, 'Towards equal opportunities? Women in Britain since 1945', in Terry Gourvish and Alan O'Day (eds), *Britain Since 1945* (Basingstoke: Macmillan, 1991), p. 187.

68 For an analysis of the wartime disputes over equal pay, see Harold L. Smith, 'The problem of "equal pay for equal work" in Great Britain during World War II', *Journal of Modern History* 53 (1981), 652–72.

69 RCN/13/EB/1/1.

70 RCN/17/4/39, press cuttings, *Catholic Herald* 9 April 1948.

71 The dissenters were Dame Anne Loughlin, Dr Janet Vaughan and Lucy Nettlefold. *Report of the Royal Commission on Equal Pay 1944–46* Cmd 6937 (London: HMSO, 1946), pp. 188–90.

72 *Royal Commission on Equal Pay*, p. 196.

73 For details, see Harold L. Smith, 'The politics of Conservative reform: the equal pay for equal work issue, 1945–1955', *Historical Journal* 35 (1992), 401–15.

74 A fourth-year male student nurse earned more than a female staff nurse in her tenth year and more than a female ward sister in her first year.

75 Some hospital authorities gave way over this type of advertising. See RCN/13/EB/1/2, F. Goodall to Mrs F. Popplewell, 11 Aug 1948; H. C. Hart to F. Goodall, 15 Sept. 1948.

5

The work and training of a nurse

The government hoped in vain that women who volunteered or were conscripted as auxiliary nurses during the war would undertake further nurse
training and remain in the profession. The Ministry of Labour noted dispirit-
edly in 1948 that many 'were only awaiting the day for their compulsory
service to end, so that they might leave to take up clerical or Civil Service
posts'.[1] Nursing, with its low pay and inflexible traditions, so heavily criticised
in the Wood report, obviously did not attract them. The new grade of state
enrolled nurses for nursing assistants did not solve the problem, and once the
initial 'bulge' of untrained service nurses was placed on the roll, their numbers
slowly declined.[2] Neither the work nor the title was attractive, and the pay was
even lower than for registered nurses. The Ministry considered various ways
of reducing the nursing shortage. As well as male nurses, overseas students
and part-time nurses were possible fields for recruitment. Male nurses, desperately sought by the understaffed mental hospitals, increased in numbers
slowly, in spite of incentives for male nurses leaving the Forces. Hospitals were
permitted to recruit 'aliens' from abroad, but by 1951, only 4 per cent of the
annual intake of students came from this source, and there was a high drop
out rate.[3] The search for part-time workers (mainly married women) was
more successful in that the proportion of part-time hospital nurses in England
and Wales rose from 13 per cent to nearly 20 per cent of SRNs between 1949
and 1957. There was a similar rise in the proportion of enrolled nurses working
part-time, from 26 per cent to 36 per cent, but their numbers overall were
diminishing.[4] Whereas the first war altered social attitudes about the types
of work that women could do, and the second relaxed objections to married
women working, neither change was rapid. The social role of women
was changing, but a generation that saw domesticity shattered during the
war was not anxious to discard traditional views of women's domestic
responsibilities.

The College too was torn between traditional and new forms of nursing.
While nursing textbooks became increasingly technical in content, they still

defined the personal qualities of a nurse in nineteenth-century terms. The nurse should be accurate, punctual, tactful, patient, truthful and cheerful. She should also have good powers of observation, and a professional manner. The hospital staff were a 'well-disciplined army', and the nurse must defend the reputation of her hospital 'as loyally as she would the reputation of her own home'.[5] These virtues, usually associated with the Nightingale legacy, were emphasised in the College's celebration of Founders Day in 1950, with the official adoption of its coat of arms featuring a shield with the sun and stars to denote day and night service, the open book of learning, a Roman lamp symbolic of nursing and the motto *Tradimus Lampada* – we hand on the torch. Although it aimed to defend nurses' interests in the workplace, the College's determination to assert nurses' professional status sometimes led it into defending conditions unacceptable to the trade unions, including low pay for student nurses and long shifts without overtime pay. This reinforced a conventional public image of the nurse as heroic in war, self-sacrificing in peace. With membership restricted to state registered nurses, the College could not claim to speak for a majority in the profession, and its membership began to fall, from a peak of 46,008 in 1948, to a trough of 39,991 in 1953. The trade unions were offering a more attractive agenda for change in the hospitals.

The College did not find traditional virtues particularly effective in its negotiations with government, and there was an undercurrent of official hostility towards it in the Conservative administrations of the 1950s. Some Conservative politicians believed that the nation could ill afford the expense of the NHS, and the College did not conform with their plans for running hospitals economically. If more nurses were needed, then they should be at the cheaper and less trained levels of the nursing hierarchy. The College, demanding longer training, higher educational qualifications for nurses and equal pay, was a potential threat. Nor was the Ministry of Labour as amenable as in Ernest Bevin's time. It began to chafe against funding places on College training courses for industrial nurses, and argued that a government department should not subsidise industry. It questioned the course's value:

> the case, on strict merit, for continuing to keep [the course] going seems, at best, doubtful but . . . dropping our support at the present time when occupational health is receiving so much attention would lead to attacks which might, in practice, be difficult to answer convincingly.[6]

The subsidy therefore survived for political reasons.

Industrial relations

The College also had to fight to defend its position as a negotiator against a number of government departments, particularly the Ministry of Labour.

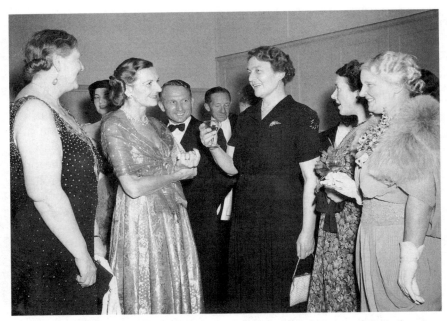

5.1 Annual general meeting, London (left to right): L. Duff Grant, president; Countess Mountbatten; D. Bridges; F. Goodall, general secretary; A. Woodman, chair of council, June 1950.

Wartime industrial regulations had banned strikes and lockouts, and compelled trade unions and employers to seek compulsory arbitration to resolve disputes. These regulations, which were renewed every year, also applied to professional bodies. Although the government was in favour of strict control over industrial relations, the wartime regulations imposed penal sanctions that were politically unacceptable in peace, and Churchill's government decided to relax them. In August 1951, a new Industrial Disputes Order ended the ban on strikes and lockouts, and enabled both employers and unions to demand compulsory arbitration through a new Industrial Disputes Council. But under the new regulations, only unions registered under the Trade Union Act of 1913 could request arbitration. The BMA, the Royal College of Nursing and many other professional associations were excluded, not being registered as unions. The College immediately called an informal meeting of all professional organisations on the Whitley Councils in the NHS, and wrote to the Ministers of Health and Labour requesting that the new regulations apply to professional bodies also.[7]

The Minister of Labour, Sir Walter Monckton, was conciliatory, and admitted that the exclusion of professional organisations was an oversight. He promised to amend the Industrial Disputes Order, but a year later, nothing had been done. The main obstacle was the Ministry of Health, which, facing a large pay claim from consultants, was unwilling to strengthen the position of NHS employees. An unforeseen consequence was that the trade unions, which now included NALGO, mounted a campaign to recruit nurses, arguing that only registered unions could represent them effectively.[8] Frances Goodall, supported by the Royal College of Midwives and the Association of Hospital Matrons, met officials from the Ministry of Health in November 1951, but received no encouragement, and after this meeting the Minister of Health refused all requests for an interview on the subject. Goodall continued to lobby the less hostile Ministry of Labour, with the aid of her formidable ally from the 1930s, the Conservative MP, Irene Ward. Miss Ward wrote profusely and bluntly to Monckton, arguing that it was intolerable that trade unions should have rights that were denied to professionals. The Minister replied rather feebly that the Ministry of Health had hamstrung him, but Irene Ward was not placated:

> your letter confirms my suspicions that other Government departments are prepared to ride rough-shod over the Royal College of Nursing, and . . . if we do not get your undertaking implemented within a short space of time, I shall be on the public warpath.[9]

The subject was indeed raised in parliament, without result. A bombardment of letters from these two strong-minded women provoked a series of exasperated memoranda from the Ministry's officials, who admitted privately that they were on weak ground: 'Minister – Irene Ward & Miss Goodall are having another go at you' and, in March 1954, 'I thought we had tired them out, but we shall clearly have to continue our delaying action'. At this point the dispute was still raging, and the officials' tactic was to defuse their tenacious critic in the Commons, whose lobbying was by now extensive:

> Correspondence with Miss Ward about the amendment of the Industrial Disputes Order has been a running sore for longer than I care to remember. If the Home Secretary feels under an obligation to deal specifically with the last paragraph of Miss Ward's letter of the 16th July, I can only suggest that you serve up some rehash of the blandishments we have long tried on her.[10]

The dispute fizzled out because the government allowed the Industrial Disputes Order to lapse in 1958. It had existed uneasily alongside the older Industrial Court, which still acted as arbitrator if both employer and employees requested it, and as will be seen, the College had recourse to this from time to time. The College worked through the Whitley Council in pay negotiations, and the system was not put to any serious test in the 1950s. Rather, the College concentrated on questions of professional status,

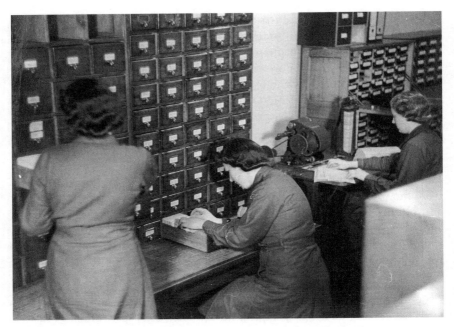

5.2 Membership records staff, College headquarters, London, March 1952.

and on rethinking the role of the nurse at a time of rapid technological change. Nevertheless, the situation revealed weaknesses in the College's legal position in industrial relations that gave the trade unions a decided advantage.

The Nuffield report: defining the role of nurses

The hospitals, and nurses' duties within them, were changing, and this required readjustment by the Ministry of Health and the College. The Ministry's aim was to move the increasing patient population through the hospitals rapidly, and major advances in surgery and pharmaceuticals made this possible. The time-consuming nursing techniques of former days, emphasising the hygiene and comfort of the patient, were now accompanied by complex post-surgery management and drug regimens. In early 1953 the Nuffield Provincial Hospitals Trust published *The Work of Nurses in Hospital Wards*, based on research begun in 1948.[11] The Trust, encouraged by the Ministry and the College, carried out this research as part of its mission to make the National Health Service more effective. It tried to answer a question posed in the Wood report: 'what is the proper task of the nurse?' Wood could not answer this question satisfactorily in the absence of any quantitative analysis of nurses' duties.

Without hard evidence, it was impossible to determine what kind of nurses were required, and to what level they should be trained. The chairman was H. A. Goddard, director of a management consultancy firm, who also chaired the management side of the Nurses and Midwives Whitley Council.

The research subjected nurses to the kind of time and motion study usually associated with industrial workers. Teams of researchers, none of whom was a nurse, surveyed twelve general hospitals responsible for nurse training, including nine former voluntary hospitals and three municipal hospitals. They studied twenty-six wards where two observers recorded for a week all activity over twenty-four hours, and interviewed all grades of staff. In order to quantify their results, they divided nursing into two types, basic and technical. The former involved all nursing care devoted to the well-being of patients, whatever their illness, and the latter all the specialised nursing tasks for specific diseases. Ward activity was divided into nursing time and non-nursing tasks, and the survey concluded that 43 per cent of ward activity was spent in basic nursing, 17 per cent in technical nursing, and the remaining 40 per cent in other tasks such as administration and domestic work. This meant that of the time spent on actual nursing, two thirds was devoted to basic nursing, and only a third to technical nursing, though the latter had a higher input from the more experienced nurses. Domestic duties turned out to be less onerous than many expected. In the most extreme case, a first-year student might spend an hour a day on dusting and cleaning, but the average was about thirty-five minutes, and less for senior students.[12] Rather, the main problem was that routine and avoidable tasks took up too much time, mainly because of the antiquated state of many hospitals and lack of equipment in the wards. Older hospitals were often poorly designed for minimising effort, even in such straightforward matters as the placing of wash-basins. Nurses wasted time in moving scarce items from ward to ward, or undertaking jobs that could be done by labour-saving devices. The report's attention to detail was striking: 'Three of the wards (one surgical, one medical, and one geriatric) had no other sterilising apparatus than a fish-kettle on a gas ring'.[13] Students sometimes had to sterilise bedpans, a task that in better-equipped hospitals was done mechanically. These problems arose from the low level of financial allocation to the hospitals, which remained cash-starved until the 1960s.[14] The report also concluded that the most experienced nurses did much of the administration, and they delegated routine care of patients to the less skilled because 'the accepted function of the trained nurse is not to nurse the patient herself, but to see that he is nursed'.

To the key question 'what is the proper task of the nurse?' Goddard replied that bedside nursing was the proper task of the state registered nurse.[15] By this he meant the direct care given to all patients, whether 'basic nursing' or 'technical nursing'. The report favoured a team approach, with a trained nurse in charge of a small group of assistants and students, and responsible for the whole care of a manageable number of patients. Under present conditions, each nurse performed specific tasks for all patients, such as doing a ward round taking temperatures, rather than becoming involved in the total care of each patient, and ward sisters delegated most of the routine work to others, retaining administration and the more technical tasks for themselves. To break down this specialisation, the Nuffield report recommended that ward sisters have clerical assistants for repetitive paperwork. By concentrating a small number of nurses on a small group of patients the team would perform all the duties for that group. This came close to a 'holistic' concept of hospital nursing, though the word was not in vogue at that time. To meet the obvious objection that these measures required more trained nurses at a time when recruitment was stagnant, the report contended that efficient use of existing labour would minimise this problem.

The report had a mixed reception, and many of the issues it raised are still being debated. Although all agreed that the report was the first piece of serious research into nursing, its recommendations were contentious. *The Hospital* thought its conclusions were the least satisfactory part, and that it was unrealistic to propose that all bedside care should be in the hands of state registered nurses, particularly when, according to the evidence, much of this care did not demand their special skills.[16] However, one of the problems was the declining numbers of enrolled nurses. In many wards the sister had no trained assistant, and had to delegate responsibility to students or untrained staff. When the report was debated in the House of Lords, Lord Woolton, for the government, stated that while the number of full-time trained nurses in England and Wales had increased from 40,000 to 47,600 in the last four years, and that student nurses had increased from 42,000 to 50,000, the number of enrolled nurses had dropped from 12,000 to 11,500, and untrained staff had risen from 16,000 to 25,000. He added that it was inevitable that there should be considerable wastage in nursing, but if the wastage were caused by marriage it could not be regretted: 'Marriage would continue, probably to the great advantage of the nation'.[17] Lord Moran, the eminent medical peer who chaired the NHS committee on consultants' pay, argued that it was essential to make the best use of nursing skills, and urged hospitals to implement nursing by group assignment, as recommended in the report. He also recommended that hospitals procure the simple items that would lighten nurses' tasks.

The *Nursing Times* ran a series of articles on the Nuffield report, and in May 1953 the College organised a three-day study conference for sisters, tutors and matrons to discuss it, led by Goddard himself.[18] Sir Ernest Rock Carling, governing trustee of the Nuffield Provincial Hospitals Trust, opened the conference. He hoped the report would mark the beginning of 'a renaissance of nursing thought', and argued that 'a profession that does not include research as part of its function is not complete, because it is only by research that the body of scientific knowledge peculiar to each profession can be built up'.[19] At Goddard's suggestion, the College appointed a group to respond to the report, led by Gertrude Williams, a distinguished social economist at Bedford College. Mrs Williams noted that the College also hoped the research would be the first of a series of such investigations into nursing. In the future, nursing skills must be maximised because the nursing shortage was likely to be permanent. She did not accept the College's usual argument that if nurses' pay was high enough, the shortage would end:

> Nursing is no longer the only profession that satisfies the kind of people who want to work in the field of human relations . . . there is sometimes a temptation to think that if only nurses' conditions were made sufficiently attractive, the problem of recruitment would be solved . . . you cannot create a pool of workers who do not exist.[20]

At the end of 1953 the College published its comments on the Nuffield report. Not surprisingly, the College agreed with Goddard that modernising the wards was a high priority, and also that team nursing was the way forward. But it did not accept that basic nursing and technical nursing were distinct tasks. Rather, a nursing procedure that would be basic and straightforward at one stage of illness might require a high level of skill at another, such as moving a patient who had recently undergone major surgery. The College also disputed the report's use of the term 'administration', preferring to describe this as essential ward management.[21] The ward sister's role incorporated all aspects of the patient's well being, and thus management *was* the proper task of the trained nurse. The College even cited Florence Nightingale's work in training an elite cadre of nurses to supervise reform in the hospitals. This administration was part of the proper function of the nurse. Goddard's division between nursing and administrative duties is still contentious, but he was advocating the employment of fairly junior clerical staff to relieve nurses of routine ward administration, not that the sister's or the matron's authority be supplanted by administrators.

The Nuffield report was particularly revealing over the lot of the student nurse. The newspapers, always happy to champion this group, responded with headlines such as 'Student nurses in hospitals, negligible training alleged'.[22] One of the fundamental problems of nurse education was relating instruction in nursing theory to practical training in the wards. The traditional assumption that student nurses could acquire good practical experience simply by working in a ward was no longer sufficient. The Nuffield teams observed that the time spent on formal instruction in the wards ranged from eleven hours to seven minutes weekly. Ward sisters were too busy to make time for teaching, and instruction of student nurses was secondary to care of patients. Due to staff shortages, student nurses were left in charge 22 per cent of the time during the day and frequently in charge during the night, sometimes alone. Ward sisters determined the allocation of students' time, and no sister tutor entered any of the wards studied, even though all the hospitals in the study were training schools. The report concluded that student status was an empty name, and if it existed at all, it was 'as an attitude of mind on the part of student nurses themselves'.[23]

In Scotland the Standing Nursing and Midwifery Advisory Committee also responded to the Nuffield report, with particular emphasis on student nurses.[24] Its response demonstrates that within the College there was a variety of opinion over the level of education desirable for a nurse. Margaret Lamb, education officer of the Scottish Board of the College, took a major part in the discussion. Like several of the educationalists in the College, she believed that a cadre of nurses with higher education was necessary for the development of the profession, though at that stage there was no suggestion that nurse training was itself a university discipline. The SNAC accepted, as did the College, that the future development of nursing and nurse training lay in the team method of nursing. In response to the criticism that little direct teaching was done by ward sisters, the SNAC proposed the introduction of a new group of clinical instructors. These would link the ward sister to the nurse tutor and would train student nurses in the wards, under the general direction of the ward sister. Like so many proposals for reform, this was hindered by the hospitals' manpower needs, and clinical instructors were introduced slowly, in the more prestigious hospitals.

The SNAC in Scotland also drew up an experimental scheme to train students for the general register in two years by withdrawing them from ordinary ward duties. They also proposed a revised course of training extending over three years but including wider experience than under the existing GNC syllabus. As previously noted, the College in Scotland enjoyed a much closer relationship with the Scottish Department of Health than the College in London had with the Ministry of Health. Their suggestions were followed up in 'the Glasgow experiment' at the Royal Infirmary, funded by Nuffield. Between 1956 and 1963, three groups of students undertook a more comprehensive syllabus over two years. They were not part of the ward staff, and, as the Nuffield report had advised, their training needs determined their ward activities. They took their examinations at the end of two years, but had to spend a year in practical nursing before registering.[25] The Glasgow experiment provided much-needed information about the effects of separating nurse teaching from routine ward duties. Compared with a control group of students who spent more time in the wards, the Glasgow group were somewhat tentative and less skilled in nursing practice when they began their ward duties, but significantly, the drop out rate was minimal. But this was a small-scale experiment, and Nuffield was covering the cost of taking the students out of the wards. Extending such a programme nationally would be very expensive.

Twelve months after the publication of the Nuffield report *The Times* drew attention to the lack of progress on its recommendations despite a series of conferences and much discussion.[26] Frances Goodall was quick to respond that 'there has been nothing passive about the way the nursing profession has received the report'.[27] The College had referred the report to its 174 branches, held two study conferences, appointed a working party and submitted comments to the Ministry of Health. Rosemary White argues that the College misunderstood the Nuffield report, and was out of sympathy with it because team nursing would have ended the 'officer' role of the ward sister. Goddard thought of teams as small groups in which all had multiple nursing tasks, and it would not be necessary to have a sister in each ward at all times to direct the teams. The College certainly did not welcome the suggestion that SRNs spend more time on basic nursing, for although technical nursing occupied less ward time than basic nursing, it was a growing area, for which the ward sister was responsible. The College's response is understandable in the context of the 1950s. The College claimed to be 'realistic' in its approach, though White does not accept this as a virtue.[28] Goddard was convinced that reform of nursing routines would permit a shift to team nursing without requiring more trained staff, and wished to apply principles of industrial management to nursing. Undoubtedly, modernised wards, up-to-date equipment and extra clerical staff would have streamlined the nurse's duties. Yet all of these required expenditure that was not forthcoming. In competition with medical demands for new operating suites, radiography, pathological laboratories and other costly equipment, nurses' needs tended to take second place.

The Nuffield report coincided with the first major government survey into the costs of the NHS, the Guillebaud report, which appeared in 1956. In spite of the Treasury's hope that this report would offer ways of containing the rising cost of the NHS to the Exchequer, Guillebaud revealed that the NHS, far from being recklessly extravagant, was absorbing less of the national output than in the previous decade.[29] The Treasury, however, was determined to exercise tight control over NHS expenditure, and was very sceptical of the argument that investment in new hospitals would reduce running costs. As Gladys Carter, now research fellow in nursing at the University of Edinburgh, noted, it was unreasonable to expect the regional hospital authorities to deal fairly with student nurses unless there was a replacement for their cheap labour. Student nurses, she contended, should be treated like medical students, and responsibility for them should be handed over to the Department of Education.[30] The fundamental difference between Goddard and the College was that he assumed that basic nursing would take far less time once hospitals and nursing routines were modernised – a classic managerial strategy. The College, accustomed to a world of hospital economies, did not believe that any reduction in tasks defined as domestic would proceed fast enough to allow trained nurses to share the basic nursing tasks, even if more clerical assistance were available. If student labour were withdrawn, more trained nurses must be recruited, and the College did not see how this could be achieved without meeting long-standing demands for better pay and status for nurses.

The College gave its own vision of the way forward in 1956, when it published a substantial policy document entitled *Observations and Objectives*.[31] This identified the social changes affecting the profession, including the expanding demands of the NHS, competition from other professions in a time of full employment, and the shrinking pay gap between skilled and unskilled workers. It was essential to cast the recruitment net wider to include part-time nurses and older workers. *Observations and Objectives* accepted the Nuffield criticisms of the poor state of hospital wards, and referred approvingly to the principle of team nursing, though its notion of a team was rather different from Goddard's, since it was based on wards rather than small-group nursing. The College was reluctant to waste the skills of highly trained nurses on routine tasks, and tended to see the whole ward as a team, which should include state enrolled nurses with their shorter training, nursing auxiliaries for very basic nursing duties, and ward orderlies for domestic tasks. Students should be part of the team only according to their training needs. The College believed that the assistant nurse, so useful during the war, was the key to the labour shortage.[32] Now it wanted to see SEN status improved, and more respect for their training and functions. These suggestions reflected some fundamental changes in the College's viewpoint, since it had previously been worried that part-time (usually married) staff who lived out would disrupt conventional shift patterns. In demanding more respect for the assistant nurse, the College was also changing its position in relation to a group to whom membership of the College was still denied because of their less rigorous training.

On education and training, the College recommended two distinct levels, one to staff the nursing service and one to prepare a cadre of leaders. At this time, hospital management committees pressed to have their hospitals approved as training schools for state registration, in order to secure the labour of student nurses. Yet at a time of shortage, small and badly organised training schools could not require more than basic educational standards of their recruits. Faced with an alarming nursing shortage in 1939, the Ministry of Health had forced the GNC for England and Wales to suspend its requirement of a minimal educational standard for trainee nurses, and after the war it refused to allow the GNC to reinstate it. The College deplored this, and wanted entrance tests and individual assessment to indicate whether a student should take SEN or SRN training. The College wanted to reduce the number of training schools for registered nurses because some were of poor quality, and to increase those for enrolled nurses. Trainees for the SEN roll, known as 'pupils' rather than 'students' to distinguish them from those training for the register, spent much of their time in practical training on the wards. But hospitals and many other organisations needed senior nurses in administrative and teaching posts. To secure future leaders for the profession, some members of the College, particularly in its educational section, became more interested in university degrees in nursing. They did not intend that all nurses should go to university, but believed that university degrees would attract an elite of educated women who might otherwise be drawn into other professions. This view reflected the changing position of middle-class women, who were attending university in larger numbers after the war. As previously noted, the age of entry for nurse training deterred girls who needed to work as soon as they left school, although the Ministry had lowered the entry age to seventeen and a half during the war. The College's growing interest in university education would certainly not end the class bias implicit in its views of nurse training.

Observations and Objectives also raised the long-standing problems of nurses' pay, pensions and working hours. A note of self-congratulation crept in over the College's achievements in representing nurses in this area, for 'not so long ago, a deputation of nurses to a government department was something of a concession granted only in response to urgent request'.[33] Now their advice was actively sought on nursing and related matters, and consultation between the College and government departments had become so frequent that many points were adjusted without formalities. This was overly optimistic for, while the Ministry of Health was prepared to listen to the College on uncontroversial matters, it was by no means welcoming when the College intervened over issues involving finance.

If the Ministry was un-cooperative in financial questions, it was no more conciliatory over the status of nursing in the NHS. The College estimated that no more than 300 nurses were involved in running the NHS through membership of the standing advisory committees of the Central Health Services Council, Regional Hospital Boards and other bodies. They had established no firm presence in management. Further, the matron's administrative position in the hospital service was insecure. In hospitals where she was recognised as head of the training school and nursing service, she attended meetings of the hospital management committee. Yet in many hospitals, especially mental hospitals, the matron did not have equal status with the heads of administration and medicine, and was excluded from management decisions. In public health there was a similar lack of consistency in accepting a nurse as head of the nursing service with full responsibility for her own staff and department.

The Nuffield report raised important questions about the allocation of duties in hospitals, noting that each hospital had its own procedures in dividing responsibilities between the staff. The College was disturbed that nurses were increasingly taking on work previously done by doctors. While younger nurses welcomed the challenge of new technical procedures, senior nurses often believed that these tasks were a distraction from their nursing duties. The usual assumption was that the two professions had separate tasks, though in fact the relationship between doctor and nurse in the twentieth century involved a constant transfer of duties. Many tasks, such as monitoring blood pressure, were originally done only by doctors, but by the 1950s were routinely performed by trained nurses, and the boundaries of responsibility were (and are) constantly in flux. The College was by no means averse to giving nurses greater responsibility in medical procedures, for these were proof of the professional status of nursing. But the College had to take account of legal issues. Nurses could be sued for any mishap that occurred if they performed tasks outside their accepted sphere, and a nurse who exceeded her responsibilities also risked disciplinary action by the GNC. Nursing ethics stressed obedience to the medical staff – although nursing textbooks often suggested tactful strategies for deflecting misguided requests – but the College paid insurance for the legal defence of its members, and clarity was needed for financial reasons. In 1953 the College produced a memorandum 'on the legal position of the nurse who undertakes procedures outside her professional scope'.[34] This set out the problem facing nurses who, due to shortages of medical staff, were asked to carry out procedures not covered by their training, particularly intravenous injections. The College decided that the most practical guide to the registered nurse's duties was the syllabus of the General Nursing Council. If a nurse went beyond this, the doctor or the hospital authorities should take legal responsibility. The College considered that the only professional negligence for which a nurse should be liable was incompetence in standard nursing tasks. It was concerned that between filling in domestic gaps at one end of the scale and taking on quasi-medical techniques at the other, the nursing role was being eroded to the detriment of the patient.

In February 1954 the College called a conference with representatives of the BMA, the Medical Defence Union, the Society of Medical Officers of Health and the Institute of Hospital Administrators, to see if any progress could be made towards establishing the legal position of the nurse.[35] It was clear from the discussion that opinions differed on the boundaries of a nurse's duties. Robert Forbes, secretary of the Medical Defence Union, said that there must be teamwork between doctor and nurse and it was difficult to draw a demarcation line. While there were certain duties that the union recommended should be performed by doctors, they were aware that outside the hospital, nurses working in clinics were frequently instructed to immunise, to read the results of certain tests, to give anaesthetics and to perform minor operations. Frances Goodall reported the College's view that the nursing profession needed more than reassuring words – they needed to know where their ulti-mate responsibility lay. Another nurse participant argued that there were two views of nursing: the first assumed that the nurse would fill in the gaps for the doctor, and the second that all her energy should be devoted to her nursing work. The drawing of blood, she argued, did not require great skill, and people other than nurses could be trained to do it, but running a ward and ensuring the well-being of twenty to forty patients was a greater challenge, though not usually credited as such.

The College circulated its views on the legal position of the nurse to all hospital authorities, which greatly annoyed the Ministry of Health. Another flurry of irritable correspondence followed. The Ministry considered that the College had no right to contact hospital authorities without consultation, and that only the Ministry could instruct the hospitals in such matters. It also doubted whether the College accurately reflected the views of the medical profession. Invoking the 'thin-end-of-the-wedge' principle, one official argued that if all the professional organisations, from the Royal College of Physicians to the almoners, were to follow the College's example, chaos would ensue. The chief nursing officer, Elizabeth Cockayne, was instructed to speak unofficially to Frances Goodall along these lines.[36] The Ministry privately conceded that the College had a case, and that nurses were increasingly being called upon in technical procedures that were properly the doctor's province. The Department of Health for Scotland was anxious about the planned tubercu-losis campaign in Glasgow, which would require nurses to give BCG injections and perform Mantoux tests. They feared litigation if any accidents occurred.[37] The Ministry of Health replied that as long as employers had a clear idea of the nurse's responsibilities, there should be no problem.

> We agree that such employment is wrong in principle, but do not think it desir-able to lay down any hard and fast rules as to what a nurse can or can't do e.g. by reference to what the student nurse is taught, which is what the RCN suggest. The decision whether it is right for a nurse to undertake certain procedures must largely depend on the personal judgement of those under whose direction she works, and may vary with individual circumstances.[38]

The College refined its position a little, and no longer insisted that only the GNC syllabus should define the nurse's role. In any case, the syllabus did not change fast enough to accommodate new medical procedures. In 1958 the College issued a press release:

> the College acknowledges that the scope of duties to be undertaken by the trained nurse is not necessarily circumscribed by the syllabus of the General Nursing Council, but where it appears necessary for her to undertake duties carrying additional responsibility, the College is concerned to ensure that special arrangements are agreed and safeguards established.[39]

If medical staff trained nurses in new techniques, and supervised them, then a new responsibility could be accepted. A discussion between the College and the BMA led to a joint statement in 1961 on the duties and position of the nurse. They agreed that certain duties were outside the province of the nurse and should be undertaken only in an emergency. They recommended setting up local committees of medical and nursing staff to agree the boundaries between the two professions. If both sides accepted new duties for the nurse, these must be approved by her employer, who was legally responsible for her actions.[40] Rapport with the BMA led to regular liaison meetings. From time to time it was necessary to reach ad hoc decisions, as in 1961, when the Medical Defence Union sought an urgent meeting to discuss responsibility for marking limbs or digits with an indelible pen before amputation. The union had recently to deal with twelve claims from patients who awoke from the anaesthetic to find that the wrong part of their body had been removed. The College firmly maintained that the marking of limbs should be a doctor's responsibility, and agreed with the Medical Defence Union that doctors should mark the limb in the presence of a senior nurse, who would make note of it, and check it before the operation.[41] Similar co-operation was needed to ensure that no instruments or swabs were left inside the patient after an operation. To reinforce this message, the College co-operated with the Medical Defence Union in making a training film in 1964 entitled *Make No Mistake*. But divisions of labour were almost impossible to enforce in the hectic routine of the NHS wards, and current studies show that nurses and doctors make their own tacit arrangements in each hospital.[42]

By 1957 the College was disappointed that the Nuffield report had not produced much improvement in the hospital wards, and organised a three-day conference on 'Work study and the hospital service'. Work studies were much in vogue, and many in the profession saw them as a solution to everyday problems. In Monica Baly's words, the Nuffield report 'introduced nurses to the mysteries of flow and string charts' and encouraged research into nursing practices.[43] By providing evidence to assess the best use of staff and equipment, these studies would help to reduce the drudgery of overworked nursing staff. The conference aimed to demonstrate to hospital administrators how work study had increased efficiency in industry, and speakers included experts from ICI and other firms. Over 250 representatives came from numerous organisations, including government departments in England and Scotland, the Northern Ireland hospitals authorities, hospital administrators, doctors, matrons and nurses in administrative posts. Iain Macleod, the Minister of Labour, opened the conference.[44] Although the College sometimes had difficult relations with departments of state, it was not a body that government could ignore. Its conferences attracted large and prestigious audiences, and were widely reported in the press.

The Nuffield report stimulated the College's interest in research. This was not new, for since the 1920s the College had collected data, such as the results of questionnaires on unemployment among nurses in the 1930s. A small amount of statistical work was carried out for the Athlone and Wood reports. The Sister Tutor Section of the College participated in the job analysis undertaken by the Nuffield Trust, and in 1952 the council appointed a small group to consider how nursing research should be undertaken. After the Nuffield report, several experiments tried to find alternative means of carrying out non-nursing duties. The Standing Nursing Advisory Committee also set up a research project to study the group assignment of patients to teams of nursing staff. Other bodies took an interest in nursing research. In 1953 the University of Edinburgh accepted a grant from the Boots Pure Drug Co. to establish the first nursing research fellowship in a British university. The Dan Mason Medical Research Trust also funded research into nursing, and in 1956 Gertrude Ramsden, its research organiser, produced its first research report, on wastage among trained nurses, followed in 1960 by a second on the work of staff nurses. *Observations and Objectives* also made the case for research, and the College considered establishing an authoritative research body to study the problems of the nursing profession.[45] Lack of funds prevented this, but in 1958 the College appointed a research officer, Marjorie Simpson. A College tutor in industrial nursing, she took three years out to study for a degree in sociology, and on return moved into research. She began a long College-funded project to investigate the salary structure of nurses and midwives in the NHS.[46] This was conducted with advice from a working party chaired by Dr Marian Bowley, a well-known economist at University College, London. The partnership indicated the College's growing interest in social science techniques.

Although the College could not afford to undertake major research projects at this stage, individual members conducted useful small-scale research on their own initiative, seeking piecemeal funding where they could find it. At the College's AGM in July 1959, Gertrude Ramsden discussed with Marjorie Simpson the problems facing nurses who wanted to do research. The outcome of their conversation was the informal Research Discussion Group of College members interested in or actively engaged in research, and the forerunner of the RCN Research Society.[47] Only a small minority of nurses had university degrees – possibly no more than 334 in England and Wales – and none had doctorates.[48] The group decided to hold meetings for the exchange of ideas and research techniques, and for stimulating interest in research among nurses. The first meeting took place at Gertrude Ramsden's home in London and was attended by ten people. A notice then appeared in the *Nursing Times* inviting other nurses engaged in research projects to contact Simpson.[49] The group met in members' homes, but the College paid for secretarial help,

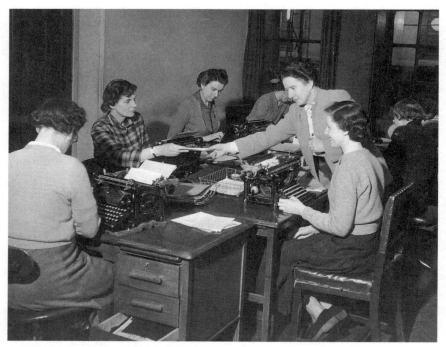

5.3 Typing pool, College headquarters, London, March 1952.

stationery and postage. Outcomes from this group included publications by
Doreen Norton on care for the elderly, and Margaret Williams on surgical
dressing techniques in industry.[50]

The Education Department and nurse training

The College had failed to persuade the Ministry of Health of the need for
post-registration training to meet the growing demand for specialised nursing
skills, and so it began an ambitious programme to expand its own courses.
To many members of the public in the early 1950s the College was probably
most visible in its well-advertised fundraising campaigns. Its methods were
the traditional ones employed by the College's founders and the old voluntary
hospitals, to attract donations with the support of royal and aristocratic
patrons.

Queen Mary was patron of the College until her death in 1953. In 1944 her
granddaughter Princess Elizabeth became the first president of the Student
Nurses' Association, and female members of the royal family, including Queen
Elizabeth and the Duchess of Kent, visited Henrietta Place from time to time

and attended College functions. In 1949 the College set up an Educational Appeal Fund to raise £500,000 for the College's training courses. It justified the need for public contributions in the following terms: 'the State can make but a partial contribution to the nurse's education and training . . . she must look elsewhere for that wider training and guidance'.[51] The College astutely secured as president of the appeal the dashing figure of Edwina, Countess Mountbatten. Lady Mountbatten had much experience of nurses from her extensive war work with the Red Cross. After the surrender of Japan, she followed her husband into dangerous territory in Burma with medical teams to locate and assist internees and prisoners-of-war. Her commitment to the College was sincere and energetic. She launched the appeal in May 1950, gave a personal donation of £500, and continued to support College fundraising after this appeal ended until her death in 1960.[52] Each local branch had a target to meet, and in the years that followed, local newspapers ran regular accounts of fêtes, bazaars, garden parties, whist drives, fashion shows, balls, football matches, dinners and exhibitions in aid of the appeal. Lady Mountbatten opened many of these, as did other aristocratic supporters, including the Duchess of Gloucester. Local organisers realised that other types of celebrity would attract public attention, and film stars began to appear at these functions, from established favourites like Douglas Fairbanks, to the rising Rank starlet Diana Dors.[53]

The most successful national event was the Royal Film Premiere, an early occasion of its kind, when Princess Elizabeth and Prince Philip cut short their holiday in Balmoral to attend a screening of *The Lady with the Lamp* in September 1951. Herbert Wilcox's film starred his wife Anna Neagle, who specialised in playing British heroines. She had portrayed Queen Victoria and Edith Cavell, and Florence Nightingale was an obvious addition to her repertoire. The interests of the College and the film's distributors happily coincided. Proceeds from the premiere in Leicester Square were devoted to the Educational Fund, and huge crowds gathered to see the arrival of the Princess in superb evening dress, Neagle and her co-star Michael Wilding, and a glittering audience who had paid handsomely for their seats.[54] The film then had simultaneous premieres in Cardiff, Belfast, Edinburgh and several large cities abroad, with the takings also going to the appeal. Massive publicity encouraged many local cinema managers to hold their own more modest premieres for the same cause. The two stars took their roles very seriously, and visited several infirmaries as well as attending local premieres. The combination of royalty and the film's regal actress was irresistible, especially to the women's magazines, and only a few heretical publications dared suggest that the film was 'long, slow, without movement . . . and completely lacking in romance'.[55]

As a result of all these activities, the appeal raised £358,000, and was ceremonially wound up in January 1954. This was less than the College had hoped, but was an impressive sum. The appeal also cemented relations between the College and the royal family. When Queen Mary died, the recently crowned Queen Elizabeth II agreed to become patron of the College, while her sister Princess Margaret replaced her as president of the Student Nurses' Association. Princess Margaret, following her grandmother's example, liked to visit the College for afternoon tea, but these occasions became less formal and much smokier.

The College's Education Department, the main beneficiary of these appeals, was responsible for post-qualification training courses, and was recognised by the Ministry of Education as a major establishment for further education. At this time there was a clear demarcation between the professional and the educational sides of the College's work, and Mary Carpenter, the director of education, reported directly to council and not to the general secretary. Elaine Wilkie, who joined the Education Department in 1947 as a health visitor tutor, remembered that the education staff tried to maintain a distance from the College's professional work, because their courses were not for members of the College only, but for all nurses. Every morning the College staff met for 'letters', when the general secretary distributed the post to the various officers for their attention. On these occasions the education staff always said that they had nothing to report.[56] By 1950 the staff consisted of six full-time tutors. Eleven full-time and part-time courses were offered, together with refresher and postal courses. Each course had a College lecturer and an external examiner and there was a large panel of visiting lecturers from universities and the business world. Full-time courses included the training of health visitors, industrial nurses, ward sisters and nursing administrators, but the majority were training courses for sister tutors, and for tutors in other branches of nursing. The department also had an international reputation, with students from overseas taking its courses. After the war the number of overseas students, particularly from the Dominions, increased steadily. They were usually senior nurses selected by their governments to take post-qualification courses at the College. The Education Department ran special courses requested by the Colonial Office for overseas nurses, such as a one-year course for fifteen West Indian ward sisters in 1950, and another in 1952 for twelve ward sisters from the West Indies, Malaya, Singapore and West Africa. Each year study trips were organised in Britain for foreign nurses (in 1951, eighty Norwegian nurses visited London), and British nurses were sent abroad on study tours.

Throughout Mary Carpenter's period as director of the Education Department, the student group maintained its international character, and the department worked in co-operation with the Ministry of Overseas Development, the British Council, and other national and international organisations. Some of the nursing staff of the World Health Organization were former students, and the WHO invited Carpenter to be a short-term consultant in several countries. In 1959–60 she was awarded a fellowship from the Rockefeller Foundation and went on a study tour in the United States and Canada. The average number of students on full-time courses was 150 but each year the number increased. Carpenter believed it was important for senior nurses to understand the relationship of their work to others in the hospital structure, and started the ward sisters' course to equip staff nurses for their new roles in the NHS. The syllabus of each course was continually reviewed and updated. The Advisory Board, set up in 1944, monitored the department's work. The College set its own educational standards without interference from hospitals or government, although in 1949 it applied to the Ministry of Education for a grant towards its educational work. The Ministry inspected and approved the College's facilities and in future the College received an annual grant from this Ministry.[57] The College got off to a good start with the Ministry of Education, but the Ministries of Health and Labour viewed its courses less cordially. The latter's somewhat churlish attitude towards the training of industrial nurses has already been noted, and in the mid 1960s the Ministry of Health was not enthusiastic about the proliferation of College courses. The Ministry of Education was happy to support local education authorities who wished to offer courses leading to a diploma from the College, but the Ministry of Health was discouraging:

> the R.C.N. (Educ Side) is not at all forthcoming in bringing the Dept into discussion about the content of its many PG courses. I would like to feel that we kept at the centre of this further development from the outset.[58]

The Ministry of Health intended to interrogate hospitals about the usefulness of the College courses, and, following its usual principle that the hospitals were its own territory, warned the Ministry of Education not to contact hospitals directly, for 'this is better done by us'.[59]

The library continued to expand alongside the Education Department. At a time when many schools of nursing had few educational pretensions and no libraries, the College library met a real need. Postal loans were almost as numerous as books borrowed in person, and a system of group borrowing was instituted to allow training schools to borrow a small collection of books for an extended period. The appointment of Alice Thompson as librarian in 1949 began a period of steady expansion for the library. Her interest in the history of nursing led her to build up the collection as the 'library of nursing', the main national collection of nursing literature. She collected all English language nursing journals dating back to their origins in the late nineteenth century, a pamphlet collection encompassing a wide range of subjects related to health, women and nursing, and a large number of nursing textbooks. The library now holds the largest collection of nursing literature in Europe. Believing that a nursing library was an essential part of the educational resources of a school of nursing, Thompson produced a leaflet in 1952 stating the need for nursing libraries in hospitals. She advised on how to start and run a small library and recommended that schools of nursing include library funds when submitting a budget to the Area Nurse Training Committees. She realised that few nursing schools could afford the services of a qualified librarian and that the responsibility would fall to the sister tutors, and so she encouraged them to contact her for assistance. In 1963 she started courses in library techniques for nurse tutors. Aware of the expansion of nursing knowledge, she played a key role in supporting the small group in the 1950s who became pioneers of nursing research in the United Kingdom. Thompson's personal contribution to nursing research was the preparation and publication of a bibliography of nursing literature.[60]

The College's educational work was not confined to London, and local branches could set up their own courses. The decentralisation of the Education Department began with a new Education Centre in Birmingham. Birmingham was particularly active in supporting nurse education and welfare, assisted by the Birmingham and Three Counties Trust for Nurses, established in 1922 with financial support from the Cadbury family and local College members. The Trust had a nurses' club and educational centre in Hagley Road, Edgbaston, with residential facilities for retired nurses, who were often poorly provided for, but it was in constant financial difficulties.[61] In 1950, again with generous support from the Cadbury family, a second house was purchased in Hagley Road and gifted to the College. The Birmingham Education Centre opened in July 1953. Support from the NHS locally assisted in the cost of altering and equipping the centre and guaranteed a sufficient flow of nursing students for its courses. The first task of the centre was to organise refresher courses in public health, occupational health and nurse training. In the first ten years the number of students steadily increased from 250 to 800 per year and the centre built up a network of visiting lecturers from the University of Birmingham, the hospitals and local public health departments. Jean McFarlane, one of the public health tutors on the staff of the College in London, was appointed education officer at Birmingham from 1963 to 1968. She recalled that although she was answerable to the Director of Education in London, she could set up new courses in response to local demand, such as accident and emergency nursing, and care of the elderly.[62] The Birmingham Centre launched her career, for she became director of the Education Department of the College in 1968, and in 1974 was appointed the first professor of nursing in England, at the University of Manchester. She was, ultimately, one of a very small group of nurses who reached the House of Lords.

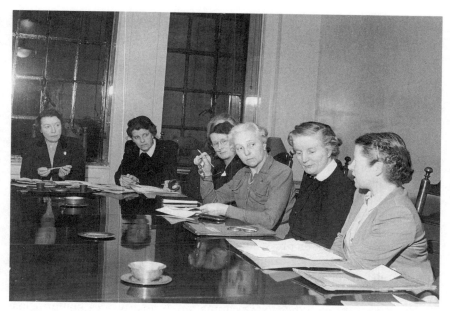

5.4 Meeting of heads of departments, headquarters, London (left to right): F. Goodall, general secretary; M. Carpenter, director, Education Department; B. Adams, financial secretary; Mrs Blair Fish, public relations officer; W. Christie, secretary, Sister Tutor Section; M. Knight, secretary, Public Health Section, March 1952.

Further education for nurses

For a decade, inquiries into nursing had stressed the need for a wider basic training. By the 1950s the traditional British nurse training system, developed in the Nightingale wards of the previous century, was no longer appropriate. The demands being placed on nurses were changing, as medical techniques for earlier diagnosis of disease led to more frequent hospitalisation. Surgery was becoming more specialised, and diseases previously regarded as incurable, such as tuberculosis, were responding to new forms of treatment. Patients recovered faster and spent less time in hospital, and the rapid turnover of patients affected the workload of nurses. More attention to the patient's environment and mental health brought curative and preventive medicine closer together, also changing the character of nursing. As more people became involved in a patient's care, both inside the hospital and afterwards, ward sisters had more responsibility in co-ordinating their work.

Nursing education struggled to keep pace with these changes, and by the 1950s the reputation of British nursing seemed to be losing ground internationally. In the United States and Canada, university and college courses in nursing were more common. In Britain the universities refused to recognise nursing as an appropriate subject for higher education, and many nurses did not welcome the advance of the theoretical content of training at the expense of the practical. The previous high reputation of British nursing came from its disciplinary apprenticeship system and its emphasis on service, and some feared this would be lost in an academic training. As the College's growing body of literature on the subject showed, a possible solution was to remove nurse training from the hospitals, with their insatiable labour demands, without abandoning the apprenticeship system altogether.

Many of those working in nurse training believed that the main cause of high wastage among students was their low standard of education. For twenty years after the Ministry of Health suspended the GNC's minimum standards in 1939, no educational requirements were demanded of recruits. Hospitals applied their own standards, and while the prestigious teaching hospitals could insist on a good school education, many smaller training hospitals, relying on student labour, pressed their matrons to accept candidates who had difficulty passing the state examination. This led to a decline in the educational levels of nursing students and created problems for the sister tutors, whose job was regarded in many hospitals as nothing more than pushing the student nurses through the GNC examination. In 1951 two leading principal sister tutors, Marion Gould of the Nightingale Training School, and Joan Bocock of the Royal Free Hospital, argued that the hospital training schools under the NHS were pushing standards down.

> Shortages will never be overcome by reducing the standard of candidates to the nursing profession, or by exploiting during training those who have come forward . . . [it is] only a matter of time before we regress to the standard of Sairey Gamp and Betsy Prig.[63]

Nurse training also required well-trained tutors. In an effort to raise the standard of tutors, the GNC from 1946 required that they be registered only after completing one of the prescribed tutors' courses at the Universities of London, Birmingham, Manchester, Hull or Leeds. But hospitals did not have to employ qualified tutors, and the number of nurses taking these courses remained very low. For many years the normal route into nurse teaching was to take the Diploma in Nursing offered by the University of London. This was a postal course and attracted the more academic women in nursing. Margaret Lamb recalled the pleasure she had in studying for the diploma. She had a hunger for learning that was difficult to satisfy at that time.

> They sent you the papers and they corrected them, like the Open University. I loved that. I enjoyed all this learning . . . I took extra subjects. You could do an extra subject like teaching and that was where I excelled . . . I enjoyed doing that course.[64]

Concerned about the lack of candidates for tutors' courses, the Ministry of Health considered shortening the courses to make them more attractive to hospital authorities, who had to release their staff for training. While the Ministry and the professional organisations were pondering the content and length of the courses, the University of London announced its intention to extend its diploma course from one year to two. The Ministry of Health then decided on a comprehensive study of the function, status and training of nurse tutors.[65] Dr Janet Aitken, a principal medical officer at the Ministry, chaired the investigation, and those involved were mainly matrons and principal tutors, with some representatives from medicine and higher education, including Mary Carpenter and Margaret Lamb from the College. Their report, published in 1954, argued that the nurse tutor should be an educator with broad knowledge and wide experience. It compromised on the length of nurse training, concluding that two years was too long to be out of the hospital, and recommended a course of five terms, or twenty months.[66] 'Schools of nursing', based on several hospitals, would ease the shortage of tutors and provide some career progression for them, for small training schools were uneconomic, and could not provide satisfactory training. Hospitals unable to obtain student nurses of a sufficient educational standard should give up their status as an independent training school and either become a part of a group training school or convert to a training school for enrolled nurses. A debate on a suitable title for the heads of nursing schools masked continuing anxiety about whether final authority over students in the wards lay with their training schools or the hospital matrons.[67]

The Sister Tutor Section offered its own ideas on the subject.[68] It believed that the shortage of teachers would continue as long as hospitals undervalued the role of the sister tutor and regarded student nurses as cheap labour. It was concerned about the quality of candidates for the tutor courses, alleging that some had no desire to teach and were selected by their hospitals because they had proved unsuitable in administration.[69] (Another common perception was that nurses who had injured themselves in lifting patients were shunted into teaching.) The section believed that experience as a sister on a teaching ward was essential for sister tutors. At the time, the GNC required only that candidates for sister tutor posts had at least three years post-registration experience, but it now increased this to four years, of which two should be as a ward sister. Although hospitals were reimbursed the salaries of nurses seconded to the tutor course, applicants were few, and some provincial courses had to be discontinued. The Education Department of the College extended its own one-year course for sister tutors to two years in 1952.[70] By 1959 the University of London was still the only university in England to offer a diploma course for sister tutors. Some nurses feared that becoming a sister tutor would take them away from the wards, while others, with little formal education themselves, were reluctant to train as teachers, and were not confident in their communication skills. As one critic argued, it was difficult to teach a young nurse 'the art of social gumption' that would enable her to become a leader.[71]

When the register for sister tutors opened in 1946, there was no training course for them at a Scottish university. Margaret Lamb approached the Faculty of Medicine at the University of Edinburgh proposing a course leading to a university certificate. The university agreed, and a one-year course was started in 1946. Supervision of the course was left almost entirely to the Scottish Board of the College, and students attended most of their lectures in College premises. When the University of London extended its tutors' course to two years in 1951, the organisers of the Scottish course had to reconsider the length of their own course, as the GNCs operated a reciprocal recognition of tutors' qualifications. Shortly afterwards, the first research fellowship in nursing, funded by Boots, was attached to the Department of Public Health and Social Medicine in Edinburgh, under the geneticist Professor Albert Francis Crew, a strong advocate of university education for nurses. Gladys Carter, the first research fellow, was asked to report on the Scottish nurse tutor course with a view to raising its standard and to consider the 'desirability and the possibility of instituting an academic degree in nursing'.[72] Carter, Lamb and Crew hoped that the revised tutors' course would be an academic base for advanced nursing education in the University of Edinburgh. Their cause received an unexpected boost when Lady Mountbatten announced, to a startled academic audience on the occasion of receiving an honorary degree from the University of Edinburgh in January 1954, that it was her fervent wish that the University of Edinburgh might be the first British university to award a degree in nursing. This, however, was not easily arranged.

While Carter was working on her study, Professor Crew negotiated with the university, the nursing organisations and the Department of Health for Scotland to extend the course to eighteen months, and to require university entrance qualifications of the students. Crew approached the Rockefeller Foundation about funding for the new course. The concept of a department of nursing within the Faculty of Medicine took shape and the Rockefeller Foundation agreed to provide funding for five years. The Scottish Board offered to pay the salary of one tutor in the department and to provide temporary classroom accommodation in their premises at Heriot Row. However, they had all misjudged the animosity of the Faculty of Medicine towards nursing as a university discipline. Crew was unable to persuade them to accept a nurse teaching unit in their faculty, or in any other, and it was only under pressure from the principal of the university, who did not wish to lose the Rockefeller grant, that the doctors were forced to accept a nursing studies unit in another faculty. The College advised that it should be located in the Arts

Faculty, because the students would be taught through the university's Department of Education.[73] The Nurse Teaching Unit, established in 1956, later grew into the Department of Nursing Studies. The Scottish experience revealed anxiety in the medical profession, the hospitals and among nurses themselves over academic education for nurses. While the College's educational work relied on a small group of nurses with higher education, there was no agreement about the future of nursing in the universities. From its earliest days the College had welcomed links with the universities for specialised post-qualification courses, but even the Scottish innovators believed that the role of universities in general nurse training would be confined to a nursing elite.

During this time, the College received many complaints about the educational standard of student nurses. Some were said to be unable to calculate drug dosages. Matrons were pressured to recruit unsuitable candidates, including women from overseas with poor English who were barely literate.[74] At a meeting with the GNC in 1954 the Minister of Health confirmed that his primary concern was to staff the hospitals, and that the standard of the nurses' training was secondary. He was influenced by hospital authorities, which argued forcefully that an educational entrance test would reduce the number of recruits. In November 1952 the GNCs announced that they wanted a minimum educational qualification of two O-levels for entry to nurse training, and that the standard of their new curriculum, to be introduced by January 1954, would take account of this. In response, the Luton and Hitchin Hospital Management Committee, who were facing the possibility of having to close wards because of the decline in nursing recruits, asserted their 'profound disagreement with the policy of the General Nursing Council and such other bodies as are concerned with the formulation of high policy in nursing affairs'.[75] They complained that the GNC must be oblivious to the practical needs of the hospital service and its patients if it considered that the time was right to reinstate an educational standard. The GNC was accused of trying to make nursing an academic profession and of forcing nurses to spend time in the classroom at the expense of the wards. On top of this, the GNC declared its intention to restore the minimum age of entry to nurse training from seventeen and a half to eighteen years. The outraged Hospital Management Committee believed that these policies would be disastrous for the provincial hospitals:

> [by] subordinat[ing] all other considerations to an overriding desire to establish the nurse in training solely as a student, in no sense an employee of the hospital, and undertaking only such nursing duties as were necessary to her training. The absurdity of such a course is clear enough to those concerned with the management of general hospitals. Nothing is to be gained by persisting in an illusion and a frank recognition of the real position of the nurse in training is long

overdue. For so long as 75 per cent of nursing work in the ward is undertaken by nurses in training, and for so long as the major part of their time is spent on giving service to the hospital, as distinct from receiving tuition, the real status of the nurse in training is something between that of an apprentice and one serving articles, and not that of student. Indeed, the old title of probationer nurse was far more accurate than that of student nurse.

Once again the Minister was persuaded by the hospital authorities, the GNC in England was over-ruled, and the profession had to wait another decade before a minimum educational standard was reinstated.

The acute shortage and low morale among nurse tutors continued, and in 1957 the GNC in England consulted representatives of the professional organisations over the regulations for the approval of hospitals as nurse training schools. They recommended a method that would eliminate the smaller schools and raise the standard of training for both registered and enrolled nurses. They proposed a two-tier system of nursing with SRNs forming the higher level and SENs the majority of the workforce. The new system would require reintroducing a minimum educational level for student nurses, who must possess at least two O-levels, or take a special GNC examination. Without this hurdle there was no reason why any recruit would choose enrolled nurse training, since status and career prospects were better for SRNs.[76] The Ministry of Health favoured reducing the number of student nurse training schools for SRNs and increasing pupil nurse training schools for SENs, but it was not until 1959 that the Minister finally agreed to the reintroduction of a minimum educational test, and this was to be delayed until July 1962. The hospitals again objected strongly, but this time, the combination of the GNC and the College persuaded the Ministry to give way.[77] Given the expansion of compulsory secondary education, a requirement of two O-levels did not seem excessive. New regulations for training schools, requiring a minimum of 300 beds before they could be recognised for SRN training, came into force in 1964.[78]

The Sister Tutor Section of the College continued its battles with the Ministry, and called on the services of leading personalities in the field, such as the principal sister tutors Annie Altschul from the Bethlem Royal and Maudsley Hospitals, and Muriel Hill from the London Hospital. *The Nurse Tutor, A New Assessment*, was published in 1961 showing how little had been achieved in the 1950s.[79] In the UK most training schools continued to be of the Nightingale model, centred on one hospital, with the matron the head of both the nursing service and the training school. In some schools the position of the tutor was equivocal and her advice was either not sought or ignored. This traditional concept of nurse education, combined with a lack of resources, low professional status and poor promotion prospects, meant that many tutors had no job satisfaction. Their desire to break away from the control of the matrons was evident in the recommendation that the principal tutor of a large school should be known as the director of nurse education. Those favouring reform of nurse education believed that British nurses were falling behind their international colleagues. A comprehensive curriculum had already been established in other countries while the British system continued to require nurses to take a series of training courses and certificates in order to qualify in specialised fields of nursing, resulting in many nurses spending years in post-qualification training. British Columbia even rescinded its reciprocal recognition of British nursing qualifications with the GNC because of the alleged inferior quality of nurse education in Britain. Gladys Carter drew attention to the hospital authorities' conflict of duty between their patients and their student nurses. She believed that the Department of Education would be in a stronger position to enforce standards of entry and education than the Ministry of Health, which had to prioritise the hospitals' demand for staff. At the same time, Brian Abel-Smith and Richard Titmuss questioned the economic grounds of making the National Health Service financially responsible for training nurses, especially as so many went abroad after completing their training.[80]

While the hospitals had great difficulty in coming to terms with nurse education, public health nurses had more success in forging links with the universities. Nurses were often attracted to public health work by the independence it offered, and by the challenges of a rapidly developing field. They were much in demand by the World Health Organization and other bodies attempting to rebuild international public health standards after the war. The College had several leading activists among its members and staff, including Olive Baggallay with her experience of international relief programmes, Irene Charley working closely with the Department of Social and Preventive Medicine at the University of Birmingham, Marjorie Simpson, occupational health tutor and then researcher at the College, Elaine Wilkie, health visitor tutor at the College, and Ada Woodman, chairman of the College council from 1949 to 1960 and a superintendent health visitor. Within public health these women were making links with new university departments of social and preventive medicine that were happy to embrace nursing, unlike the medical faculties. In these departments the first steps towards a full university education for nurses were made at Edinburgh and Manchester. Wilkie believed that public health nurses broke the mould of nurse education in Britain and recalled that when this group met they 'were striking sparks off each other'.[81]

Throughout the 1950s various experimental training schemes began, including several that combined nursing with health visiting. Known as integrated training schemes, they required students to spend five years qualifying, first as a general trained nurse and then as a health visitor. For example, training at the Nightingale School at St Thomas's Hospital could be combined with health visiting at the University of Southampton.[82] A more famous experimental training scheme started at the University of Manchester in October 1959. This was not just another attempt to integrate general nurse training with public health, but aimed to provide a university education in nursing. Under Professor Fraser Brockington at the Department of Social and Preventive Medicine, the course had a wide curriculum. Brockington believed that a proportion of nurses needed a university education in order to fill senior positions, and that clinical nursing practice called for a deeper study of the behavioural sciences, social studies and social medicine that only a university could provide. On completion, the students qualified as state registered nurses and were awarded the University of Manchester diploma in community nursing. Brockington argued that the course effectively demonstrated that 'the student can be taught in hospital with true student status and supplementary to the service needs'.[83] The public health nurses thus began a drive towards training outside the wards that began to gain wider currency within the College.

By the end of the 1950s, the College outlook was more research oriented, and more academic in its approach to nurse education, although the reformers made little headway in convincing the Ministry of Health that nurses needed more training away from the wards. Their determination to create a nursing leadership through higher education may have looked back to the College's elitist origins, but the College was also being pushed in this direction by an NHS structure that paid scant attention to nurses' needs, and sometimes relegated matrons to an inferior position in hospital management. Only a well-educated and assertive leadership could maintain nurses' interests against other competitors for resources in the NHS, and the history of struggle with government and hospital managements in the 1950s reveals how little attention nurses received. While nurses' time was cheap, it could be wasted on unnecessarily labour-intensive tasks, even if the solution lay in providing such inexpensive equipment as trolleys, bed curtains and moveable screens.

What's in a name? The birth of the RCN

Any reader consulting the College's publications will be struck by the various titles it has used since its foundation. These reflect significant changes in its relationship with other nursing organisations. Although essentially a story of internal politics, it shows how the College raised its status in the profession internationally. Relations with the National Council of Nurses of Great Britain and Northern Ireland were important here, because they affected the College's international profile and its name. Behind the changes of the 1960s was a long history.

The NCN was older than the College, and laid the first claim to international recognition. In 1899 Mrs Bedford Fenwick and members of her campaign for state registration founded the International Council of Nurses. Based on the model of the International Council of Women, it was to be a federation of national nurses' associations. Few such associations existed at that time, and the ICN hoped to encourage them. Bedford Fenwick and her close friend Isla Stewart, matron of St Bartholomew's Hospital, also founded the NCN as an organisation to represent the nursing associations of Britain, and in 1904 the NCN affiliated to the ICN at its second international congress in Berlin. By the time the College appeared in 1916, the ICN was well established and Bedford Fenwick, founder of the ICN, president of the NCN and a leading suffragette, dominated a forum that regarded her as a living legend.

As noted in chapter 1, Bedford Fenwick was implacably hostile to the College, partly because it would not join her battle for state registration, and partly because she disapproved of the mixed nature of the College council. In 1923 the College tried to persuade the ICN to accept it as a member without going through the NCN, but while the ICN welcomed the College as the largest organisation of nurses in Britain, its constitution prevented any country from having more than one representative, and the NCN already filled this place. In the mid 1920s the College was permitted to affiliate to the NCN, but with both the College and the NCN claiming to speak for British nurses the relationship was very strained. Lack of trust between the College and the NCN meant that British nurses did not speak with one voice, and the College was often unhappy about decisions taken by the official delegates to the ICN.[84]

During the war the NCN ceased to function and the College took over as Britain's representative at international conferences. But the NCN re-appeared after the war with a revised constitution, and once more claimed to speak for British nurses at home and abroad. At the same time, new international health agencies were emerging, most notably the WHO from 1948. The College wished to participate in these, but it first needed to clear the small, but extremely determined NCN from its path. Although the College was the largest of the NCN's constituent bodies, the NCN's new constitution ensured that the College could not control it. The College was restricted to eight delegates to the NCN and was easily out-voted, even though it was paying the largest annual subscription. An additional grievance was the voting rights of the hospital leagues affiliated to the NCN.

The leagues consisted of nurses who had trained at the same hospital, and by 1946 their activities were mainly social. Of the forty-eight organisations in the NCN, fifteen were professional organisations and thirty-three were hospital leagues. The College objected to these small bodies deciding NCN policy, which then appeared as the British view at international gatherings. The NCN retorted that the College was not a fully representative body, because it did not include nurses on the supplementary registers, such as mental health and fever nurses.

Throughout the 1950s the two organisations argued over who should speak for British nurses at the ICN. Bedford Fenwick had subsidised the NCN, and it fell into financial difficulties after her death in 1947. In 1948 the two sides were still irreconcilable, and Frances Goodall wrote to Katherine Armstrong, president of the NCN:

> you will agree that an entirely different position has grown up in the country so far as nurses are concerned since 1939. This is largely due to . . . the nationalisation of the health service which has resulted in the setting up of the Whitley Councils for nurses and midwives. During this period the College has come to be recognised as the chief negotiating body on behalf of nurses by the government.

Armstrong replied:

> the Royal College of Nursing cannot have a balance of power appropriate to its large membership, as you suggest it should, . . . if this were done the National Council would cease to have any real individuality and become merely a shadow of the College . . . unless the College accepts this . . . it should come out of the National Council. To my mind the Royal College of Nursing can only become the National Council by gaining the confidences of all the member bodies to such a degree that these other bodies ask the College to do so. I feel that the constant demand of the College members themselves to take it over merely puts off the day when this position can arise, if it is to be the eventual outcome.[85]

In 1949, the Branches Standing Committee of the College voted to withdraw from membership of the NCN. The *British Journal of Nursing*, still hostile to the College, commented that the College was 'hankering after autocracy' and that its withdrawal would cause many to rejoice.[86] The College council decided to postpone action while the two sides negotiated. Little progress was made and the College became increasingly uneasy over incidents at international gatherings when British delegates were ignored or the nature of their representation was criticised.[87] At the 1957 ICN Congress in Rome, the matter came to a head. College delegates were embarrassed when the British group failed to vote together, and the College decided that the situation could not continue.[88]

At this point two distinguished nurses, Mabel Lawson and Florence Udell, assumed positions of influence in the two organisations. They were both involved in international health agencies. Lawson, elected president of the NCN in 1957, had been deputy chief nursing officer at the Ministry of Health for the previous sixteen years and a member of the GNC. Udell's work for the United Nations has already been mentioned. She was chief nursing officer at the Colonial Office and then nursing adviser at the Ministry of Overseas Development. Lawson and Udell encouraged the two sides to reconsider. At a joint meeting in February 1958 it was obvious that both sides desired a unified professional body for British nurses. The College's Royal Charter was an impediment to change, since any alteration in the College's name or functions required approval from the Privy Council. The College wanted to keep the prestige of a Royal Charter, and the NCN was equally anxious to share it. Negotiations continued slowly for another four years. Eventually it was agreed that the Royal Charter would be the basis of the new organisation. The College and the NCN amalgamated in May 1963.

After immense argument about every combination of words in its proposed title, the new organisation took the unwieldy name of *Royal College of Nursing and National Council of Nurses of the United Kingdom*. For everyday purposes this was reduced to Rcn, with a capital 'R' for Royal, and lower case 'cn' for both College of Nursing and Council of Nurses. The College used these initials both on paper and in everyday speech, and encouraged members to do the same in order to fix them in the public mind.[89] Lawson was the first President of the new body and was succeeded by Udell. In 1973 the title was changed to *Royal College of Nursing of the United Kingdom*, or RCN, but few noticed the change of case. During the 1960s the press often referred to the merged body as the Royal College of Nursing, or RCN (in capitals), and the public accepted it as such. The merger required Letters Patent from the Privy Council, which agreed that the College's functions were primarily educational and that the Royal Charter was still appropriate. Other professional associations like the BMA were not eligible for a Royal Charter, because 'a professional society whose primary object is the promotion of the interest of its members rather than the acquisition and dissemination of knowledge . . . is not eligible to receive permission to use the title "Royal".'[90] But even as these words were written, the traditional image of the nurse was being challenged, and the RCN was beginning very forcefully to promote 'the interest of its members'.

To avoid confusion, the chapters that follow use the current title RCN rather than the short-lived Rcn.

Conclusion

Although the College council was traditional in its composition and many of its ideas, the College needed to defend the status of nursing in the early years of the NHS. Its legal status as a negotiating body was questionable, and although its status had been much enhanced during the war, it could not depend on a favourable reception in government departments when its views differed from the prevailing desire for NHS economies. The continuing nursing shortage led governments to seek the cheapest solution in staffing the hospitals, usually through employing less qualified staff. This led to much debate on the nature of nursing, and the amount and type of training required, and the Nuffield investigation into nurses' work in the hospitals brought these questions into sharper focus. As noted in chapter 1, the College founders were reluctant to separate the professional from the vocational ideal in nursing, though neither of these terms was clearly defined. By the 1950s, these vague aspirations did not fit easily into the Nuffield world of time and motion studies.

The College was not monolithic in its response to these challenges. The College council saw nurse training as divided between the classroom and the ward, but the ward was still the sister's domain rather than the tutor's. From its inception the College had argued that student nurses were trainees, not cheap labour, but to most hard-pressed ward sisters, they were a necessary part of the labour force. The 1950s were the last great demonstration of the College's capacity to raise funds for its educational activities through the Victorian strategies of charitable campaigns fronted by royalty and the aristocracy, but the College's educationists were beginning to negotiate for a closer relation between nurse training and higher education, though at this period it would affect only a minority of nurses. The first major breach with tradition came from the public health nurses, who demanded a more specialised training outside the hospital wards. By the early 1960s the College was operating under a new name, and its views were also changing in a number of important ways.

Notes

1 TNA LAB 8/1305.
2 Abel Smith, *Nursing Profession*, p. 233.
3 TNA LAB 8/62, extract from the minutes of 18th meeting of N[ational] A[dvisory] C[ouncil], held on 30 January 1953.
4 White, *Effects of the NHS on the Nursing Profession*, p. 205.
5 Jessie D. Britten, *Practical Notes on Nursing Procedures* (Edinburgh: E. & S. Livingstone, 1957), pp. 5, 9, 11.
6 TNA LAB 18/619, minutes of meeting on the training of industrial nurses.
7 TNA LAB 43/189, F. Goodall to I. Ward, 16 April 1953.
8 TNA LAB 43/165, F. Goodall to Minister of Health, 11 Feb. 1953.
9 TNA LAB 43/189, I. Ward to W. Monckton, 4 May 1953.
10 TNA LAB 43/189, memo on letter from I. Ward to the Ministry of Labour, 16 July 1954.
11 Nuffield Provincial Hospitals Trust, *The Work of Nurses in Hospital Wards* (London: Nuffield, 1953), pp. 28, 37.
12 Ibid., p. 74.
13 Ibid., pp. 35, 54.
14 Webster, *Health Services Since the War. Vol. 1*, pp. 341–3.
15 Nuffield, *Work of Nurses*, p. 133.

16 RCNA, folders of press cuttings, Nuffield Job Analysis, *The Hospital* 49, 3 March 1953.

17 *The Times* 13 May 1953, p. 3.

18 *NT* editorials 1953, 21 Feb. p. 173; 28 Feb. p. 203; 7 March p. 225; 14 March p. 254; 21 March p. 281.

19 *NT* editorial 16 May 1953, p. 477.

20 'College conference on the job analysis', *NT* editorial, 5 Dec. 1953, p. 1233. See also pp. 1238–40.

21 Royal College of Nursing, *Comment on the Nuffield Provincial Hospitals Trust Job Analysis of the Work of Nurses in Hospital Wards* (London: Royal College of Nursing, 1953), p. 8.

22 *The Times* 20 Feb. 1953, p. 3.

23 Nuffield, *Work of Nurses*, p. 145.

24 *The Work of Nurses in Hospital Wards, Report by the Standing Nursing and Midwifery Advisory Committee on the 'Job Analysis of the Work of Nurses in Hospital Wards' Prepared by the Nuffield Provincial Hospitals Trust* (Edinburgh: HMSO, 1955).

25 R. I. Weir, *Educating Nurses in Scotland: a History of Innovation and Change: 1950–2000* (Penzance: Hypatia, 2004), pp. 16–18.

26 'Poor response to criticisms', *The Times* 22 Feb. 1954, p. 3.

27 Letter from F. Goodall, *The Times* 3 March 1954, p. 9.

28 White, *Effects of the NHS on the Nursing Profession*, pp. 203–6.

29 For an account of Conservative policy, see Webster, *Health Services Since the War. Vol. 1*, pp. 204–11, and Tony Cutler, '"A double irony", the politics of National Health Service expenditure in the 1950s', in Martin Gorsky and Sally Sheard (eds), *Financing Medicine. The British Experience Since 1750* (London and New York: Routledge, 2006), pp. 201–20.

30 Letter from G. Carter, *The Times* 3 March 1954, p. 9.

31 Royal College of Nursing, *Observations and Objectives: a Statement on Nursing Policy* (London: Royal College of Nursing, 1956).

32 Ibid., p. 4.

33 Ibid., p. 18.

34 RCN/28, Royal College of Nursing, 'Memorandum on the legal position of the nurse who undertakes procedures outside her professional scope', Feb. 1953.

35 RCN/28, Royal College of Nursing, *Conference on the legal position of the nurse who undertakes procedures outside her professional scope* (1954).

36 TNA MH 55/2615, 'Duties and position of the nurse'. Memorandum 26 April 1954.

37 TNA MH 55/2615, Dept. of Health for Scotland to Minister of Health, 18 June 1953.

38 TNA MH 55/2615, D. Emery to Miss Watson, 23 Oct. 1953.

39 RCN 17/5/1, press release, 20 Oct. 1958.

40 Royal College of Nursing, *The Duties and Position of the Nurse* (1961). See also TNA MH 55/2626, C. Hall to E. Powell, 16 Feb. 1961.

41 CM 19 Jan. 1961, pp. 25–7.

42 For a full study, see Davina Allen, *The Changing Shape of Nursing Practice. The Role of Nurses in the Hospital Division of Labour* (London and New York: Routledge, 2001).

43 Baly, *Nursing and Social Change*, p. 216.
44 *NT* 22 Nov. 1957, pp. 1321–2, 1324–6.
45 CM March 1954, pp. 106–7, Memorandum on the suggested function and scope of a Nursing Research Council.
46 Discussed in the next chapter.
47 June Clark, 'Nursing research', in Baly, *Nursing and Social Change*, pp. 313–14.
48 Estimated by the GNC. Marjorie Simpson, 'The early days in nursing research', RCNA C261/8/4/2.
49 *NT* 9 Oct. 1959. A report went to council setting out the group's proposals, and was welcomed by council, CM Oct 1959.
50 D. Norton, *Looking After Old People at Home* (London: National Council of Social Service, 1957); M. M. Williams, *Report of a Survey of Some Current Surgical Dressing Techniques in Industry* (London: Royal College of Nursing, 1961).
51 RCN/28, Educational Fund promotional literature.
52 *NT* 25 March 1960, p. 387.
53 The College's fundraising activities are covered exhaustively in RCN/17/4/42 and RCN/17/4/43.
54 RCN/17/4/43, press cuttings, *Sunday Pictorial* 23 Sept. 1951.
55 RCN/17/4/43, press cuttings, *The People* 28 Sept. 1951.
56 RCNA T45, interview with Elaine Wilkie, 1992.
57 CM Oct. 1949, p. 347. The first grant was for £3,000.
58 TNA MH 165/138, memo by N. Power, 6 July 1965.
59 TNA MH 165/138, memo by F. D. Walker, 25 June 1965.
60 Alice Thompson, *A Bibliography of Nursing Literature 1859–1960* (London: Library Association, 1968).
61 McGann, *The Battle of the Nurses*, p. 213.
62 RCNA T18, interview with Baroness McFarlane of Llandaff, 1987.
63 'Developments in nursing education', *Medical Press* 19 Sept. 1951, pp. 296–9.
64 RCNA T17, interview with Margaret Lamb, 1987.
65 This was a joint committee of the Ministry of Health, the Department of Health for Scotland, and the two national GNCs.
66 The two educationalists on the committee disassociated themselves from this recommendation.
67 Ministry of Health, Department of Health for Scotland, the General Nursing Councils for England and Wales and Scotland, *Report of the Committee Set Up to Consider the Function, Status and Training of Nurse Tutors* (London: HMSO, 1954), p. 8.
68 *Memorandum on the Nurse Tutor, Function, Scope, Responsibilities and Conditions of Service* (London: Royal College of Nursing, 1954).
69 RCN/28, Royal College of Nursing, *Memorandum on the Selection of Nurses for Secondment to take Nurse Tutor Courses* (1955).
70 The course began in 1947.
71 *The Lancet*, 26 Nov. 1949, p. 16. The words were those of Dr Josephine Brew, LL.D, education adviser to the National Association of Girls' Clubs and Mixed Clubs.
72 RCNA pamphlet collection, G. B. Carter, 'A study of the course for nurse tutors organised by the Royal College of Nursing (Scottish Board) leading to the certificate awarded by the University of Edinburgh to nurse tutors' (unpublished, n.d. [1956/57]).

73 Carter, 'A study of the course for nurse tutors'; Rosemary Weir, *A Leap in the Dark, the Origins and Development of the Department of Nursing Studies, the University of Edinburgh* (Penzance: Jamieson Library, 1996), pp. 9–12.

74 CM Sept. 1950, p. 310; May 1952, p. 195; also RCNA, folders of press cuttings: Nursing Education 1950–52, 'Royal College's action on standards in arithmetic', *Hospital and Social Service Journal* 11 July 1952.

75 RCNA pamphlet collection, Luton and Hitchin Group No. 2 Hospital Management Committee, *Some Current Problems of Nurse Training*, 10 June 1953.

76 White, *Effects of the NHS on the Nursing Profession*, pp. 108–11.

77 Abel-Smith, *Nursing Profession*, p. 226. See also Penny Starns, *March of the Matrons: Military Influences on the British Civilian Nursing Profession 1939–1969* (Peterborough: DSM, 2000), pp. 67ff.

78 Bendall and Raybould, *History of the General Nursing Council for England and Wales*, pp. 190–2.

79 Royal College of Nursing, *The Nurse Tutor, A New Assessment* (London: Royal College of Nursing, 1961).

80 B. Abel-Smith and R. H. Titmuss, *The Cost of the National Health Service in England and Wales* (Cambridge: Cambridge University Press, 1956), p. 10.

81 RCNA T45, interview with Elaine Wilkie, 1992.

82 RCNA pamphlet collection, H. M. Williams, 'The integrated nurse/health visitor course. A report of the first five years of the experimental course organised by the University of Southampton and the Nightingale School, St. Thomas' Hospital' ([Southampton University], 1962).

83 RCNA pamphlet collection, Fraser Brockington, 'A university course in nursing: a report on the first 4 years of the University of Manchester experimental course in nurse education' (typescript, 1964), pp. 20–1.

84 Letter from Olive Baggallay, *BJN* March 1938, p. 79.

85 RCN/5/1/N/20/8.

86 Editorial, *BJN* Aug. 1949.

87 RCN/5/1/N/20/8.

88 Daisy C. Bridges, *A History of the International Council of Nurses 1899–1964, the First 65 Years* (London: Pitman Medical, 1967), p. 192.

89 *AR* 1965, pp. 19–20.

90 TNA HO 28/89, memo from R. J. G., 23 Jan. 1963.

6

The 1960s: a decade of discontent

Between 1960 and 1972, membership of the RCN more than doubled, from around 43,000 to nearly 90,000.[1] During this period the RCN changed from a relatively small organisation, open only to women on the general nursing register, to a more inclusive body. At the same time, its involvement in labour relations became more prominent, and the RCN used its growing membership and favourable public image to confront governments in ways never envisaged by its founders. While political and economic pressures forced it into national pay campaigns, its new general secretary had a significant role in responding to these new challenges, and in expanding the College membership. In 1956, Frances Goodall's retirement was imminent, but the College had to advertise twice before appointing Catherine Mary Hall to replace her. After working with Goodall for a year, Hall succeeded her at the age of thirty-four.[2] A former member of the RCN's staff described this as replacing the 'velvet glove' with the 'iron rod'.[3]

Catherine Hall was the only child of a high-ranking police officer in Sheffield, and attended a private boarding school. Her parents held the fairly common view that nursing was not a good career for an educated girl, and her mother would have preferred her to stay at home when she left school. Failing this, her parents insisted that she take secretarial and domestic science courses to equip her for office work or marriage; but the war broke down parental opposition, since nursing seemed a better option than conscription. In 1940, aged seventeen, she began pre-training in the Sick Children's Hospital in Birmingham, where she worked through air raids and slept in the basement. She needed to work near home because of her mother's ill health, and so trained at Leeds General Infirmary, where, as in many hospitals, students had to attend lectures after a full stint of nursing duty. 'In retrospect', she remembered, 'it was abysmal . . . they stood up and gave a very formal lecture and you were expected to scribe and scribe and produce your own notes and so it went. It was not really being educated, it was being taught'.[4] By 1950 she was night superintendent at the infirmary, but took advantage of the scholarships offered to a few promising nurses, firstly by the governors of the infirmary, and then by the RCN, to study nursing education and administration. She travelled in the USA and Canada, and then studied at the College. At the early age of twenty-eight, she became assistant matron at the Middlesex Hospital. As a northerner, not trained in one of the prestigious London hospitals, she needed exceptional qualities to impress the Middlesex governors, who usually appointed their own trainees to senior posts. Her parents' expectation that work would be a temporary phase before marriage proved unfounded. Questioned many years later by an intrepid interviewer, Catherine Hall told of a broken engagement, and of the many young men of her generation lost in the war. She remained unmarried, and devoted her energies to the RCN for twenty-five years.[5]

Handsome, solid and imposing in appearance, Catherine Hall soon established her authority in Henrietta Place. Officials in the Ministry of Health may have hoped that her conservative manner indicated a less tenacious character than her predecessor's, but they rapidly learned not to underestimate her. She had remarkable powers of organisation, and commanded the complete loyalty of her staff. She had the difficult task of negotiating on behalf of the RCN during a period of rapid inflation in prices and wages, and of increasing trade union militancy. Public employees were particularly vulnerable to the nation's frequent economic crises as governments struggled to counter budgetary problems with 'stop-go' spending policies; and the RCN had to compete with unions armed with more powerful weapons in wage negotiations. Catherine Hall believed that only a large and inclusive organisation could defend its members' interests. The first step was to open membership of the RCN to male nurses.

New members

The RCN's decision to admit men followed, slowly, on legislation that altered the nature of the general register. Most civilian male nurses worked in mental hospitals and mental deficiency institutions, and did not have a general training. In 1945, the Ministry of Health estimated that there were about 10,000 men employed in such institutions in England and Wales with only 2,000 in other types of hospital.[6] Of the latter, around 1,300 had a full general training.[7] The Nurses Act of 1949 abolished the separate register for male nurses, and placed qualified men on the general register. A further Nurses Act in 1957 discontinued the supplementary registers for specialised nurses, though it divided the general register into separate sections for them. Consequently, mental and mental deficiency nurses now appeared on the general register, though the GNC and RCN opposed this, since mental nurses (renamed psychiatric nurses) often had a lower standard of school education than nurses

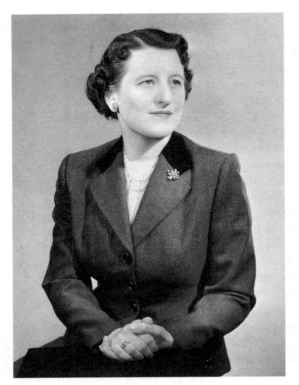

6.1 Catherine Hall, general secretary 1957–82.

accepted for training in the larger general hospitals.[8] The RCN's reluctance to include male nurses was rooted in the belief that, like the enrolled nurses, they threatened the professional status of the College because of their shorter training.[9] The voluntary hospitals were able to impose their own educational standards, even if these were not compulsory under the GNC's regulations, but the mental hospitals rarely had a choice in selecting staff.

It is debatable whether the RCN's Royal Charter actually excluded men from membership. Individual applications from male nurses with a general training were turned down from 1949 onwards, the RCN's lawyers advising that, since the Charter assumed that only women could be on the general register, male membership was not contemplated.[10] Yet the Charter did not specifically prevent the council from accepting suitably qualified men, if they wished, and indeed, the council had discretionary powers over whom they admitted to membership. There were deeper feelings involved. The Association of Hospital Matrons, in particular, was not happy about male nurses moving into general nursing, believing that 'it was a custom of the country that female nurses only should work in medical and surgical female wards and that patients would in the vast majority of cases object to any other practice being adopted'.[11] The matrons were anxious not only about sexual propriety, but the inconvenience of employing male nurses who would be restricted to male wards. They preferred to deploy staff freely to meet the unpredictable demands of the hospital service, and some matrons avoided difficulties by simply refusing to accept male students in their training schools. At this stage, men were also excluded from hospital or community nursing posts that required midwifery training. So strong were gender stereotypes in nursing that men who entered general nursing were objects of suspicion for two contradictory reasons: either that they intended to cause havoc with the female students or that they must be homosexual, or they would never have chosen such a career.[12] At this stage there was apparently no fear that males would usurp the managerial role of senior nurses in general hospitals, partly because of their restricted roles in general hospitals, and partly because of persistent snobbery. The RCN council and the Association of Hospital Matrons consisted of middle-class career women, usually unmarried, and feared no male challenge. An official in the Ministry of Health apparently agreed:

> Without being in the least snobbish I think everyone would agree that male nurses in general are not, as yet anyhow, drawn from the same social stratum as the women who become leaders of the profession. There may be exceptions, and I know that qualities of leadership need not depend on social rank but, in the main, this is a fair generalisation.[13]

During the war, the military medical services had brought male and female nurses into the same sphere, where they worked together without difficulty. But state registered male nurses called up for military service often found they were not given the opportunity to use their professional skills in the same way as female nurses. Men enrolled in the Royal Army Medical Corps complained of being treated differently from their female counterparts, of not being promoted to the appropriate rank, of being reduced to acting as batmen to officers, scrubbing barrack room floors, window cleaning or gardening.[14] Despite this, many male nurses and orderlies of the Royal Army Medical Corps returning to civilian life looked for positions in nursing, and the government's relaxed standards of entry to the profession allowed them to do so. In 1946 the Ministry of Health, much preoccupied with the nursing shortage, issued a circular encouraging the employment of more male nurses. TB and mental hospitals had desperate staffing problems, but men were encouraged to apply to general hospitals also. Frances Goodall commented on the Ministry's circular before publication, doubting whether hospitals had adequate training facilities for men. She argued that separate accommodation would have to be provided for them, but did not wish to segregate them from the normal life of the training schools.[15] The number of full-time trained male nurses in the NHS increased from 9,515 in 1948 to 12,145 in 1955.[16] The ratio of female nurses to male in all sectors, including students and pupils, was ten to one. Complaints of being passed over for promotion in favour of women continued, and the Society of Registered Male Nurses also alleged that male nurses were systematically discriminated against in government departments and the nationalised industries.[17] By 1960 little had changed for men in nursing, but their numbers continued to grow.

Frances Goodall allegedly said that men would be admitted to full membership of the RCN 'over her dead body', although she had encouraged the setting up of the Society of Registered Male Nurses and its affiliation to the College in 1941.[18] Catherine Hall did not share her opinion, and planned to enlarge RCN membership in order to increase its political influence and woo nurses away from the trade unions. In 1957 the Branches Standing Committee voted to accept all male nurses on the general register, but the council objected, fearing loss of professional status, but also that 'the College might well be subjected to Trades Union influence from within'.[19] It was possible, though not very common, for nurses to belong to both the RCN and a trade union, and the council seems to have been anxious about fifth-column infiltration by male nurses whose loyalties were elsewhere. The affiliated Society of Registered Male Nurses pressed for full membership, and this led to heated internal debates throughout 1959. Catherine Hall's views finally prevailed in the council, and active members plainly agreed with her, for at an extraordinary general meeting of the College in June 1960, they voted overwhelmingly to open membership to 'all persons of either sex whose names are on a Register of Nurses established by Act of Parliament'.[20] This decision also opened membership to nurses who were registered on the supplementary parts of the register. So important was this decision, that voting by proxy rather than personal attendance at the meeting was permitted for the first time in the RCN's history, although only about one sixth of the membership cast a vote.[21] The Privy Council amended the RCN's charter to include men, and at the same time, seats on the council were formally restricted to members of the College.[22] This was already the informal practice. Between 1916 and 1928, members of the council (of either sex) automatically became members of the College. The Charter removed this right, but still permitted non-members to be elected on to the council. The 1960 changes ended the original council structure that included patrons like Arthur Stanley; but they also assisted the merger with the National Council of Nurses, which firmly opposed governance by anyone other than members of the profession. Within a year, the first male nurse was voted on to the council. He was Albery Verdun Whittamore, aged forty-five, chief male nurse at Horton Psychiatric Hospital.

Many critics have commented that the effect of promoting equality of the sexes, in the RCN and in the NHS more generally, was ultimately to promote a disproportionate number of men to positions of leadership in a largely female profession. Numerous sociological explanations have been offered for this, particularly the gendered expectations of professional and bureaucratic systems, into which the complex responsibilities of working mothers do not fit.[23] Catherine Hall, reflecting on this in her retirement, believed that the crucial change had not been the arrival of men, but the diminishing proportion of senior single women in the profession. One of her earliest actions in the RCN was to persuade the council to take up the case of married nurses, and encourage them back to work, for it was becoming obvious that nursing could no longer rely on unlimited supplies of unmarried women.[24] The result was not exactly as she had planned:

> I've got no hang-ups about men being in senior positions, but there is no doubt that the number is disproportionate because you now have such a high percentage of married women.[25]

The rapid rise of male nurses in administrative posts at least scuppered the old assumption that their lowly origins made them unfit for leadership, and modern discussions of the subject tend to focus on gender inequalities rather than social class.

The arrival of male nurses in the RCN did not bring an immediate increase in membership and the College, apparently, wanted to digest them slowly rather than 'in bulk'. About sixty men joined the College in 1960, and the Society of Registered Male Nurses did not disband.[26] The Cowdray Club, originally intended for professional women, deliberated long before admitting men, then allowed them into associate membership in 1968.[27] Although College membership increased slightly between 1960 and 1962, it then declined until 1968. Male nurses did not flock to join. Many were already members of trade unions, particularly the Confederation of Health Service Employees. This union was founded in 1946 with around 40,000 members from an amalgamation of older unions representing employees of the mental hospitals and poor law institutions. It rapidly expanded its membership among NHS staff. It recruited male nurses, enrolled and assistant nurses, student and pupil nurses and ancillary staff, all of whom were excluded from the RCN, and unlike the RCN, COHSE was run largely by men.[28] It is difficult to calculate the union density of nurses because of the fluctuating and divided nature of the workforce, but assuming that the quarter of a million nurses recorded in the 1951 census of England and Wales is an accurate indication of the size of the profession, then the combined *national* membership of the RCN and COHSE in that year (under 100,000), indicated that less than half of the nation's nurses belonged to a union.[29] This was close to the national average of around 45 per cent of union membership for all employees, though less than in largely male heavy industries.[30]

Leavened by an active group of men, the RCN became more interested in defending the professional interests of male nurses. Their Ward and Departmental Sisters Section was renamed the Sister and Charge Nurses Section. Male nurses pointed out that modesty was not confined to women, and that male patients were often embarrassed when intimate procedures, such as shaving body hair before an operation, were carried out by young women. In extreme cases, shaving might have to be done after the anaesthetic was administered. One male nurse's memories of the imperious attitude of certain senior female staff may be exaggerated, but reflects a fairly widespread folk memory in that generation of men:

> Male nurses literally came on requisitions. It was common for the ward sister to send a chit to the nursing office: 'Please send six toilet rolls and three male nurses for shaving'.[31]

Before the Second World War, district nursing and health visiting were regarded as women's work. After the war, with labour shortages in these posts as in all sections of the profession, men were recruited, but their role was restricted because they were denied training in midwifery. Not all jobs were open to them, and they were restricted to male patients.[32] In 1965 the Scottish Board reported to the RCN council their view that men should be accepted as health visitors, and that a suitable course in midwifery should be designed for them.[33] By the following year several local authorities were willing to employ male nurses in this capacity, and in Aberdeen a special training course for male health visitors began. The Council for the Training of Health Visitors also indicated that statutory approval was likely to be given to male health visitors. The RCN council, in common with other professional organisations, approved this in principle and agreed to admit male nurses to their health visitors' course. Qualifications in district, psychiatric or mental subnormality nursing were accepted instead of obstetric training; and male students would receive the College's certificate until the Council for the Training of Health Visitors could award its own.[34] Opinions were divided over obstetric training for men, however, and it was not until 1971 that the council and the annual meeting of the RCN Representative Body (RRB) voted that male and female students should have the same training. The Ministry of Health gave official approval at the same time.[35] At first, the RCN's cautious view was that male students should learn obstetrics for use only in emergencies, and not to equip them for becoming male midwives, but by 1973 it was pressing the Central Council of Midwives to accept men. June Clark, a health visitor in Reading, and a future president of the RCN, expressed the views of younger nurses to the 1971 RRB:

> I am not an advocate of women's lib but I am an advocate of equal opportunity for all and I think nursing for too long has been held back in its professional development because it has been a female oriented profession.[36]

In 1975 the Sex Discrimination Act permitted men to train and work in midwifery, under certain restrictions that were lifted in 1983. There was also an element of feminine self-interest in the RCN's changing attitudes towards male nurses. As men entered areas of nursing previously confined to women, the issue of unequal pay came into sharper focus.

Trade union allegations that the RCN could not speak for anyone other than its own small membership confirmed Catherine Hall's desire to make the RCN more inclusive. A debate began on whether to offer membership to enrolled nurses, who, if trade union minded, were joining COHSE or the National Union of Public Employees. In April 1965 the Birmingham branch recommended to the RCN council that enrolled nurses be admitted to membership, as the branch thought it desirable that all trained nurses should be members of 'one national professional association'.[37] There was much disagreement over whether such a move would woo enrolled nurses away from the trade unions. Enrolled nurses had their own professional body, the National Association of State Enrolled Nurses, and this, while happy to be affiliated to the RCN, objected strongly to the RCN taking over its members.[38] RCN branches were invited to give their views on the inclusion of enrolled nurses and students, and were also much divided, some believing that a more inclusive organisation would strengthen the RCN in pay negotiations, others fearing that professional standards would be eroded, and that the proposed new members might be able to outvote the old.[39] For many older members of the RCN, permitting enrolled nurses to join would destroy the RCN's image as a professional body for fully trained nurses. Social class, though rarely mentioned, was still an issue, since the SRN/SEN qualifications were still believed to distinguish middle-class nurses from working-class ones. But the RCN leadership was determined to proceed, and, to break the deadlock with NASEN, the RCN proposed to accept enrolled nurses as members without further consultation. The enrolled nurses' leaders realised that it was impossible to hold out against the much larger forces of the RCN, and agreed to disband NASEN, on condition that the RCN establish a separate enrolled nurses' section, and that NASEN staff be taken into RCN employment.[40] When this was put to a vote at the Annual Meetings in 1969, members overwhelmingly supported admission for enrolled nurses, and the RCN duly negotiated amendments to the Royal Charter. Members of NASEN joined the RCN as a group in 1970, and pupil nurses were offered membership of the Student Nurses' Association.

The RCN decided against giving students full membership, although it risked losing them to the more inclusive trade unions. If students were recognised as employees, rather than learners, the NHS would have another excuse to treat them as cheap labour and neglect their training needs. The effect of large numbers of student members with full voting rights was unpredictable.

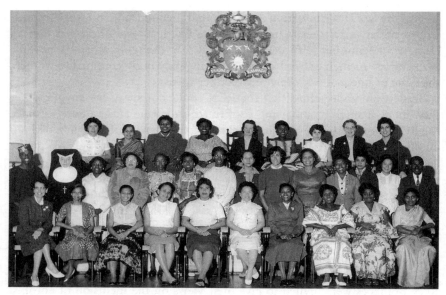

6.2 International students, September 1960.

The RCN compromised by incorporating the Student Nurses' Association into the College in 1968, and giving students all membership privileges except the right to vote in ballots or at College meetings. Students could not vote in council elections, but were represented like other sections of the College, and could speak and vote at the RCN Representative Body. Princess Margaret, the Patron of the Student Nurses' Association, became a patron of the RCN, joining her mother and sister. The RCN knew that students often regarded it as a stuffy organisation, and that it was difficult to interest them in branch activities. The Student Nurses' Association held a series of critical discussions on the failure of communication between students and the College. They noted that trade unions, through their shop stewards, could offer 'on the spot' help to individuals experiencing problems in the workplace.[41] The RCN used 'key members' in the hospitals and elsewhere to negotiate on behalf of its members. These were members in clinical positions who were willing to recruit and disseminate information, but they were volunteers. The union structure, with a fully developed system of local shop stewards, had considerable advantages over the RCN arrangements.

Reorganisation

During the 1960s, the structure of the RCN changed substantially both at the centre and the regions. The first change was in its handling of public relations, to which Catherine Hall gave high priority. She wanted to keep members better informed about the College and to reach out to new recruits.[42] A full-time information officer, Lt. Colonel Douglas de Cent, was appointed in 1963. His background was an unusual mixture of military, consular and sales management experience. The RCN was becoming more aware of the importance of the media, for an organisation that could not resort to trade union tactics had to rely on public support in making its case for improved pay and conditions of work. In 1965 the council noted that the new arrangement was working well.

> A very close and satisfactory liaison has been created with the broadcasting services in general, and with the BBC in particular. The advice of the Rcn is often sought now on routine matters and there has been an increasing tendency to consult over the production of special programmes which have a nursing implication. Coverage of Rcn activities in News and Current Affairs programmes has been highly satisfactory.[43]

The RCN still employed a press-cuttings agency, and Catherine Hall, like Frances Goodall, replied rapidly to correspondence or comments in the press.

The second priority was to take account of growing specialist interests in nursing. The RCN's affairs were becoming too complex for the council to handle in detail, and its separate committees, each with a full-time secretary, took more responsibility. In its early days, the RCN relied on local branches to recruit new members and support its fundraising activities. The branches, usually based in larger hospitals, did not meet all needs and so the professional sections were set up as forums for special interests. These sections emerged piecemeal, some based on occupational groups and others on specialised functions. In 1960 there were five of them: Sister Tutors, Public Health, Ward and Departmental Sisters, Private Nurses and Occupational Health. Members of each section met locally to discuss their specialist interests and passed resolutions to a Central Sectional Committee, elected from the total UK membership of that section. This arrangement was not unique to the RCN: from the 1920s trade unions of workers with diverse occupations had developed a similar type of branch and section structure. The structure had difficulties in adapting to specialisation in nursing practice, as shown when nurse administrators requested permission to establish a specialist section in 1960. The council wanted the new section to be open to administrators in all fields of nursing, but dual section membership had been ruled out since the beginning.

The problem of dual membership led to a series of lengthy internal investigations into the relations between branches and sections, and the debate reflected tension in the profession between general and specialist interests. Many branch meetings to discuss College affairs were attended mainly by retired members, with a local matron presiding in uniform. The sections, consisting of active specialists, threatened to eclipse the branches, and there was no consensus on how to integrate the two. While specialists wanted to meet and discuss common interests, the branch structure in theory enabled the College to speak for all nurses and provided a focal point for nursing opinion in each area. As Monica Baly, the Western area organiser, pointed out, if nurses met only in specialised groups, the profession would be divided:

> the public health nurses meeting in a clinic saying that hospital nurses don't understand them, ward sisters sitting in nurses' homes knitting, complaining that the branch is full of matrons, the occupational health nurses drinking tea in chilly meetings in a factory, and the tutors spending hours discussing their status in a classroom.[44]

After much argument, in 1966 a new structure for general and special interests was adopted. Although the aim was to produce a simpler and more flexible structure, many thought that the new arrangement was as complex as the old.[45]

Members insisted on retaining the parallel system of branches and sections. This was expensive, and the council decided to end capitation payments to these groups. Sections were removed from the branches and organised into area groups of varying size according to the needs of each specialty. Each section had its own elected national committee, meeting twice a year, and its members represented their section on the new RCN Representative Body. Section committees advised the council on professional matters in their own field, and dual section membership was permitted. Branch membership became optional, as in the early years of the College, and the minimum acceptable branch size was reduced to twenty members. Branch executive committees were replaced by more informal arrangements, and each branch could elect a representative to the RRB. Branches were expected to promote the RCN in their district and encouraged to appoint a public relations officer. By 1973 the branches were still seen as ineffectual, playing little part in the College except once a year in the RRB.[46] The branches were often regarded as a tea party for senior and retired hospital staff, but as the RCN's pay campaigns showed, branches could be activated when required. Although branches became more independent, they were weakened by the loss of capitation fees, and were distanced from the College staff, particularly the area organisers.

The third priority was to make RCN government more open. The RRB, which first met in November 1967, replaced the Branches Standing Committee. This was the most successful of the reforms, providing the RCN with a more democratic forum for its growing membership. Douglas de Cent was largely responsible for transforming the Branches Standing Committee into a public window for the RCN. He believed that if the press attended the business part of the meetings, the RCN could reach a large audience. By projecting the RCN as a lively and powerful body, open meetings would aid recruitment by breaking down the image of the RCN as 'unbusinesslike, starchy, authoritarian, out-of-touch, remote and reactionary'.[47] The new RRB had more streamlined procedures and wider powers than the old Branches Standing Committee. Delegates, including branch and section representatives, had a free vote after debate. Resolutions and subjects for debate could be submitted from many sources, central and local. All members of the RCN could attend, together with council members and the RCN staff, although only representatives had the right to vote. The first meeting attracted 278 voting members, representing 183 branches and the seven section committees, while over 100 members came as observers. Thirty-four motions were debated including the structure of the NHS and standards of nursing care. The RRB met for the second time in Cardiff in 1968 as part of the Annual Meetings, and delegates discussed the treatment of psychiatric and geriatric patients, following the publication of damning criticism of NHS standards in Barbara Robb's *Sans Everything*.[48] The RRB sent telegrams to the Prime Minister and the Minister of Health urging more financial support for these services, and sending telegrams to government became something of an annual tradition.

The trade unions had annual congresses with vocal participation from their members. Compared with this, the indirect representation originally favoured by the RCN was likely to discourage younger and politically active nurses, the group most likely to be attracted elsewhere. The RCN began to move along a more democratic route by amalgamating the Annual Meetings with the meeting of the RRB, and the whole event was renamed the Annual Congress and Exhibition. Annual conferences of the sections were replaced by one large clinical conference on a theme of general interest, with speakers who were experts in the field, whether nursing, medical or political. In October 1969 Baroness Serota, the Minister of State for Health, opened the first congress, in Harrogate. The RRB meeting occupied three days, concluding the week-long congress. Following the tradition of the Annual Meetings, social activities were as important as the professional events, and included a civic reception, formal dinner and church service. Profits from the exhibition were intended to underwrite the whole enterprise, although members had to be reminded that their support was needed to ensure this.[49] Like other medical meetings, the congress was also supported by commercial displays from pharmaceutical and other companies, who saw the advantage of attending such gatherings.

Another major reorganisation was the creation in 1962 of a Welsh Board. Members in Wales decided on this when the College proposed reducing their council members from three to two. In 1959 the RCN in Wales had approximately 800 members in fifteen branches, divided between two of the English area organisers for administrative purposes. Mary Davies, one of the first health visitor tutors in the Welsh National School of Medicine, began the movement for a separate board, in an impassioned plea at a meeting of all the Welsh branches in Aberystwyth. It was unusual for the Welsh branches to meet together, since the north and south usually kept within their separate domains, but they now agreed to unite in their request for a Welsh Board with a prestigious headquarters building and its own post-registration programme of courses and conferences. Welsh members were disadvantaged in their access to College courses, which were offered in Scotland and Northern Ireland as well as London. In response to a Welsh deputation in 1959, the RCN council approved a Welsh Board in Cardiff in principle, but refused to take a firm decision for two years for financial reasons.[50] Welsh members were not daunted. Led by two dynamic nurses, Eileen M. Rees, matron of the Cardiff Royal Infirmary and member of the RCN council, and Miriam Gough, the principal tutor at the same hospital and member of the GNC for England and Wales, they started a national Welsh appeal. The RCN council stipulated that before they launched the appeal they must raise £20,000 from Welsh nurses. The Welsh leaders set up a Nurses' Appeals Committee and agreed that each member would give a shilling a month. By September 1962 they had raised £27,000 and went on to organise their national appeal.

A Welsh Board was appointed and held its first meeting in Cardiff in November 1962, with Olwen Caradoc Evans as its first secretary, though she resigned shortly afterwards and was replaced by Hetty Hopkins, senior tutor at the Cardiff Royal Infirmary.[51] The main appeal was launched in September 1964, though the cautious RCN council stipulated that it must be confined to Wales. Backed by a committee that included leading figures from the Welsh medical establishment, the Welsh nurses stirred up national enthusiasm for 'their' Royal College of Nursing. Fund-raising fever mounted, Welsh companies and local authorities gave generously, and Hetty Hopkins drove all over Wales in her Morris Minor, collecting shillings and inspiring Welsh nurses who had never heard of the College.[52] The target of £250,000 was exceeded within two years. With the support of Dr David Morgan, of the University Hospital, a site for the new headquarters building was purchased on the edge of the site for the new university hospital. The national pride of Welsh members in building their own headquarters was matched by a wider response from the Welsh public, not least the architects and the builders of the new headquarters, who gave their services free. *Ty Maeth* (House of Service) was opened by Princess Margaret in October 1965, having been completed within fifteen months. When Hopkins retired in 1978 the membership within Wales had risen to 5,000 and the Welsh Board had six members on the RCN Council.[53] A tutor to the Welsh Board was appointed at the end of 1966 to develop the educational programme, and the Welsh Hospitals and Health Services Association gave £500 annually towards scholarships for post-registration nurses. In 1964 the council decided that the constitution of the three national boards should have a common format, and the Committee for Northern Ireland changed its name to the Northern Ireland Board. Like the reorganisation of sections and branches, the new Welsh Board maintained local support for the RCN. Its successful fund raising also showed the continuance of a long standing tradition of public support for nurses.

After the merger with the National Council of Nurses, an International Department was set up to deal with international issues and representation on the International Council of Nurses. The Labour Relations Department also emerged at this time. The College had had a Labour Relations Committee from 1948 with Sir Frederick Leggett, formerly of the Ministry of Labour, as chairman, and during the 1950s and 1960s it was largely concerned with the work of the Nurses and Midwives Whitley Council.[54] The College's influence in the Whitley Council was increased when the secretary of the staff side, Mary Elizabeth Davies, joined the College staff in 1955, and continued to work in both posts. Davies, who was not a nurse, had a legal training. She married Keith Newstead, the first male nurse appointed to the College staff, and is better known in the RCN as Betty Newstead. She became the first labour relations secretary of the College and stayed until her retirement in 1975.[55] The Labour Relations Department prepared submissions to the Whitley Council and kept under review the salaries and conditions of service of all nurses. Aided by the seven area organisers, the department also advised individual members on employment problems, represented them at inquiries or industrial injury tribunals, provided legal assistance if necessary and handled cases covered by the Indemnity Insurance Scheme.[56]

All these bureaucratic changes signalled the RCN's determination to operate more effectively in the regions and open its discussions to a wider section of the membership. Critics of the RCN still argued that it was too remote and dominated by hospital matrons, but the 1960s' reorganisation was a conscious effort to change not only the RCN's name, but also its image in the nursing profession. The Welfare Advisory Service, established in 1969, can be seen in the same way. This service, funded by private donations, assisted and advised nurses with personal problems, whether or not they were members of the College. Since its beginning the College had acted as a conduit of donations for the whole profession, and it was the body to which donors naturally looked. A welfare adviser was appointed to provide counselling help to nurses and in the first year over 500 cases were dealt with. By 1972 there were two qualified social workers. Problems fell into five categories: health, employment, personal and family, accommodation and financial. Retired nurses needing help were the main applicants, but as the service became better known more nurses in full-time employment sought advice.

Some of the tensions in the profession during the 1960s were also reflected in changes to the *Nursing Times*. Its circulation reached almost 18,000 by 1960, when the College's share of the profit was over £10,000.[57] In the same year, a new editor arrived. Peggy Nuttall regarded the RCN as an excessively conservative body, and was not content to let the journal remain an uncritical vehicle for its views. She introduced lively, provocative articles and encouraged nurses to submit their own clinical studies. These changes proved very popular and circulation increased further. Nuttall resented having to submit her leaders to the RCN for approval, and although this was largely a formality, she decided it was time to break free.[58] From 1961 the editor took full responsibility for the content of the *Nursing Times*, and the RCN provided material for a monthly supplement devoted to its own activities. A suggestion that the *Nursing Times* should no longer style itself 'the official journal of the Royal College of Nursing' was not accepted, but in 1967, when the contract with Macmillan came up for renewal, the publishers were not prepared to continue it on the existing terms. By this time the circulation of the *Nursing Times* was catching up with the *Nursing Mirror*, the market leader, and Macmillan no longer needed to rely on the College to guarantee a readership. Macmillan offered to publish a quarterly RCN newssheet as well, but made certain conditions, including first refusal of all College material. The RCN rejected these proposals, and accepted an alternative bid from Johnson & Johnson, who offered to sponsor a College newspaper, the *Nursing Standard*. From 1968 this was distributed free to all members six times a year.[59] So ended a forty-year relationship with Macmillan, to the publisher and editor's regret. Over the previous twenty years, the *Nursing Times* had contributed £142,000 to the College, a lifeline to an organisation whose finances were often precarious.[60] The *Nursing Times* continued to prosper, taking over the declining *Nursing Mirror* in the 1980s. The more independent position of the major nursing journal did the RCN no harm. Although the *Nursing Times* editors sometimes criticised the College, they gave extensive coverage to its activities and shared its interest in promoting nursing research. RCN congresses were reported in detail. Accounts of garden parties and whist drives were replaced by debates over contemporary issues such as abortion, contraception and drug abuse, subjects on which the profession, like the public, had divided views.

The 1962 pay campaign

The first test of the new publicity machine came in 1962. In the later 1950s health services employees received small but regular pay rises, and these slightly narrowed the pay gap between students and qualified nurses. Nevertheless, from 1955 to 1960, nurses' wages fell from 68 to 60 per cent of the national average.[61] The Conservatives under Harold Macmillan won the general election of 1959 comfortably, having paved the way with strategic tax cuts. In this climate of generosity, the new Minister of Health, Enoch Powell, began work on a hospital plan for major expenditure on 200 new hospitals and renovation of older ones. But by 1961 the British economy was struggling to cope with rapid inflation, a balance of payments deficit and a sterling crisis. The government's desperate remedies included a 'pay pause' for public employees, ostensibly until national productivity improved.[62] Postal and railway workers reacted by striking, and unionism among public employees increased. Nurses were particularly unlucky, because the slow-moving Whitley Council was still deliberating their settlement when the pay freeze began. They were also disadvantaged by the large size of their profession, for even small pay rises for nurses cost the NHS dear, and nurses could hardly demonstrate an increase in their productivity without reducing services to patients. In April the government announced a 2.5 per cent pay rise for the public sector, though it undermined its own policy by agreeing to an increase of up to 9 per cent for the dockers, whose threatened strike would damage the economy. The government thought of 2.5 per cent for nurses in terms of its cost to the NHS – about £3.3 million. The RCN thought of it in terms of a nurse's pay packet – a few extra pounds a year.

The RCN and COHSE launched separate but co-operative attacks on the government's pay freeze, the RCN favouring a press campaign and pressure on MPs, COHSE preferring large demonstrations. The RCN was not in favour of street rallies, fearing to alienate the public, but organised a mass writing campaign to the Prime Minister and MPs using black-bordered envelopes. COHSE had fewer inhibitions, and sponsored national and regional demonstrations, culminating in a grand march through London. They also staged a mass lobby at Westminster.[63] COHSE's general secretary Jack Jepson began to talk of a ballot on strike action. The public, when confronted by a demonstration of uniformed nurses, naturally lumped them all together, regardless of affiliation, and cheered them on. More worryingly for the government, a number of other unions, including Liverpool dockers and workers at the Ford plant at Dagenham, began to hold token strikes in support of the nurses' claim, or to donate an hour's pay towards the cost of their campaign.[64] One recipient of these donations was a somewhat disconcerted RCN, which was nevertheless gratified by this proof that the public identified it as the nurses' representative. Within a few weeks, over £1,000 had been donated, and was used to subsidise local campaigns.

The RCN was well used to enlisting support from all political parties. Dame Irene Ward, once again opposing her own party's policy, attacked the government vigorously, and chaired a meeting of over 1,000 nurses at the RCN's Cowdray Hall. The press was very sympathetic to the nurses, and ninety-three Conservative backbenchers signed a motion urging the government to 'review, as soon as economic circumstances permit, the salary structure of the nursing and midwives' profession'.[65] Even this mild reproof embarrassed the government, and the Labour Party initiated a parliamentary debate on nurses' pay on 14 May. The seven-hour debate was memorable for the deep unease shown by many Conservatives at the government's treatment of the nurses, and for the remarkable sentimentality displayed on all sides of the House. Member after member related anecdotes of their sufferings in hospital (revealing a variety of medical conditions), and praised the devoted care of the nurses. Mothers, wives and daughters, past and present members of the profession, were invoked in evidence of its self-sacrificing virtues. The Labour MP Laurence Pavitt contended that men would not become nurses because male students had no accommodation in the hospitals and had to pay commercial rents. He recounted the affecting story of a student nurse, 'Mr Philpot', which provoked a sardonic interjection from his radical colleague Willie Hamilton:

> [Mr L. Pavitt: Mr Philpot] has given me his pay slip, showing £9.14.2d. He is a third-year student and he tells me that he pays £4 in rent, £2 for electricity and £3.10s for food. The total of his bills is £9.14s: balance in hand, 2d. Mr W. Hamilton: He has never had it so good.[66]

Some Labour MPs took sides between COHSE and the RCN, arguing that nurses needed a 'real' trade union to represent them rather than a professional association. Others felt that nurses were a special case, requiring the chivalrous support of male unionists. Ray Gunter stated:

> as a trade union leader . . . I do not want to see the nursing profession dragged into the roughness of industrial disputes. I do not want to see either male or female members of that profession having to talk the language which some of us have to talk.[67]

To all these emotional outbursts, Enoch Powell replied in his glacial fashion that the nation's economic needs must be paramount, and that there was currently no shortage of nurses; while the financial secretary to the Treasury spent so long defending the government's incomes policy that the future Prime Minister James Callaghan heckled him with shouts of 'What about the nurses?' Although the government majority held firm, the Cabinet was discomfited by the backbench revolt, and met to discuss a way of conciliating the nurses without compromising its pay strategy.

RCN and COHSE representatives on the staff side of the Whitley Council were frequently at loggerheads with each other about their ultimate aims in the pay dispute, and particularly about the wage differential between students and qualified nurses. COHSE wished to reduce this, while the RCN concentrated on trying to raise the salaries of qualified nurses. COHSE also believed that the RCN was over-represented on the council, especially because Frances Goodall, although retired from the RCN, was still chairman of the staff side, and also chaired the RCN's Industrial Relations Committee. Nevertheless, the two organisations continued to mount joint protests, including a rally at the Albert Hall that attracted 7,000 nurses. Kenneth Robinson, the Shadow Minister of Health, and Jo Grimond, leader of the Liberal Party, were among the speakers. RCN members from many parts of the country began to arrive in Westminster in large groups to lobby their local MP, though this initiative did not originate from RCN headquarters but from nurses in Manchester, and the tactic was widely copied. Branches were encouraged to use their initiative in rousing public support.[68] The government's misery was compounded by independent decisions of arbitration tribunals, awarding civil servants, hospital almoners and psychiatric social workers pay rises well above the recommended 2.5 per cent. COHSE held a ballot on nurses' willingness to strike, and a clear majority endorsed a resolution supporting strike action in principle, but refusing to strike on grounds of conscience. The staff side of the Whitley Council then took the nurses' case to arbitration, and the industrial court awarded an interim increase of up to 7.5 per cent, which the government accepted on the pretext that it was time for a general review of nurses' grades and responsibilities.

The 1962 dispute had a number of lessons for the RCN. It effectively divided the Conservative Party and gained press and parliamentary support, but local branches were sometimes prepared to use more dramatic tactics than RCN headquarters expected. COHSE appealed more directly to the public through its widely reported, and often theatrical demonstrations. COHSE also caused alarm by balloting on strike action, and then acquired moral credit for voting against it. Although, like the RCN, it was not prepared to strike, it gained the reputation of being ready to fight its members' claims by all available means. This was at a time when industrial militancy and union membership among public employees was rapidly increasing, and the unfortunate result for the RCN was that while its own membership remained stagnant, COHSE's membership among female nurses rose.[69] The events of 1962 also revealed a deep reservoir of popular sympathy for nurses, because the public persisted in regarding them as a special case. Translating this goodwill into practical action was difficult, for the public could admire nurses' 'angelic' role while resisting any tax increases to support the NHS. As a result, nurses' pay did not keep pace with the cost of living during the 1960s. Nevertheless, the RCN felt that the dispute had been handled well, and the council thanked Catherine Hall and Betty Davies for their effective public presentation of the RCN's case.

Another feature of the dispute was significant. Before the 1960s, the nursing shortage in the NHS was undisputed, and invariably featured in any discussion of nurses' pay. Yet in 1962 Powell used the argument of market economics – there was no nursing shortage, therefore pay must be adequate. His political opponents claimed that hospital beds were being closed for want of nurses, but Powell revealed that the Ministry of Health kept no statistics on this, and he argued that the overall number of nurses was increasing.[70] In fact, there was no official view of what a hospital establishment should be. Health authorities made their own decisions over staffing within the limits of their budgets and recruited low-paid ancillary staff rather than trained nurses.[71] The RCN's own investigations showed that many hospitals were having difficulty in filling senior nursing posts, and that shortages were often regional, or particularly serious in certain areas of nursing. One issue briefly surfaced in the parliamentary debate and disappeared again: the recruitment of nurses from overseas. Powell's Ministry actively encouraged this, though the focus shifted from 'aliens' (Europeans) recruited after the war to immigrants from the Commonwealth. The Ministry was coy about the statistics, but one estimate suggests that by 1965 around 35 per cent of nursing staff had not been born in Britain.[72] Hence Powell could deny that there was a nursing shortage, even though British nurses were emigrating in large numbers, attracted by higher wages overseas. Immigrant nurses were frequently offered a lower level of training and shunted into areas of nursing where recruitment had long been difficult, particularly psychiatric hospitals and geriatric wards. The RCN's reaction to these events will be discussed later, but the 1962 debate showed that the nursing shortage was no longer a clear-cut issue, but one that raised difficult questions of how to define a 'nurse', and what level of training was desirable.

The RCN was also forced by an adroit manoeuvre from the trade unions on the Whitley Council to reconsider its opposition to overtime pay for nurses. Overtime pay was a standard union demand, but the RCN had long opposed it, arguing that it would side-step the more important issue of low pay in the profession, and preferring to lobby for an overall salary increase of £50 a year in return for nurses agreeing to flexible hours. The RCN also believed that overtime pay would confirm the hospitals' view of student nurses as cheap labour, and encourage students to spend more time in the wards at the expense of their studies. The trade unions refused to accept the RCN's authority to speak for psychiatric nurses and enrolled nurses, and the management side of the Whitley Council was happy to grasp at overtime payments as a cheaper alternative to an overall pay rise. At an agitated RCN council meeting, Catherine Hall explained the dilemma. If the RCN refused the offer of overtime pay on behalf of staff nurses in general hospitals, these nurses would be much aggrieved if they were the only excluded group, and there was no guarantee of a pay rise for them.[73] The RCN also feared to alienate student nurses, some of whom were finding the radical atmosphere of COHSE or the National Union of Students more congenial. All members of the College council were in principle against overtime payments, but after a lengthy discussion, they decided by eleven votes to ten to instruct their representatives on the Whitley Council to vote in favour, except in the case of student nurses, while recording the RCN's displeasure. The management side of the council did not agree the unions' terms, and during the delay, the RCN carried out a referendum of its members that showed a substantial majority in support of overtime pay. Enrolled nurses polled by the National Association of State Enrolled Nurses made the same choice. Students were more divided, though generally in favour of overtime pay, and many agreed with the RCN's argument that overtime undermined their student status. The council agreed in January 1966 to accept overtime in accordance with the members' wishes, except for student nurses.[74] The RCN's faith in the Whitley Council was shaken by these events, and it began to consider alternative forms of negotiation.

Nursing education and nursing structures: the Platt and Salmon reports

While the most publicised actions of the RCN in the early 1960s concerned nurses' pay, education remained a central concern. The first part of this chapter argued that the RCN was becoming more inclusive, yet the College's stance on nurses' training seemed to indicate the opposite. From its beginnings, the RCN had pressed for a delayed entry into a relatively lengthy training, and a basic educational standard for entrants. These demands ran counter to the hospitals' labour requirements, and led to allegations that the RCN was interested only in educating an officer class of middle-class women. Unions like COHSE resented the RCN's claim to represent nurses in pay disputes, while the BMA was sceptical of the RCN's professional credentials, objecting that nurses should not be over-educated. The RCN was caught between the conflicting requirements of trade unionism and professionalism, with the danger that its educational and labour relations departments would operate without reference to one another. In daily practice there was some truth in this: the education staff saw themselves as serving the whole nursing profession; while the professional organisation side served College members only. Nevertheless, in RCN policy the two areas were closely related, since the RCN always saw nurses' status and pay as linked to their standards of education and training. In the 1960s, as educational and professional opportunities for women widened, the RCN became even more concerned with the quality of nurses' training. Its views were certainly hierarchical, as are those of most professional bodies. The BMA, for example, claimed to speak for all members of the medical profession, although there was a great gulf between the affluent consultant and the recently qualified houseman. Doctors, nurses, teachers, lawyers and other professions accepted the notion of hierarchy; but they aimed for a ladder of promotion that would (in theory) give opportunities to all who gained the basic qualifications. This was also the view of the 1960s Labour governments as they opened new universities and expanded higher education. Later critics argued that inequality, rooted in social class, was not overcome by the expansion of higher education; but in the optimistic 1960s a meritocratic society seemed within reach.

The RCN was also sensitive to international influences. In 1957, the International Council of Nurses recommended a broad general programme as a basis for the teaching of specialties in nursing care. The RCN council welcomed the ICN policy and supported the principle of one basic course of nurse training. In 1959 it announced its intention to set up a special committee to consider nurse education in the light of developments since the Horder reports, 'taking into account present trends and future needs in order that the profession itself may retain the initiative in determining policy'.[75] Progress was slow, and it was not until November 1960 that the council agreed the terms of reference and membership of this committee, which was large, high-powered and multi-disciplinary, with experts in general education, sociology, medicine, public health, hospital administration, nurse education and nursing service. The RCN knew that if it hoped to influence government, the committee and its chair must command respect. Catherine Hall became adept at capturing eminent personalities to give their time freely to the RCN, though finding a chair for such an intensive investigation was not easy.[76] The RCN's choices were, in the order named, Sir Ifor Evans, provost of University College, London, Sir John Wolfenden, vice-chancellor of the University of Reading, and Sir David Hughes Parry, professor emeritus in English law, University of London; but none was available. At length Sir Harry Platt, a former president of the Royal College of Surgeons and emeritus professor of orthopaedic surgery at the University of Manchester, agreed to act as chair, and the committee held its first meeting in February 1962.

The Platt Committee planned a major overhaul of nursing education based on five considerations. The first was the existing system's failure to produce sufficient numbers of registered nurses for the needs of the health service. The committee did not share Enoch Powell's view that the supply of nurses was sufficient, and noted the high levels of wastage among nursing recruits. The RCN attributed this to the labour demands of the hospitals taking precedence over the educational needs of students, many of whom gave up before qualifying. Secondly, the growth of the NHS and the complex demands of modern medicine meant that more highly trained nurses were needed. Thirdly, nursing education must adapt to social change and improved educational opportunities. It should be comparable with the training provided by other professions, and sufficiently flexible to deal with demographic change. This meant career breaks to raise a family, and an educational system that welcomed mature students. The Robbins report on higher education (1963) pressed for an expansion of higher education, with a higher participation of women, and nursing would have to attract recruits against this background. The fourth factor was the changing attitude of patients, who were more critical of the care they received, as shown in the emergence of patients' associations. The Platt Committee believed that shortage of staff and antiquated buildings contributed to this dissatisfaction, but patients also resented the authoritarian organisation of hospitals with their inflexible ward routines. Nurses of the future would need to understand sociological and psychological problems in order to adapt to change. The fifth factor was the need to assess experimental schemes in nurse education. Most experiments during the previous decade had been modifications of the traditional system of nurse education, leading to registration on more than one part of the register, but schemes at Manchester, Edinburgh, Glasgow and St Thomas's had shown that full-time nursing students could be trained for registration within two years. These experiments also indicated that nursing could be taught in the universities.

As they proceeded, the Platt Committee became convinced of the urgency of their work and decided to publish their recommendations for reform of basic nursing education as a first report. They then intended to examine advanced education for nurses in a second report, but lack of funds prevented this.[77] Sir Harry Platt and the other medical members of the committee presented their interim report to the RCN council in January 1964.[78] Central to the report was the committee's concept of the nursing team of the future, which somewhat resembled the RCN's response to the Nuffield report of the 1950s. At the head of the team would be the ward sister, who would be a SRN or university graduate, then the staff nurses, also SRNs, then enrolled nurses, the mainstay of the nursing team, then the third-year nursing students and pupils. First- and second-year nursing students would be on the ward for carefully planned nursing experience and would contribute a limited amount of service, while ancillary workers would undertake duties that the committee defined as not essential for nurse training.[79] Nursing students would spend two years in independent schools of nursing, during which time they would gain practical experience in the hospital and community services, and then sit the final state exams. In their third year, still pre-registration, they would be members of the nursing team in a hospital. The overall number of student nurses would be smaller, but the committee believed that wastage would also fall in response to more stimulating training and less routine ward labour. In contrast, the training of pupil nurses (the future SENs) would be on apprenticeship lines, with two years' practical training on the wards similar to the existing training for student nurses. The number of pupil nurses would be increased and their status would be improved. They would no longer be identified mainly with the chronic sick and geriatric hospitals. Although SENs would have a different educational standard from the student nurses,

experienced enrolled nurses would have more responsibility and the opportunity to progress to the status of registered nurse. The committee, as in so
many earlier investigations, wanted to see nursing schools independent of the
hospitals and proposed that they be funded by Exchequer grants channelled
through Regional Nursing Councils. The General Nursing Councils, the statutory bodies, would retain their powers of inspection of new schools of nursing.

   The RCN council generally supported Platt's recommendations, showing
some movement in their position since the Wood report, as discussed in
chapter 4. They were still divided over the proposed separation of the nursing
schools from the hospitals, some members expressing the familiar view that
the high standard of British nursing had been achieved because the nursing
school was part of the hospital. The Platt Committee pressed for immediate
publication of its report, since the Robbins report was being rapidly implemented. Mabel Lawson, president of the RCN, chaired the subsequent council
meetings when the report was discussed in detail. She had been chair of one
the working groups within the Platt Committee, having considerable influence on the report's contents. After much discussion, all but two members of
the council voted in favour of the report, the main point of disagreement
being the loss of labour in the wards if students were not an integral part of
the staff. The College officially launched the Platt report, *A Reform of Nursing
Education*, at a press conference on 17 June 1964. The first print run was sold
out within a week and a further 5,000 copies were printed.[80] The report had
good coverage in the national and provincial newspapers and on BBC television and radio. The College wrote to all MPs, bringing the main points of the
report to their attention, and questions were asked in the House of Commons.
To make sure the proposals were fully understood the College organised a
major conference in October, to present the report to an invited audience of
800, comprising doctors, nurses, educationalists, representatives of local
authorities, hospital management committees, regional hospital boards, professional organisations, trade unions and government departments. The
general secretary wrote to the branch secretaries asking them to arrange local
meetings to discuss the report and offered to send speakers from the Platt
Committee. Major regional conferences were organised over the following
months at which key members of the committee discussed the report. The
Scottish Board, after holding its own conference, reported that they, along
with representatives of the Association of Hospital Matrons and the Scottish
General Nursing Council, were having informal discussions with the officers
of the Scottish Home and Health Department.[81] From articles in the nursing
press and reports of the conferences organised by the College it seems that
the nursing profession welcomed the Platt report and accepted the principle
of separating nurses' education from work on the wards. This principle had
been rejected by the RCN in 1947 when proposed in the Wood report, but by

the 1960s nurses at many levels believed that the needs of modern medicine were more complex than the old apprenticeship system could support. Despite this shift of opinion in the profession, and all the activity to publicise it, both the GNC for England and Wales and the Ministry of Health were slow to respond. It took the former over a year, and the latter two years, to reply.

The medical profession's reaction was more rapid and predictable. The BMA denied that the existing system of nurse training was inadequate. While conceding that there might be a need for a review, they were reluctant to remove student nurses from the bedside, and were not convinced that the educational background of nurses was significant in nursing care. Experience had shown, they argued, that academic ability did not necessarily produce the most efficient nurse.[82] Dr Dennis Barker argued in *The Guardian* that nurses' recruitment was hindered not because the profession's image was too low but because it was already academically too high. In his opinion the Platt reforms envisaged a system of training like that of medical students, and would produce nurses incapable of giving a patient a bed pan.[83] The response of the hospital authorities was more mixed. Some accepted that reform of nursing education was necessary but believed that the Platt reforms were impractical because of staffing problems. Others thought the recommendations too close to the academic American system, and that separating the schools of nursing from the hospitals would undermine the practical basis of British training.[84] In Scotland, where a larger proportion of school leavers went into higher education, Platt's scheme had more support. The nursing sub-committee of Glasgow Royal Infirmary accepted the principle of separating training from nursing service, and agreed that students did not get sufficiently varied nursing experience while they were working on the wards.[85] They had no difficulty in accepting the recommended minimum educational requirement of five O-levels for students, since a high proportion of their own student nurses had already reached this standard.[86] The health services unions were hostile. In the *Health Services Journal*, Jack Jepson of COHSE attacked the report for its 'elitist philosophy', and argued that the Platt reforms would reinforce class distinctions between registered and enrolled nurses.[87] The unions regarded student nurses as employees and believed they would be disadvantaged financially if treated as full-time students. The College and the unions had long disagreed on this point, the unions arguing that the low wages paid to nurses in training kept the wages of ancillary workers down, while the RCN contended that student wages were equivalent to maintenance grants.

Catherine Hall kept the Ministry of Health informed of the progress of the Platt Committee, presumably hoping to prevent a repetition of the events of the 1940s, when the Ministry had ignored the Horder Committee's recommendations. When the Platt report was published, she requested a meeting with the Minister to discuss it, but this was refused while the Ministry consulted other relevant bodies. One of these was the General Nursing Council for England and Wales, which took fifteen months to publish its response.[88] The GNC, a conservative body, was content with its own measures to improve nurse training. These included the reintroduction of a minimum educational requirement, a new syllabus, efforts to increase the number of tutors and clinical instructors, and encouragement of experimental schemes of training. The GNC believed that patients' needs must sometimes take precedence over students' education, and was unwilling to contemplate drastic changes in the staffing of the wards. They criticised Platt for unrealistic assumptions about the numbers of candidates with five O-levels who would be prepared to train as nurses. The GNC also rejected most of Platt's proposals on nurse education, though they acknowledged that the absence of degree courses in nursing was preventing British nurses from obtaining positions of international standing, and supported further investigation into this.

The College was outraged at the GNC's attitude, and attacked it for lack of vision:

> the Platt Committee can only express its serious concern at the seeming com-placency of the statutory nursing body and on the effect which this can well have on the future of British nursing and the part which British nurses will be able to play in the development of the Health Service in this country and in making a contribution to nursing in overseas countries.[89]

The RCN council felt that the GNC was concerned mainly with self-justification.[90] Nursing education had to be sufficiently challenging to break down the widespread belief of parents and teachers that anyone with five O-levels was over-qualified for nursing. If nursing could not compete with other careers then it would have to accept candidates deemed unacceptable by the more demanding professions. The RCN believed that when educational standards were raised for admission to professional training, more people wished to enter. In July 1965 the general secretary took the opportunity of her regular report to the Branches Standing Committee to convey her chagrin at the GNC's 'disappointing and depressing' response. 'These comments did not even damn with faint praise, instead they put forward the view that drastic reform was neither necessary nor desirable: they defended the present system.'[91] Delegates called on the Labour Minister of Health, Kenneth Robinson, to implement the Platt report immediately, and Catherine Hall again requested a meeting. Once more Robinson postponed meeting the College's representatives until his formal consultation process ended. By the time the official GNC response appeared in October 1965 the GNC's position was wavering. Just before publication, the GNC held its five-yearly election, and six members of the new council moved that the previous council's dismissal of the Platt report be reconsidered.[92] By this stage it was too late.

The Minister finally met the College's representatives on 20 July 1966, the same day that his response to Platt was conveyed to the House of Commons in a written answer. His statement, after two years' consultation with the hospital service, the medical profession and the statutory nursing body, was a blow to the RCN. He rejected the principles of the report and agreed with the GNC that there was no need for drastic reform of nurse training.

[The Minister] does not share the Report's implied view that the average registered nurse today is of insufficient calibre for the demands the present and future hospital service is likely to make on her . . . He has certainly received no volume of evidence either from medical organisations or from those concerned with the administration of the hospitals, that the average registered nurse, serving in the average staff nurse or sister post, is proving inadequate for her responsibilities. On the contrary the British nurse seems to enjoy a very high reputation both at home and abroad.[93]

Robinson generally supported the GNC's arguments and did not accept that higher educational requirements for nurse training would attract better-educated students. Entry requirements for trainees might be raised gradually as general educational standards improved. He rejected Platt's recommendation that recruitment of student nurses be reduced to 12,000 annually. Rather, he argued that two or more registered nurses were needed on each ward, not so much for their technical skill, but for their experienced judgement. He also rejected the proposal to set up nurse training schools under regional councils. This recommendation was criticised from all sides because, apart from the cost, student nurses and their teachers might become isolated, without a base in either the hospitals or the colleges of further education. The Minister made some token gestures to encourage experimental training courses, though the RCN publicly criticised his response.[94] Catherine Hall wrote to Robinson:

once again history has repeated itself in relation to nursing education and considerations of short-term expediency rather than of sound long-term planning lay behind the official view that has now been conveyed to the Rcn.[95]

The RCN's support for Platt, never entirely unanimous, has been dismissed by historians as either naïve or elitist.[96] Platt was, in any case, overtaken by proposals for new management structures in the NHS that had different implications for nurse training. Nevertheless, the RCN believed that the Platt report continued to influence new approaches to nursing education. By 1968 there were schools of nursing offering courses linked with universities, preparing students for both state registration and a university degree or diploma. There were special shortened courses for university graduates; a part-time course for mature women was being introduced where students would be supernumerary to service; and negotiations for a university degree in nursing were almost complete.[97] The RCN was perhaps unrealistic in terms of the cost of its proposals, but it was the only large organisation working to reform nurse education to keep abreast with changes in hospital management and national educational standards. By contrast, COHSE and the medical profession, from their different standpoints, made assumptions about nurses' capacity for education based largely on gendered views about what a 'women's profession' might be expected to achieve.

The Ministry soon discovered that hospital training schools could not be improved because of a shortage of qualified tutors, a problem that linked the debate on nursing education to nurses' pay. Although the number of unqualified tutors increased substantially in the 1960s, the number of qualified tutors was static, around 1,150, for the tutors did not receive pay that reflected the extra years spent in training.[98] Poor working conditions and lack of status led to an exodus of qualified tutors, some giving up nursing to take better paid posts in colleges of further education. An already volatile situation was aggravated early in 1968 by the publication of the report of the Prices and Incomes Board on the pay of nurses and midwives. The board accepted that there was a shortage of tutors, but assumed that this would end if their working conditions were more agreeable, and it adopted Platt's idea of larger, more specialised regional training schools to replace the current small ones.[99] It then noted rather feebly that this would have to wait until finances permitted. Tutors' status and pay were not specifically addressed, although the staff side of the Whitley Council had specifically requested this. The RCN was not impressed, and argued that the report downgraded the status of tutors relative to administrative nursing staff, while reinforcing the apprenticeship image of student nurses. The RCN council, backed by the RRB, called for a reappraisal of the career structure for tutors.[100]

The board's report was the last straw for many tutors, and the South Wales Tutor Group called on the RCN to hold a referendum of all tutors asking if they were prepared to withdraw their services if there were no improvement in their conditions and salaries. Some teaching hospitals provided very poor facilities for classes, and the tutors felt undervalued by the hospital authorities, including some senior nursing staff, who resented the removal of students from the wards to attend lectures. The RCN was committed to a no-strike policy where patients were concerned, but a withdrawal of tutors' services raised different issues. The RCN's lawyers advised the council that such action was inconsistent with the Royal Charter and might jeopardise the RCN's charitable status.[101] Instead, after consultation with the other professional bodies, a joint deputation went to the Minister of Health, who immediately appointed a nurse tutor working party. Comprising five representatives each from the RCN and the GNC for England and Wales, and six from two government departments, the working party's remit was to study current and future education and training needs of student and pupil nurses, and the role of nurse teachers. Kathleen Raven, Elizabeth Cockayne's successor as chief nursing officer at the Ministry of Health, was chairman. She believed that nursing needed major changes and planned to use the working party to explore the possibilities.[102] Aware of unrest among nurse tutors, the working party decided to publish an interim report setting out general principles and recommending some short-term measures to relieve the shortage of tutors. The report appeared in 1970, by which time the Ministry of Health had been replaced (in 1968) by the Department of Health and Social Security (DHSS). The department, interested mainly in solving the immediate problem of the disappearing tutors, believed that the working party was following the Platt Committee by pursuing unrealistic objectives, and wished to disband it as soon as possible. The report had a limited circulation, but only at the insistence of the RCN, since the department was reluctant to publish it at all.[103]

The working party knew that it was difficult to predict the type of nurse that would be required in the future. While certain basic nursing skills would always be needed, nurses' training would have to keep pace with clinical developments in hospitals, the extension of group medical practice, and more specialised nursing in the community.[104] The preparation of the student nurse should be flexible, a studentship *and* an apprenticeship, with experience in both the community and the hospital. As the demand for qualified nurses was likely to outstrip supply, the training system should be suited to all abilities, and the working party recommended a modular system of training for student and pupil nurses.[105] The underlying principles of the Platt report therefore continued to flicker, even though forcefully rejected by government a few years previously.

Another issue that, in the RCN's view, was linked to the problems of nurses' education and pay was their role in hospital management, since the hierarchical traditions derived from the nineteenth century could not keep pace with changes in the hospital service.[106] By the end of the 1950s it was difficult to attract suitable candidates for senior posts and in 1959 the College council set up two inquiries, one on salary structures, the other on nursing administration. The first, in spite of five years of investigation and considerable expense, was abortive, as the complex questionnaires into pay and conditions could not be analysed effectively.[107] The second inquiry was completed in 1961, but by this time the government had decided to conduct its own investigation, and announced the appointment of Brian Salmon as chairman of a committee to 'advise on the senior nursing staff structure in the hospital service, the administrative function of respective grades and the methods of preparing staff to occupy them'. Salmon, chairman of Lyons Catering Co., was expected to bring a managerial approach to hospital administration. The 1962 pay dispute caused delay, and the Salmon Committee did not start work until

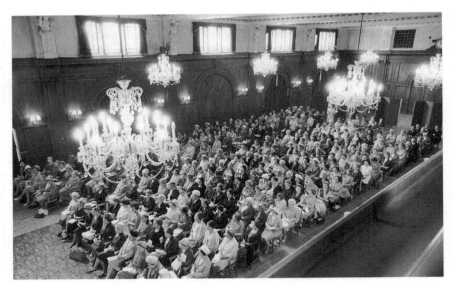

6.3 Annual general meeting, golden jubilee, London, 1966.

November 1963.[108] In the meantime a special committee of the RCN was collecting further evidence, and this appeared in 1964 as *Administering the Hospital Nursing Service, a Review.*[109]

The RCN's report accepted that the administrative framework of nursing was out of date. The structure was not attractive to new recruits, and evidence from the profession showed that nurses had little inclination to fill the posts at the top of the administrative ladder, such as matron, chief male nurse, deputy or assistant matron, or night superintendent. These positions compared unfavourably with other administrators in the NHS. Comparatively low salaries were equated with low status, and the image of the nurse manager was of an individual beset by many problems, never completely off duty, yet without the satisfaction of close contact with the patients. Within the clinical structure the ward sister's post had undergone the greatest changes as a result of the advances in medicine and surgery, the ever-increasing speed in the turnover of patients, and the mounting complexity of administration. An experienced ward sister was at the pinnacle of clinical nursing, yet she could not progress further without moving into an administrative post. The RCN considered this a waste of her skills, and contrasted her position with that of the medical profession, where clinical consultants were better rewarded than administrators.

The Salmon report, published in 1966, recommended a new structure of nursing posts in the hospitals. Nurses in senior management posts (chief and principal nursing officers) should play a major part in formulating nursing policy in their hospital group. Nurses in middle management (senior nursing officers and nursing officers) would work out the detailed application of policy in individual hospitals or specialised units, while the ward sisters, charge nurses and staff nurses would carry policy into practice. The report emphasised that management training for the new grades of nursing administrators was essential, and it proposed a national committee and regional nursing committees to organise this. The Salmon Committee was surprised that the nursing profession occupied a secondary position within the health service and that the right of nurses to speak on nursing policy was ignored when the NHS was established.[110] Salmon attributed this to 'a seeming inability on the part of nurses to assert the rights of their emergent profession'.[111] This was unfair, given the prevailing prejudice against women as managers. When viewed against the background of the equal pay campaign of 1944–55, and the comparable problems of women in the civil service and other professions, nurses were not unique in failing to push their way into management. Additionally, nurses had to contend with many in the medical establishment who preferred deferential nurses to managerial ones.

With the appointment of the Salmon Committee there was little reason for the RCN to publicise its own report on the reform of hospital nursing administration, and it put its resources into co-operating with the Salmon Committee. It submitted written, oral and statistical evidence, and Catherine Hall had many friendly and informal meetings with Brian Salmon.[112] Consequently, the RCN received the Salmon report very favourably, believing it to be consistent with the principles of its own report, *Administering the Hospital Nursing Service*.[113] If the new structure were implemented, nurses could influence policy at the highest level in the health service. The RCN promoted discussion of the report in many regional conferences addressed by members of the Salmon Committee. The only serious disagreement was over nursing education, for the RCN regretted that the Salmon Committee did not adopt Platt's recommendations on separating nurses' education from work in the wards.

The Minister of Health and the Secretary of State for Scotland accepted Salmon's recommendations, and pilot schemes were scheduled for 1967 and 1968. The Salmon Committee regarded such schemes as essential to test the new system, and intended to modify it in the light of experience. However, in the autumn of 1968 the government announced that the new grading structure must be in place in all hospital groups by the beginning of 1969. This was a direct result of the report of the Prices and Incomes Board, which demanded early implementation because two different salary structures for nurses in the NHS would be unacceptable. The profession was also calling for acceleration of the new grading structure with its higher rates of pay, and the RCN membership voted overwhelmingly for it at the meeting of their representative body in July 1968. In retrospect, Salmon considered that the government's decision to roll out the new structure without pilot studies was 'outrageous', since his committee regarded these as integral to the whole scheme.[114]

Hospital authorities often disliked the Salmon reforms because of the expense of training nurse administrators and the cost of replacing them on the wards. But the most vocal opposition came from the medical profession. Despite many consultations between the royal medical colleges and the Salmon Committee, the doctors were convinced that Salmon would ruin the health service. They believed that the best nursing staff would move into administrative posts, to the detriment of clinical work.[115] The RCN tried to defuse medical opposition, and arranged meetings and joint conferences with the BMA. One such conference, attended by over 700 doctors, nurses and administrators, met in November 1970, with the theme of 'Harmony in management'. It discussed the implementation of the Salmon structure and the similar recommendations for new managerial structures for the hospitals' medical staff, which the doctors were resisting.[116] But despite these efforts, medical opposition to the Salmon reforms remained strong. J. W. Paulley, physician to the Ipswich Hospitals, wrote an article in the *Nursing Times* entitled, 'Is it too late to scrap Salmon – a charter for incompetents?' Paulley described British nurses as 'lemmings plunging to their doom' in their rush to embrace Salmon.[117] After a meeting in February 1971 with the BMA's Central Committee for Hospital Medical Services, the RCN representatives reported that the doctors persisted in speaking of the reformed structure as 'an unmitigated disaster'. The new system ranked nurses in numbered grades, and the doctors were particularly incensed over grade 7 nursing officers who allegedly spent their day 'going up and down stairs with bits of paper'.[118] The RCN had evidence that many ward sisters who became nursing officers were satisfied in their new role, and that where the new structure was introduced as Salmon intended it resulted in improved nursing care, but the medical profession refused to accept this.[119] As late as 1977, in their evidence to the Royal Commission on the Health Service, the BMA (against much evidence to the contrary), stated that the Salmon reforms had encouraged the most capable nurses to leave clinical work for administration, and that administrators were multiplying at the expense of the wards.[120]

The RCN's support for Salmon's reforms backfired in a number of ways, and caused some division in the profession. Although Salmon intended that all nurse managers should be properly trained for their new responsibilities, the rapid introduction of the new structure made this impossible and many nurses took on their new tasks without any training. Some health authorities paid little more than lip service, and a common experience that nurses recount from this period was that the title on their door was altered without the job actually changing.[121] Other authorities were heavy-handed in their managerial approach, and the matron and several senior nurses at Guy's Hospital resigned in protest. Yet the Salmon reforms undoubtedly gave nurses greater influence over policy in the health service, and June Clark believes that their real value was in preparing nurse managers for their important role after the health service was restructured in 1974.[122] Salmon's critics argued that a new class of nurse managers gained too much power in the hospitals, and that the NHS valued administrative skills more highly than clinical ability.[123] As noted at the beginning of this chapter, the main beneficiaries of the new system were a small group of male nurses, who by 1972 occupied a third of the highest administrative nursing posts.[124]

Raise the roof!

By the later 1960s, the RCN was making strenuous efforts to establish itself as the main representative of the nursing profession. Its position was uneasy, because its leadership had no wish to jettison the RCN's status as a professional association, or to endanger its tax advantages as a charity. Yet there were doubts concerning its right to act as a negotiating body in pay claims, even though it had been doing so for several decades. The RCN regularly intervened on behalf of members working for industry or local government, and had to negotiate with organisations as disparate as the Coal Board and the film industry. The RCN persuaded many employers to negotiate with it as though it were a trade union, but it lacked a union's legal safeguards against actions for damages. The South Wales tutors' request for a ballot on withdrawal of tutors' services in 1968 raised the difficult question whether, under the terms of its charter, the RCN could legally involve itself in salaries and working conditions at all, since it was a professional and educational body, not a trade union. The tutors' grievances surfaced at the close of a particularly turbulent decade in British economic and political life. The Labour government, elected in 1964, struggled to cope with a volatile economy, rapid inflation, archaic management and disgruntled workers. Trade unions were in danger of losing touch with their local branches, and inter-union disputes and lightning unofficial strikes exacerbated a tense situation. By 1968 Harold Wilson's second government, having attempted both voluntary and statutory wage controls with little success, was actively seeking ways of curbing the unions and preventing the unofficial strikes by small groups of workers that characterised this period.[125] The RCN's solicitors advised that the tutors' ballot should not be taken, because the RCN risked legal action and the loss of its charitable status if it behaved like a union.[126]

As the South Wales problem showed, the RCN, like the trade unions, was under pressure from its members. There was a growing sense of grievance over pay, especially because more powerful unions were able to circumvent government pay policy. By the later 1960s, nurses' pay was once again falling badly behind other public employees, and, as the BMA pointed out, a non-resident staff nurse might earn less than a dustman.[127] The government's prices and incomes policy restricted pay rises to 4.5 per cent. Nurses who felt that the RCN was failing to protect their interests launched their own protests. Patricia Veal, administrative sister at the South-Western Hospital at Clapham, led a growing number of militant nurses in the United Nurses' Association, and organised pay demonstrations in 1968. She was adept at capturing head-lines to criticise the government, the NHS and the RCN. In 1969, the NHS introduced a 'pay as you eat' policy, giving cash payment to nurses in lieu of free hospital meals. The sum offered fell far short of what the nurses' associa-tions considered fair, especially for student nurses. Veal picketed Whitley Council meetings and led a small, windswept group of nurses to protest in Henrietta Place. As *The Times* reported:

> She posed for the photographers using a yard broom to sweep dirt under an old bit of carpet on the pavement outside the RCN to symbolise that inside there was too much sweeping of difficulties under the carpet.[128]

The RCN was in fact planning another major pay campaign. Given the legal constraints on its activities, the RCN had to use traditional tactics: publicity and political pressure. The 1969 meeting of the RRB was memorable, not only for the decision to widen membership of the RCN, but also for its militant tone. The president, Mary Blakeley, stated that 'Morale in the nursing profes-sion is lower and dissatisfaction is more rife than it has ever been within my memory'.[129] Catherine Hall made an impassioned speech on salaries, and received a lengthy standing ovation. This was the first announcement of the 'Raise the roof' campaign, a highly organised attempt to raise public and political support for a substantial increase in nurses' pay. The campaign, while aiming at a general pay rise, was so named because of its emphasis on the upper end of the salary scale, seen as vital in motivating nurses to stay in the profession. 'Raise the roof' was also a phrase deliberately breaking with what COHSE's historian terms the 'flowery hat' image of the College.[130] The RCN's demands were complex, giving different weights to the various grades of nursing, but they prioritised qualifications and experience, and demanded an average pay rise of 28 per cent. COHSE saw this approach as yet another sign of the RCN's elitist attitudes, but the campaign aimed to improve the pay of all nurses, including those outside the hospitals. In 1969 the RCN also had a more professional team to run its campaign than in 1962.

The RCN planned a three-stage campaign. The first stage would concen-trate on national publicity and on marshalling the profession's support; the second on regional protest meetings to push the Whitley Council towards a favourable settlement; and the third would be political, with public pressure on MPs and private negotiations with government officials. Betty Newstead shared with Catherine Hall the task of negotiating with the Ministry of Health; de Cent handled public relations, and Monica Baly was called from her tasks as area organiser to the London headquarters to organise the lobbying of MPs. Local branches of the RCN soon received their battle orders, and set up action committees. A million copies of a letter stating the nurses' case were circulated for distribution to the public, to be signed and posted to Richard Crossman, the new Secretary of State for Social Services.[131] Many newspapers co-operated by printing the letter for their readers to cut out. It became standard procedure in this and later campaigns for the press to focus on the working lives of individual nurses. These were usually young, photogenic women, but local newspapers also expressed their loyalty to long-serving local nurses. A Wigan paper compared the militant tactics of the trade unions to the 'gentle voice' of Sister Dorothy Dunsford, who, after twenty-two years at Wigan Royal Infirmary, had broken with her peaceable instincts to become the local press officer for 'Raise the roof': 'It's because of dedicated people like sister Dunsford that this newspaper is backing the "More Pay" Campaign'.[132]

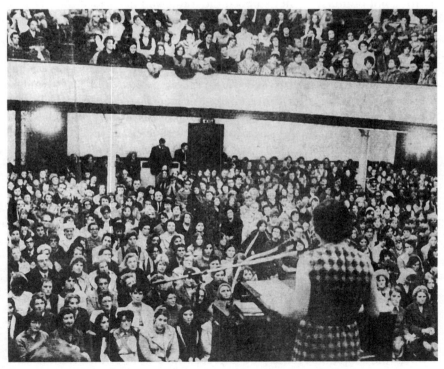

6.4 Catherine Hall, addressing meeting in Manchester, 3 December 1969.

Catherine Hall and Betty Newstead carried the campaign to the regions with meetings in Edinburgh, Cardiff, Newcastle, Manchester, Winchester, Cambridge, Belfast and Sheffield. Accustomed to low levels of branch attendance, the RCN leaders were taken aback by the passionate response from the profession. In Edinburgh an audience of 1,000 was expected, but three times this number turned up. Some 500 nurses could not get into the hall, and staged an impromptu demonstration in Princes Street, waving banners and shouting slogans. After the meeting, Catherine Hall and Betty Newstead borrowed a police megaphone and spoke to them, warning that they would forfeit public sympathy if they did not protest in an orderly manner.[133] The Manchester meeting was even more disruptive. This time, the RCN booked two overflow halls as well as the main venue, but around 6,000 nurses arrived in coaches from all over the region. On a cold, wet night, the general secretary, in a commanding check ensemble, addressed an excitable duffel-coated audience to tremendous applause. In view of the large crowd unable to get into the halls, she proposed to repeat the evening's proceedings, and those with seats were urged to give them up to those outside; but Peter Street descended into chaos. Thousands of nurses marched with banners and chanted 'Give us salaries, not peanuts'.[134] They stopped the traffic and blockaded the Granada TV station. As in Edinburgh, Catherine Hall appealed to them to go home, but was met with cries of 'Not likely!' The crowd remained good-humoured, and dispersed after an hour. Similar scenes took place in Cardiff, where 1,500 crowded into a hall intended for 900, local florists donated flowers for the occasion, and the Pendyrus Male Voice Choir greeted Betty Newstead (a Welshwoman) with 'A welcome in the hillsides' and Catherine Hall with 'Ilkley Moor'.[135] At Winchester there was more overcrowding, and the mayor pledged his support. By this stage, the press were referring to Catherine Hall as 'the General'.[136]

As in 1962, groups of workers donated an hour's pay to the campaign, sometimes with the encouragement of their employers, who also contributed. By a stroke of luck for the nurses, if not for the patient, Graham Hill, the celebrated racing driver, had just been seriously injured in a 150 m.p.h. crash. He left hospital in a wheelchair decorated with 'Fair pay for nurses' stickers, and announced his support for the nurses to a massive press reception. The publicity continued for several days as the gallant Hill treated his nurses to a private film showing and champagne party. Although the public, including even the obstructed drivers of Manchester, greeted protesting nurses with cheers and applause, the RCN leaders feared that protests would get out of control. Nursing discipline, however, meant that the RCN was not faced with the local walkouts that affected many unions where the leadership lost authority over the shop floor; rather, the unprecedented local demonstrations gave the RCN ammunition for the next stage of the campaign and gained the full attention of the public. Catherine Hall may have been surprised by the strength of feeling at the rallies, but it was a measure of her leadership that she was immediately able to take advantage of it. *The Telegraph*, one of the few papers to make the RCN a target of anti-union sentiment, nevertheless admired the success of the publicity campaign, which 'involved the public voluntarily instead of holding them up to ransom'.

> No trade union has ever before marched into battle with the names of the Queen, the Queen Mother and Princess Margaret emblazoned on its banners, so it is not perhaps surprising that the Royal College of Nursing, which is blessed with such an august patronage, has a rather schizophrenic way of slapping in a pay claim.[137]

In fact, RCN staff had to ensure that Princess Margaret was not accused of partiality. They hastily removed campaign posters from the walls in Henrietta Place before her first visit as a patron, in case the press managed to photograph her next to a militant slogan.

Unusually, the nurses had a friendly reception from the Secretary of State. Richard Crossman, appointed in 1968, astounded the nursing staff of the Department of Health by taking an interest in their work, and genuinely believed that the nursing profession was badly treated and underpaid. He wished to make a special case for nurses, though by October 1969 the government was beset on all sides by wage demands, as Crossman noted in his diary after a particularly depressing Cabinet meeting:

> the whole industrial field . . . in complete anarchy, with strikes in the motor-car industry, the whole of the coal mines on strike, including the prosperous fields, and now this madness affecting the nurses, who are steaming up at their conference at Harrogate.[138]

While the RCN was engaged in raising the roof, Crossman was instructing his department to draw up a new schedule for nurses' pay, to bring senior nurses more in line with graduate teachers. (The teachers were concurrently holding a series of disruptive actions.) He also wanted a new charter for nurses 'to make them feel we really care about them, while facing the fact that for the next few months we can do little about wages'.[139] Crossman had to battle not only with the Chancellor, who was trying to restrain government expenditure, and with Barbara Castle, who was in charge of prices and incomes policy, but also with the Education Secretary, who feared further agitation by the teachers if nurses' salaries were increased. Crossman enlisted Brian Abel-Smith, a special adviser to his department and a personal friend, to write his statement to the Cabinet in support of the nurses.[140] Professor Abel-Smith drew on his wide expertise in social administration, and his exceptional knowledge of the history of the nursing profession, to make the nurses' case. By January 1970

Crossman prevailed, on the grounds that the nurses were a historically under-paid group, and he won for them a remarkable 22 per cent increase in salary.

The pay rise, however, was to be staggered over two years. The RCN found this unacceptable at a time of rapid inflation, and began stage three of the campaign. As in 1962, coach loads of nurses arrived from all over the country to lobby their local MPs. The local press took much interest in the reaction of their elected representative to the nurses' demands, and MPs of all parties soon realised that a churlish response, publicised by offended nursing deputations, was a dangerous tactic in view of the imminent general election. Most were emollient and promised their support; but a few stood out. The Labour MP Richard Kelley told his deputation that they were too ladylike and that, as working women, they should be in a proper union, causing one of them to report to her local newspaper that 'We were all so disgusted it took our breath away . . . It was a good thing I didn't have an umbrella'.[141] The newly elected Jeffrey Archer failed to meet his deputation, and had to apologise publicly for a mix-up in his diary. Fifty MPs from all parties signed a motion in favour of the nurses' claim. The Cabinet capitulated in March 1970, and conceded an immediate pay increase of 20 per cent for one year, with another increase the next. Nurses at all levels received more pay, though the students were dissatisfied, because charges for their hospital accommodation and meals were immediately raised and eroded much of their gains.

Conclusion

Although even the record pay rise achieved by 'Raise the roof' was soon over-whelmed by inflation in the 1970s, the RCN emerged from the 1960s greatly enlarged and strengthened. Membership continued to rise, by nearly 70 per cent between 1969 and 1971, and the RCN could claim more convincingly that it represented many kinds of nurse, though other health service unions also grew rapidly.[142] New leadership and new forms of organisation expanded the RCN's appeal to a wider section of the nursing profession, including groups that the founders had excluded, particularly male nurses and enrolled nurses. Acceptance of change was also reflected – although with dissension – in the College's views of nursing education. At a time of rapid social change and expanding opportunities for women in higher education, the College council accepted Platt's view that nurse training should not be dictated by the needs of the hospitals, and should be separated from work on the wards. They were unable to convince either the government or many in the medical profession on this point.

The 1960s also set the scene for the RCN's involvement in trade unionism. The pay disputes of that time revealed a new militancy among nurses, and the RCN leadership had to respond. The sudden jump in membership after 'Raise the roof' indicates that it did so successfully. The RCN's activities were becoming ever more complex – monitoring professional standards, lobbying government over health policy, dealing with public relations, providing specialised training, and defending its members' interests in the workplace. Many people assumed, when the RCN spoke out for nurses, that it was a trade union. In Northampton, the local trades council, thinking that the RCN was a union affiliated to the TUC, proposed to support it during the 1969 campaign; but reversed this decision when an indignant COHSE representative corrected the mistake.[143] The RCN was not a trade union, and in the early 1970s its leaders had no intention that it should become one, but the politics of the times were forcing it in that direction.

Notes

1 See Appendix 2.
2 'Dame Catherine – this is your life', *NM* supplement, 21 April 1982, pp. ii–iv.
3 RCNA T330, interview with Betty Newstead, 2005.
4 RCNA T15, transcript of interview with Dame Catherine Hall, 1987, p. 5.
5 RCNA T15, p. 13. The intrepid interviewer was Anne Marie Rafferty.
6 TNA MH55/2059, memo 3 Aug. 1945. As with most statistics on nurses, these are highly suspect, and do not agree with figures produced by the Royal Commission on Equal Pay (see chapter 4).
7 Abel-Smith, *Nursing Profession*, p. 189. His figure refers to 1949.
8 The GNC was prevented from requiring specific educational standards of nursing recruits until 1962, but individual hospitals could impose their own requirements.
9 White, *Effects of the NHS on the Nursing Profession*, pp. 140–2.
10 See discussion and memorandum, CM Feb. 1957, pp. 66–7 and pp. 82–5.
11 RCN/26/1/4, Association of Hospital Matrons minutes, 19 Nov. 1947.
12 RCNA T329, interview with Frank Rice, 2007.
13 TNA MH 55/1971, memorandum 2 Sept. 1952.
14 MRC 229/6/C/CO/3/2, Guild of Nurses, memorandum respecting the position of state-registered male nurses who have been called up for military service.
15 TNA MH55/2059, F. Goodall to Ministry of Health, 28 Nov. 1945.
16 TNA MH 55/1971, Ministry of Health draft memo, 5 July 1956. Abel-Smith, *Nursing Profession*, p. 257 gives a census figure of 19,144 male trained nurses in 1951 in England and Wales. This would include nurses not employed by the NHS.
17 TNA MH55/1971, T. H. Carruthers to Home Office, 10 July 1956.
18 Trevor Clay, the first male general secretary, who qualified before men were accepted, firmly believed this, but there is no hard evidence for it. RCN/17/7/16, press cuttings, *Daily Mail* 9 July 1982. See also Catherine Hall RCNA T15, p. 14.
19 CM Feb. 1957, pp. 66–7.
20 *AR* 1960 p. 5.
21 *The Times* 24 June 1960, p. 9.

22 RCN/1/2/1/1.
23 Celia Davies, *Gender and the Professional Predicament in Nursing* (Buckingham: Open University Press, 1995), especially chapter 5. See also Joan Evans, 'Men nurses: a historical and feminist perspective', *Journal of Advanced Nursing* 47: 3 (2004), 321–8 for an overview of the arguments. For an NHS survey, see Louise R. Finlayson and James Y. Nazroo, *Gender Inequalities in Nursing Careers* (London: Policy Studies Institute, 1997).
24 CM 23 March 1961, p. 107.
25 RCNA T15, Catherine Hall, transcript, p. 14.
26 Laurence Dopson, 'When the College banned men', *NT* Supplement, 21 April 1982, p. 8.
27 Derek J. Hawes, *The Cowdray Club 1922–1974* (privately published, 2005), p. 12.
28 Carpenter, *Working for Health*, chapter 15.
29 Abel-Smith calculated 224,616 full-time equivalents from the 1951 census, but it is not clear whether all these nurses were in active employment. At that stage both register and roll listed women who probably worked infrequently or had retired from nursing, but may have called themselves 'nurses' in the census. Numbers of nurses in other unions and professional organisations were much smaller than the RCN/COHSE, though the COHSE membership also included all types of staff.
30 W. G. Runciman, 'Explaining union density in twentieth-century Britain', *Sociology* 25 (1991), 699.
31 Dopson, 'When the College banned men', p. 8.
32 Helen M. Sweet and Rona Dougall, *Community Nursing and Primary Healthcare in Twentieth-Century Britain* (New York and Abingdon: Routledge, 2008), pp. 177–8.
33 CM 18 March 1965, p. 90.
34 CM 20 Jan. 1966, p. 84.
35 CM 28 Jan. 1971, p. 33.
36 RCN/17/4/3, press cuttings, *Irish News* 26 March 1971.
37 CM April 1965, Report to Council from Branches Committee, p. 147.
38 CM March 1966, p. 160.
39 CM April 1966, p. 204.
40 CM April 1969, pp. 79–81.
41 CM April 1969, p. 31.
42 RCN/4/1945/2, Publicity and Public Relations Committee, minutes 1960–61.
43 CM Nov. 1965, p. 530.
44 RCN/4/1964/1, working party on the structure and purpose of the sections, 1960.
45 *NT* Supplement, 12 May 1967, pp. 17–19. The new constitutions came into effect in August 1967.
46 *An Exploratory Study of the Rcn Membership Structure, by the Tavistock Institute of Human Relations* (London: Royal College of Nursing, 1973), p. 16.
47 RCN/4/1964, public relations aspects of the Branches Standing Committee meetings.
48 Barbara Robb, *Sans Everything: a Case to Answer* (Nelson: London, 1967).

49 *AR* 1971, p. 26, reported a profit of £600 from the exhibition, and pointed out that this could easily become £3,000 if members took a more lively interest in it.

50 RCN/3/9/20, general secretary's reports to the Branches Standing Committee.

51 Olwen Caradoc Evans was a Welsh cartographer with an international reputation. Her papers are held at the National Library of Wales. She was a health visitor and former secretary of the RCN's Public Health Section. Hetty Hopkins was one of 'the gang of four', along with Eileen Rees, Miriam Gough and Mary Davies, who made the Welsh Board possible.

52 RCNA T101, interview with Hetty Hopkins, 1994.

53 'Nursing in Wales', Special Supplement, *NS* 12 June 1991, p. 3.

54 Sir Frederick Leggett was a retired civil servant, former deputy secretary to the Ministry of Labour 1940–45. He had an active post-retirement career as a trouble-shooter in industrial relations.

55 Keith Newstead was appointed to the College staff in 1960. RCNA T330, interview with Betty Newstead, 2005.

56 The indemnity insurance cover was up to £25,000 at this time.

57 CM July 1961, p. 276.

58 RCNA T19, interview with Peggy Nuttall, 1987.

59 The Johnson & Johnson offer was for £6,000 per year for two years in the first instance and allowed the College to raise further revenue from advertising.

60 CM 18 July 1967, pp. 208–14.

61 Dingwall, Rafferty and Webster, *Introduction to the Social History of Nursing*, p. 112.

62 Alan Sked and Chris Cook, *Post-War Britain: a Political History*, 3rd edn (London: Penguin, 1990), pp. 161–2.

63 For COHSE's tactics, see Carpenter, *Working for Health*, pp. 312–15; *The Times* 5 April 1962, p. 10.

64 *The Times* 10 May 1962, p. 18.

65 *The Times* 26 March 1962, p. 5, and 16 May 1962, p. 6.

66 *Hansard*, 5th series 659 (1961–62), 1038.

67 Ibid., 1047.

68 CM 12 April 1962, p. 151 and 17 May 1962, p. 199.

69 Carpenter, *Working for Health*, p. 315.

70 *Hansard*, 5th series, 659 (1961–62), 946–7.

71 Baly, *Nursing and Social Change*, p. 219.

72 Ibid., p. 221.

73 CM 1 Feb. 1964, pp. 86–8.

74 CM 20 Jan 1966, pp. 4–7.

75 CM April 1959, pp. 175–9.

76 CM Nov. 1960, p. 444, and March 1961, p. 84.

77 RCN/4/1964/2.

78 There was a considerable overlap between the committee and the council, with eight committee members being members of the council.

79 CM 17 Jan. 1964, pp. 5–6.

80 Over one thousand complimentary copies of the report were distributed. The cost of this was subsequently covered by the large number of copies sold.

81 CM Sept. 1964, p. 358.
82 RCN/4/1964/2, British Medical Association, 'Comments of the nursing sub-committee of the central consultants and specialists committee on Platt report', n.d.
83 RCN/4/1964/2, press cuttings, Dennis Barker, 'The case against Platt', *The Guardian* 18 June 1965.
84 RCN/4/1964/2, comments from Group Nursing Advisory Committee of South West London Hospital Group, Oct. 1964.
85 RCN/4/1964/2, Board of Management for Glasgow Royal Infirmary and Associated Hospitals, report of a sub-committee appointed by the Nursing Education Sub-committee to consider the Platt Report on the Reform of Nursing Education, n.d.
86 Scottish public examinations at this level were called O-grades.
87 Quoted in Carpenter, *Working for Health*, pp. 321–2.
88 Bendall and Raybould, *History of the General Nursing Council for England and Wales*, p. 200, state that the GNC response was published in October 1965, although the College appears to have received a copy in April. See RCN/4/1964/2.
89 RCN/4/1964/2, Royal College of Nursing, 'Main points contained in the General Nursing Council's comments and suggested replies'.
90 CM Oct. 1965, p. 395.
91 RCN/3/9/20, general secretary's reports to Branches Standing Committee.
92 Bendall and Raybould, *History of the General Nursing Council for England and Wales*, p. 201.
93 RCN/4/1964/2, written answer to question by Mr Arnold Shaw. See also TNA DT34/202, draft conclusions on the Platt report, [1966], p. 3.
94 RCN/4/1964, Platt report, and CM July 1966, pp. 294–6.
95 RCN/4/1964/2, C. Hall to K. Robinson, 25 July 1966.
96 Dingwall et al., *Introduction to the Social History of Nursing*, pp. 120–1, attacks its elitism. Webster, *Health Services Since the War. Vol. 2*, pp. 260–1, argues that government departments were generally sympathetic with Platt's recommendations, but regarded them as completely unrealistic.
97 RCN/4/1964/2, C. Hall to editor of *Hospital Magazine*, 5 Aug. 1968.
98 RCNA pamphlet collection, *Report of the Nurse Tutor Working Party* (DHSS: 1970), p. 11.
99 National Board for Prices and Incomes, *Report No. 60. Pay of Nurses and Midwives in the National Health Service*, Cmnd 3585 (London: HMSO, 1968), pp. 857–8.
100 Royal College of Nursing, *Comment by the Rcn Council on Report No. 60 of the National Board for Prices and Incomes* (London: 1968), p. 6.
101 CM May 1968, pp. 104–8.
102 RCNA T30, interview with Dame Kathleen Raven, 1988.
103 RCNA, *Report of the Nurse Tutor Working Party*, p. 11. See also Webster, *Health Services since the War. Vol. 2*, pp. 260–1.
104 RCNA, *Report of the Nurse Tutor Working Party*, p. 3.
105 Ibid., pp. 4–6.
106 White, *Effects of the NHS on the Nursing Profession*, pp. 78–9.

107 RCNA T172, interview with Marjorie Simpson, 1986.

108 Scott, *Influence of the Staff of the Ministry of Health*, pp. 169–70 and RCNA T192, interview with Brian Salmon, 1990.

109 Royal College of Nursing, *Administering the Hospital Nursing Service, a Review*, 1964. The findings of the survey were included in the report as an appendix.

110 White, *Effects of the NHS on the Nursing Profession*, pp. 52–88, for a discussion of the attitudes of the nursing profession towards the challenge from the lay administrators following the introduction of the NHS.

111 Ministry of Health, Scottish Home and Health Department, *Report of the Committee on Senior Nursing Staff Structure* [Salmon report] (London: HMSO, 1966), p. 4.

112 RCNA T192, interview with Brian Salmon, 1990. He repeatedly stressed his high regard for Catherine Hall's advice and ability.

113 Royal College of Nursing and National Council of Nurses of the United Kingdom, *Comment on Salmon* (London: RCN, 1966), p. 3.

114 RCN T192, interview with Brian Salmon, 1990.

115 Ibid.

116 'Cogwheel' was the name given to Sir George Godber's committee that argued for a management restructuring of medical services in the hospital, in a similar hierarchical manner to the Salmon recommendations. Although 'Cogwheel' reported in 1967, the doctors were sceptical of it, and it was implemented on a voluntary basis, unlike the Salmon recommendations. *Lancet* 12 Dec. 1970; Webster, *Health Services Since the War. Vol. 2*, pp. 311–14.

117 J. W. Paulley, 'Is it too late to scrap Salmon – a charter for incompetents?', *NT* 18 Feb. 1971, pp. 212–13.

118 RCN/15/1/6/1, report of a meeting of RCN representatives with the British Medical Association held 4 February 1971.

119 RCNA T334, interview with Kathie Whelan, 2007.

120 June Clark, 'Nurses as managers', in Baly, *Nursing and Social Change*, p. 285.

121 RCNA T334, interview with Kathie Whelan, 2007.

122 Clark, 'Nurses as managers', pp. 285–6.

123 White, *Effects of the NHS on the Nursing Profession*, pp. 264–5.

124 *Report of the Committee on Nursing*, Chairman Professor Asa Briggs [Briggs report] Cmnd 5115 (London: HMSO, 1972), p. 415.

125 M. W. Kirby, 'Supply-side management', in N. F. R. Crafts and N. W. C. Woodward (eds), *The British Economy Since 1945* (Oxford: Clarendon Press, 1991), pp. 247–8.

126 CM 16 May 1968, pp. 104–8.

127 RCN/17/4/1, press cuttings, *BMJ* 8 Nov. 1969. Supporters of COHSE considered such comparisons an example of the snobbish attitudes of the professions.

128 *The Times* 16 May 1969, p. 4.

129 Ibid.

130 Carpenter, *Working for Health*, p. 355.

131 This holder of this new post, involving both health and social security, had a seat in the Cabinet. Previous Ministers of Health under the post-war Conservative governments did not have a Cabinet position.

132 RCN/17/4/1, press cuttings, *Wigan Evening Post and Chronicle* 4 Dec. 1969.

133 RCN/17/4/1, press cuttings, *Scotsman* 18 Nov. 1969.

134 RCN/17/4/1, press cuttings, *Evening News* [Bolton] 3 Dec. 1969. This must have been one of the first variants of 'pay, not peanuts', the title of a later campaign.

135 RCN/17/4/1, press cuttings, *NT* 4 Dec. 1969.

136 RCN/17/4/1, press cuttings, *Hampshire Chronicle* 13 Dec. 1969.

137 RCN17/4/1, press cuttings, *Sunday Telegraph* 7 Dec. 1969.

138 Richard Crossman, *The Diaries of a Cabinet Minister. Vol. 3, Secretary of State for Social Services, 1968–70* (London: Hamish Hamilton and Jonathan Cape, 1977), vol. 3, p. 695.

139 Crossman, *Diaries*, pp. 699–700. The miners' strikes were unofficial.

140 Crossman, *Diaries*, p. 768. Abel-Smith's *History of the Nursing Profession* appeared in 1960.

141 RCN/17/4/1, press cuttings, *Doncaster Evening Post* 3 Feb. 1970.

142 COHSE's membership also increased by about 60 per cent between 1969 and 1973, though at this stage its main nursing support was still in the mental hospitals. See Carpenter, *Working for Health*, p. 33. For comparative figures with the RCN see Hart, *Behind the Mask*, p. 133.

143 RCN/17/4/1, press cuttings, [Northampton] *Chronicle and Echo* 22 Jan. 1970. The local press was frequently confused about the RCN's status.

7

A professional union

One of Richard Crossman's admirable traits as a politician was to listen to people who knew what they were talking about. Sharing a taxi with the Secretary of State on his way to a meeting, Dame Kathleen Raven persuaded him that a general review of nursing was essential.[1] The government was already planning a reform of the health service, and was concerned at the difficulty of recruiting nurses and the high wastage rate among trainees. In March 1970 Crossman announced that Asa Briggs, vice-chancellor of the University of Sussex, would lead a committee of investigation into nursing. Professor Briggs's remit was wide: 'to review the role of the nurse and the midwife in the hospital and the community and the education and training required for that role, so that the best use is made of available manpower'.[2] The committee was equally balanced between men and women, and included three doctors and eleven nurses.[3] They had four research assistants, including a future general secretary of the RCN, Christine Hancock. The committee worked energetically, taking evidence from many sources, and the RCN participated with enthusiasm.[4] Shortly after the committee began their work, the Labour Party was defeated in a general election, and when the Briggs report appeared in October 1972 a Conservative government was in office. Although Conservatives and Labour received the report respectfully, action was slow, firstly because the nursing profession was divided over it, and secondly because of NHS restructuring, which took place in 1974. Briggs wanted a single UK body to replace the three General Nursing Councils and the separate councils for midwives and health visitors. His proposal alarmed all these groups, particularly in Scotland and Northern Ireland, with their separate traditions of nurse training. The report came at an unfavourable time. Unrest among NHS employees soured relations with governments in the 1970s, and wage inflation made the Treasury reluctant to accept costly changes in the service. In 1974 another Labour government committed itself to the principles of the Briggs report, but delayed taking action until 1978.[5] The Nurses, Midwives and Health Visitors Act, the main outcome of the report, was not passed until 1979.

The Briggs report harmonised with several of the RCN's ambitions. It proposed an eighteen-month period of general training for all nurses, including enrolled nurses and midwives, leading to a Certificate of Nursing Practice. For the 'more able students' a second course of similar length would follow, leading to state registration as a nurse or midwife, and with opportunities for further specialised training. Briggs hoped to recruit nurses of all backgrounds and abilities for the general training course. Although five O-levels would guarantee entry to nurse training, the new central examining body (which later emerged as the UK Central Council for Nursing, Midwifery and Health Visiting), would have its own preliminary examination, emphasising aptitude tests as an alternative to academic qualifications. Nurse training in modular courses would give students a planned combination of theoretical and practical training in the different aspects of nursing. Although students would spend time on the wards, independent colleges of nursing would be responsible for their training. Briggs hoped to solve wastage among nursing trainees by making courses more interesting, and tailoring them to different abilities.[6] Although the dropout rate was declining, it was still about 38 per cent of recruits in 1968.[7] Because early training would be less concentrated on the hospital wards, the entry age could be lowered to 17. This still left a one-year gap between the school leaving age and nurse training, but was a long way from the seven-year gap that separated most school leavers from nurse training in the 1920s. The hospitals would no longer control nurse training, though the new colleges might still be based in hospitals. All nurses, whether aiming for the register or not, would begin with the same basic course, ending the distinction between registered and enrolled nurses at the start of their training. The RCN welcomed Briggs's proposals on nurse education, though with some reservations. Briggs supported 'cadet' schemes of nursing experience for school leavers, but the RCN wanted further education outside the hospital for this group. Briggs did not address the question of whether nurse trainees were students or employees, since he simply assumed that the NHS would continue to pay them. The RCN's main criticism was that the report paid little attention to the 'professional issue' – the expanding role of nurses and their widening responsibilities.[8]

Nearly a decade passed between Crossman's taxi ride and the 1979 Act. For the RCN, 'waiting for Briggs' was like an extended production of *Waiting for Godot* – the arrival of the titular character was much desired, but never certain. During that period the NHS was unified into new regional health authorities. Previously it was split between hospitals, local authority (community) health provision, and general practitioner services. Although the RCN was aggrieved that under the new system nurse administrators were placed on a lower pay scale than comparable administrative staff, nurses had places for the first time on the first two tiers of management, the regional and area health boards, and took part in policy-making. In Scotland, with a different NHS structure, the health boards had nurse representatives, but these could not be employees of the board, effectively limiting representation to retired or academic nurses. This caused some animosity, especially as the same rule was not applied to doctors, who were presumably seen as more independent. Briggs wanted a system of training that would prepare nurses for a more responsible role in the new NHS. Unlike Godot, Briggs finally arrived, though not quite in the shape that the RCN hoped for. The RCN's work in the 1970s must therefore be seen against this background of an expected, but uncertain, change in professional qualifications.

Industrial relations

During the 1970s, the RCN's predicament over its ambiguous status as an industrial negotiator was resolved by the industrial relations policies of successive governments. When Edward Heath's Conservative government came to power in June 1970, one of its first actions was to present an Industrial Relations Bill. This aimed to make agreements between employers and unions legally enforceable, in order to slow up the pace of wage demands and end wildcat strikes. It imposed complex obligations on trade unions and employers, and required unions to register under the Act to obtain legal recognition. Unregistered unions would face charges of conspiracy if they took industrial action, and would not have the legal safeguards of registered unions. The Bill offered rights as well as penalties: for the first time, workers could appeal against unfair dismissal, and (although this was not mandatory) the government intended to pressure large employers into giving employees a written statement of their rights and obligations in the workplace.[9] The RCN was in a difficult situation. Its leaders had no intention of turning the RCN into a trade union, but if it did not register, employers might not accept it as a negotiating body, and its members might be driven for protection into a registered union. Yet if the RCN *did* register as a union, it would lose its beneficial tax position as a charity, and endanger its Royal Charter. Charitable status was estimated as worth £100,000 a year to the RCN, and members' subscriptions would have to be increased to cover the shortfall. Catherine Hall wrote urgently to the Department of Health:

> any increase [in subscriptions] of the size calculated would, in my view meet with strenuous resistance and if implemented would involve large scale withdrawals from the Rcn . . . The fact that the services offered by the Rcn are far in excess of those offered by the traditional type of trades unions would be overlooked in such a situation.[10]

To avoid inter-union disputes and the need for an employer to deal with several unions, the Bill gave the Commission on Industrial Relations power to enforce a 'closed shop' – that is, only selected unions would be recognised in a particular workplace. Although NHS employers were very unlikely to exclude the RCN from negotiations, the RCN might lose its rights if it had only a few members in a workplace such as a factory.[11] The RCN considered setting up a separate 'front' organisation to register as a union (the BMA had already used this strategy), but this was complicated and potentially expensive. Catherine Hall and Betty Newstead immediately sought a meeting with Robert Carr, the Secretary of State for Employment, and with Sir Keith Joseph, the Secretary of State for Social Services.

Since the government's aim was to discourage strikes, Carr had no wish to drive nurses out of an organisation with a no-strike policy into more militant unions, especially since the health service unions were already in dispute over their low pay. Other professional bodies, including the BMA, were in the same position as the RCN, and the Department of Employment held a number of urgent meetings with them, but it was the rapid action and irresistible arguments of Miss Hall and Mrs Newstead that were credited with persuading Carr to amend his Bill. The amendment set up a special register for professional associations, recognising them as workers' organisations under the Act, and they would have the legal rights and obligations of a trade union. Their tax status would not change. The RCN council unanimously decided to register on these terms.[12] As the Bill passed through parliament, Labour members, led by Barbara Castle, attacked the amendment bitterly for class bias in favouring the professional bodies above the trade unions, and derided Carr for having a 'soft spot' for nurses.[13] The ill-fated Industrial Relations Act passed in August 1971, and the TUC urged unions to boycott it by refusing to register. COHSE, which registered mainly because it feared that the RCN would capture its nursing members if it did not, was ejected from the TUC.

The professional bodies also demanded representation on the Industrial Relations Commission, and the *Sunday Times* predicted that it would 'appoint a professional man, probably a doctor'. But Carr appointed Catherine Hall to the single place reserved for the professions. The RCN was delighted by this mark of respect, but other professional associations, especially the BMA, were mortified. R. L. Clark of the Association of Professional Engineers grumbled that the engineers would have preferred a medical representative, for '[doctors] have a kind of degree which makes them professional. But nurses are really just technicians'.[14] This remark neatly expressed the professional predicament of nurses. The RCN's case for higher educational standards in nursing had been repeatedly rejected, particularly by the medical profession; but nurses' right to speak for other professions was now disputed because they lacked higher education. The *Sunday Times* speculated that the Conservatives chose the RCN because it was less abrasive than the BMA, but Catherine Hall pointed out to their reporter that she had not doubled the membership of the

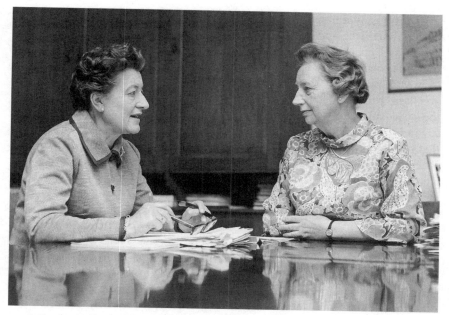

7.1 Catherine Hall, general secretary, and Winifred Prentice, president, 1974.

RCN in two years by being ladylike. The reporter was clearly disarmed by the general secretary, 'a tall mildly austere woman combining strangely a semi-military aura of the "traditional" nurse with an open and receptive mind'. [15] Her appointment did not please the trade unions that were not co-operating with the Industrial Relations Act. Another mark of official approval came in 1973 with the inclusion of Catherine Hall on the Merrison Committee of Inquiry into the work of the General Medical Council. [16] Doctors invariably took part in investigations into the nursing profession, but this was the first time that the situation was reversed.

Under the Industrial Relations Act, registered organisations had to provide representatives in the workplace, and so the RCN set up a stewards' scheme. [17] This replaced the old key members' system, which had been in place for over two decades. Stewards were elected by their RCN colleagues in the workplace, and at first they were drawn from members holding positions below middle management, because senior nurse administrators were classified as both workers and first-line management. [18] In 1976, when there were 1,041 stewards in post, this restriction was removed because many valuable stewards had to resign when they were promoted. Nurses in the higher grades could consult their area officers, who were also responsible for the stewards. This changed the nature of the area officers' work. Previously they reported to the RCN's chief professional nursing officer, and were particularly concerned with professional services and recruiting; but they now transferred to the Labour Relations Department, and reported to the labour relations secretary. The stewards, who received special training from the RCN, represented members in any dispute with their employer. As local recruiting officers, they also greatly improved the RCN's access to potential members. For the first time the RCN had a large network of accessible representatives, as the area organisers and the branches had long requested. The annual report of 1972 recorded that over 7,000 new members had joined in the previous year. The stewards' scheme contributed to the changing profile of RCN membership by creating a group trained in negotiation and not always deferential to the RCN council and staff.[19] Stewards expected to participate in decision-making, and had high expectations of the RCN leadership. The new statutory right to appeal against unfair dismissal also enhanced their position in the workplace, and gradually affected nurses' attitudes to their employers. *Nursing Times* correspondents sometimes complained of the 'permissive society' and the collapse of old traditions, but deferential habits were disappearing from the RCN along with the floral hats of yesteryear, and the annual conference grew larger and more disputatious.

Although the RCN's local organisation now resembled the trade unions, its stewards were not always welcome in local union discussions.[20] NHS management had to negotiate with several unions, and although pay levels were determined nationally, management and unions met in joint consultative committees to discuss local problems. Joint stewards' committees also met locally to co-ordinate union strategy and present a united front to their employers. In some places the RCN steward was invited to attend these meetings, and in others he or she was shunned. Because it was not affiliated to the TUC, other health services unions did not regard the RCN as a real union; and because its members included nurses in senior management, RCN stewards were sometimes suspected of being management spies. Relations between the RCN and other hospital unions became very tense in the early 1970s. Ancillary workers were hard hit by the pay freezes of the 1960s, and their wages were disgracefully low. Auxiliary nurses, hospital cleaners, and kitchen and laundry staff were usually women, and many worked part time. Like nurses, they suffered from the usual assumption that women were not breadwinners and did not need a living wage. A substantial pay rise for local authority workers in 1969 led to union demands for comparable increases for ancillary workers. As Carpenter points out, the Industrial Relations Act actually strengthened union organisation, because unions now had more stewards, and local negotiating bodies.[21] COHSE began a series of one-day strikes in 1972, culminating in a ballot in March 1973 in favour of full-scale industrial action, though this did not include its nursing members. In the hospitals, nurses had to cope when kitchen, cleaning, laundry and other services were suspended. The RCN instructed its members not to cover for ancillary staff, but in practice, if nurses believed that patients would be endangered or distressed, they did so. Some nurses in the health service unions, torn between their union duty and their professional ethics, left to join the RCN, to the disgust of the other unions. Deteriorating conditions in nurses' homes also aggrieved the student nurses. At the 1973 annual meetings, Sir Keith Joseph came to thank the RCN for its assistance during the ancillary workers' action, and was met with loud complaints about nurses' food and accommodation. Joseph admitted candidly that he was indeed one of the largest 'slum landlords' in the country.[22] These were difficult times, and although the unions won a moderate pay rise for ancillary staff, relations with the RCN remained uneasy.

The Industrial Relations Act did not survive for long, though it left a permanent mark on the RCN. Its threat to imprison workers if they defied the Act was impossible to enforce, and moving from an open vote to secret ballots on strike action actually empowered the unions. The short-term wildcat strikes of the 1960s were replaced by lengthy official disputes, particularly in the mining industry. Shortages of coal led to power cuts (though the hospitals' electricity supplies were protected), and the government imposed a state of emergency and a three-day working week. This brought down Heath's government in 1974, and Labour returned to power. But the British economy, which, in spite of many problems, had maintained full employment and steady growth since the war, was now faltering. Unemployment rose alarmingly for the first time since the 1930s. In spite of this, inflation (an international problem) also rose rapidly, leading to frantic pay claims. A number of pay settlements in 1974 averaged up to 29 per cent.[23] Once again, the wages of workers in the NHS were falling badly behind.

Barbara Castle was the Labour government's Secretary of State for Social Services in 1974. She had fiercely criticised the RCN for demanding a special register, and was tough in her dealings with the unions. She took up her new position during yet another crisis in the health service unions and growing militancy in the RCN. During her first few weeks in office, nurses staged many street demonstrations, collecting signatures for a mass petition in their 'Fair pay for nurses' campaign. Although the RCN was not co-operating with COHSE as it had in 1962, most nurses on the streets were young and willing to join any protest, regardless of who organised it. Demonstrations that had seemed new and unusual in the 1960s now seemed like a natural expression for discontented members of the profession. On 9 May 1974, a group of psychiatric nurses in Huddersfield left duty for an hour in five wards – a token gesture, but the first time that COHSE nurses had actually struck. On 13 May, forty-five RCN representatives, led by the president, Winifred Prentice, met

Mrs Castle and presented her with a detailed case, *The State of Nursing*, while several thousand nurses marched through London. Despite her flinty exterior, Barbara Castle was sympathetic. The previous week she had announced the government's support for the Briggs report, and an allocation of £18 million for the extra tutors and clinical teachers required for the reform of nurse training. The Cabinet had already agreed privately to relax their pay restraints in favour of three special cases: teachers, postal workers and nurses.[24] In her diary Barbara Castle recorded how she received a 'massive array of speakers' from the RCN, and heard their 'impressive report'. At the end of the meeting, Betty Newstead gave an ultimatum: if an independent inquiry into pay were not set up within three weeks, the RCN would instruct its members to resign from the NHS *en masse*. The RCN would then set itself up as a private nursing agency and apply for their re-engagement in the NHS as 'temporaries'.[25] Agency nurses were far more expensive than NHS employees. This was an uncharacteristically dramatic move by the RCN, and within a month the BMA threatened a similar tactic over its own claim. The RCN managed to polarise the health service unions, COHSE attacking it for not participating in the hospital disruption, and the National and Local Government Officers Association denouncing the resignation threat as 'irresponsible'.[26]

Barbara Castle persuaded the government to review nurses' pay, and Lord Halsbury, who chaired the pay review body for doctors and dentists, agreed to lead an inquiry. The government promised that any increase would be backdated to May, but despite this, and while Halsbury was deliberating, the inter-union dispute in the hospitals worsened. The RCN, the National Union of Public Employees and the National and Local Government Officers Association suspended their campaigns until the Halsbury report appeared. COHSE, which could not afford to alienate its militant wing, demanded an interim pay settlement, and when this was refused, continued with overtime bans, work-to-rule and selective short strikes.[27] The RCN council held an emergency meeting to discuss the impact on patients. In some hospitals, COHSE members withdrew their services from private patients. The Labour Party had long been uneasy about pay beds in NHS hospitals, and Barbara Castle promised to abolish them. The RCN, which, as will be seen, had its own anxieties about pay beds, nevertheless protested at the speed of the proposed change, arguing that it would cause even more disruption in the NHS and distress to patients. Unofficial street demonstrations of nurses continued, and engineers, dockers and miners held brief sympathy strikes.

Once more the nurses had much public support, and the tabloid press was a sensitive barometer of opinion. *The Sun*, though normally hostile to trade unions, invariably referred to nurses – particularly young, attractive ones – as 'angels' and supported them faithfully. Although the unions attacked the RCN for not joining in industrial actions, relations between them were never as

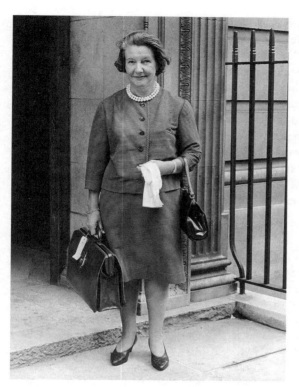

7.2 M. E. (Betty) Newstead, member of staff 1955–75 and head of the Labour Relations Department, c. 1970.

simple as they seemed. At this stage, the RCN had over 100,000 members, and COHSE around 70,000 nursing members. Christopher Hart comments perceptively that the RCN and COHSE were 'the Odd Couple', apparently in endless conflict, yet each needing the other.[28] If the government were complacent about the RCN's anti-strike policy, then COHSE would shake them up; but COHSE also benefited from the RCN's staid public image. The *Daily Telegraph*, an anti-union paper, commented, 'When a sober and responsible body like the Royal College of Nursing speaks of a "crisis of confidence and morale" within the nursing profession, it behoves the rest of us to take notice'.[29] To the public and to many unions outside the health service, all nurses were the same, regardless of training, status or union affiliation. Deeper issues of gender were still involved. Although press photographs of demonstrations usually showed a mixed group of male and female nurses, the nursing image was conventionally feminine.[30] The *Daily Express* described one protesting nurse as: 'the more-than-acceptable face of militant trade unionism [who] wears a cute little cap and breaks off from a bit of jostling with the police to smile for the camera'.[31] The unions striking in sympathy with the nurses were masculine, and made it clear that they were offering support less to fellow unionists, than to damsels in distress. Before one group of dockers walked out in support of the nurses, they discussed whether to donate a day's pay instead, but decided to strike because nurses 'were not in a position to take industrial action', whereas dockers could take care of themselves.[32]

Halsbury's committee reported in September. They provided an impressive overview of the nursing world in Britain in 1974.[33] At that stage, there were more than 415,000 nurses in the NHS, about 90 per cent of them in the hospital services, and 60,000 of them lived in hospital accommodation. Halsbury's figures showed that unqualified nurses were a growing part of the labour force:

Table 7.1 Number of qualified and unqualified NHS nurses in the UK: percentage of total in England and Wales, and in Scotland

	1968	1969	1970	1971	1972	1973
England and Wales						
Qualified nurses	47.8	48.2	48.3	47.5	46.6	46.0
Nurses in training	31.5	30.3	28.9	28.7	28.6	28.9
Other nursing staff	20.7	21.5	22.8	23.8	24.8	25.1
Scotland						
Qualified nurses	42.6	43.4	43.1	42.1	41.0	41.0
Nurses in training	27.6	25.9	24.6	25.3	25.7	24.9
Other nursing staff	29.8	30.7	32.3	32.6	33.3	34.1

Source: Halsbury report, para. 39.

The growing number of married women in the service was shown by the statistics of part-time work: 37 per cent of nurses in the hospital services, and 14 per cent of nurses in the community. Nine out of ten nurses were women. They cost the nation £510 million a year, or under 17 per cent of the NHS expenditure. Halsbury noted that the current pay claim had been dragging on for two years, and that Crossman's settlement in 1970, 'was in the nature of an exercise in the restoration of lost relationship' rather than a proper evaluation of nurses' work. The committee visited a number of hospitals, and was struck by the contrast between old and new. Nursing accommodation in some of the older homes was 'of a lower standard than can reasonably be expected by members of a key profession in an advanced society',[34] and nurses in substandard homes were charged the same rent as those in good ones. In some cases, even though the hospitals were new, the nurses' accommodation had not been renovated. Halsbury was also 'waiting for Briggs', and wanted a complete restructuring of pay grades, moving away from the complex and unloved Salmon system. He recommended higher than average pay rises for scarce staff, such as psychiatric nurses and nurse tutors. The nursing shortage was acute in London, where agency nurses were routinely employed. Management made no formal estimates of how many nurses were needed for each hospital, but acknowledged a substantial shortfall. Although the unions had fought hard for overtime pay, not much overtime work was actually done, and most full-time nurses worked a forty-hour week. Pay claims at that time were worked out in comparison with other relevant workers ('relativities'), but no other group was really comparable to nurses. Nurses' average annual pay was £1,578, compared with £2,168 for all salaried workers. Senior clinical nurses, the ward sisters and staff nurses, earned less than non-graduate primary teachers, and worked much longer hours.[35] Armed with these damning statistics, Halsbury recommended an average increase of 33 per cent for nurses, and the government and the unions accepted it.

In spite of this, the years that followed were some of the most bitter for labour relations in the NHS. The RCN, which had so long clung to its status as a professional body, decided in November 1976 to register as an independent trade union, although a meeting of the RRB a few months previously had voted overwhelmingly against this. The main reason for this sudden reversal was the Labour government's legislation on trade unions. On coming to power in 1974, Wilson's government immediately repealed the Industrial Relations Act, dissolved the Commission on Industrial Relations, and relied on voluntary agreements with the unions (the 'social contract') to keep wage demands within bounds. Consequently, industrial relations legislation had to take account of the TUC's views. The Trade Union and Industrial Relations Act of 1974 restored many of the unions' legal privileges, but to take advantage of this protection, unions had to be certified by the Registrar of Friendly Societies.[36] After some deft footwork by the Conservative opposition in a parliament where Labour had the slimmest of majorities, an amendment to the Act ensured that employers could continue to negotiate with non-certified associations, and individual workers were not forced to join a union as a condition of employment in a closed shop. At this stage the RCN's position seemed secure.

Two further measures, the Health and Safety at Work Act of 1974 and the Employment Protection Act of 1975, were important in safeguarding the rights of workers, but put pressure on the RCN. The first incorporated trade unions into the management of workplace health and safety. The second gave more protection against unfair dismissal, introduced maternity leave and required employers to give union representatives paid time off for their union duties. Nurses would benefit from these new laws, but only if they were members of an accredited body. In many hospitals, the TUC-affiliated unions continued to cold-shoulder the RCN representatives, and tried to exclude them from consultation with management. Some senior nurses joined trade unions to safeguard themselves, while remaining members of the RCN.[37] Under much TUC pressure, and with a larger majority after another general election, in 1976 the government amended the Trade Union and Industrial Relations Act to remove the 1974 amendment that recognised non-certified associations of workers. At this point the RCN council was not sure whether the RCN had the legal privileges of a union or not. Relations with the unions in many hospitals were hostile, and if a militant union insisted that management no longer negotiate with the RCN, then the more timorous hospital authorities might give in. The council took advice from a panel of lawyers and industrial relations experts, and proposed to the AGM in November 1976 that the RCN should become an independent union. To protect its charitable status, the Royal Charter, and its Royal patronage, the College would shift its non-union activities (particularly its professional and educational sections) into a Royal College of Nursing Charitable Trust. The *Nursing Standard* published a detailed warning of the consequences of failing to unionise, senior staff 'tramped the country' to convince members of its necessity, and over 10,000 members voted in favour of unionisation, with fewer than 400 against.[38] This was an unusually large vote, especially since the students, many of whom were militantly in favour of labour solidarity, could not take part. The RCN duly became a trade union in June 1977, and a set of union rules was drawn up. Rule 12 stated that the council did not have power to call on RCN members to withdraw their labour. This reaffirmed the RCN's anti-strike tradition, though the rule was not immutable. A general meeting, by a majority of two thirds, could change the RCN's policy. In 1978, the Royal Charter was adjusted to reflect the College's new position. All properties and assets formerly held by the College as a charity were vested in the new Trust, of which the College was sole trustee.[39]

Although the RCN had by force of circumstance become a trade union, its difficulties with other health service unions were not resolved. Its new status did not satisfy rival unions because the RCN stood outside the mainstream of the union movement by not affiliating to the TUC. As a union, the RCN posed a greater threat to other unions, since it was now competing directly with them for members, and the TUC constitution did not permit workers to join more than one union. Relations between the RCN and the unions reached a nadir in the late 1970s, although they shared the same grievances over the government's stringent economies in the NHS. Among the Halsbury agreements was a cut in nurses' working hours, but hospital management could not afford to employ enough nurses to take account of this, and the hospitals became short-staffed. For the first time, nurses were leaving the training schools without a guaranteed job in a general hospital. With unemployment rising, applications for nurse training increased, and the training schools had to turn candidates away. Although erosion of wages was still the major problem, union discontent also deepened because of labour shortages. In February 1977 the Mayday Hospital in Croydon was forced to close thirty-six beds after senior nurses threatened to close wards themselves if they did not have enough staff.[40] This was an unprecedented action for RCN members, and the council formally protested to David Ennals, the new Secretary of State for Social Services, about the nursing shortage. Members reported on hospital black spots where students or unqualified staff had to take charge of wards, and the press ran excited stories about the 'crisis' as hospital waiting lists grew to record levels.[41] Every year the RCN invited the current Secretary of State to attend the opening of the annual conference, which provided the occasion for a fulsome political speech; but in 1978, Ennals was loudly barracked over that year's pay rise of 10 per cent, which again failed to keep up with inflation. When Hope Trenchard, a district nurse, voiced a general anxiety about the future of the NHS, the irritated Ennals dismissed her views as 'politically motivated', and the meeting erupted in fury. After Ennals left, the RRB voted to send him a telegram demanding a personal apology to Miss Trenchard, and Ennals had to make a humiliating retraction.[42] The RRB was becoming a more political forum, causing some problems for the more conservative council, and ministers of state could no longer expect the respectful audience of former years.

A lengthy strike by ancillary workers in October 1978 caused great disruption and closed several cottage hospitals. Hospital laundries were out of action, and patients lay in paper sheets, or relied on their relatives for clean linen. In many areas, hospitals admitted only accident and emergency cases, and in Amersham the local newspaper appealed to the public to give accommodation to nurses, because their home was not being heated.[43] The dispute continued until March 1979, and was part of the 'winter of discontent' that followed the collapse of the government's attempts to restrict pay increases to 5 per cent. Although RCN members helped to keep the hospitals running, and won much public gratitude, their own pay negotiations stalled. The Treasury, already dismayed at the predicted costs of implementing the Briggs report, took advantage of the RCN's no-strike policy, expecting less resistance than in the TUC-affiliated unions.[44] Once again, busloads of nurses descended on their MPs, this time demanding 'Pay, not peanuts'. They threatened to work a thirty-five-hour week, to stick to official policy of not leaving students in charge of wards at night, and district nurses demanded to be provided with cars, rather than use their own. Catherine Hall expressed the general mood: 'Nurses see what has been achieved by the use of industrial muscle, and they wonder if this is the only language that Government understands'.[45] But the RCN did not take part in the mass day of action by public service employees on 22 January 1979, when schools closed, hospital patients had cold food, the police manned ambulances and public services shut down. Relations with government were at breaking point after interminable meetings between David Ennals and the staff side of the Whitley Council, and in February a packed RCN meeting at Westminster called for his resignation, while simultaneously rejecting a proposal to change the RCN constitution to abolish Rule 12 and permit strike action. The RCN had a publicity coup when Ennals had to go into Westminster Hospital for treatment for thrombosis in his leg. While the National Union of Public Employees threatened to 'black' him by refusing to sweep around his bed or give him tea from the trolley, RCN nurses were magnanimous, and an embarrassed Secretary of State left hospital singing the praises of his nursing staff.[46]

The widening breach between the RCN and the Department of Health seemed likely to push the College into affiliation with the TUC, and the first motion for this course of action came from student representatives at the RRB of 1977. Over the next few years, the College was deeply divided on the subject, with a substantial and vocal group, led by the Student Nurses' Section demanding affiliation at each RRB, opposed by more conservative members who feared that affiliation would drag the College into strikes.[47] The RCN leadership was pragmatic, and considered whether siding with the TUC against the government might bring more benefit to the College than remaining a chastely

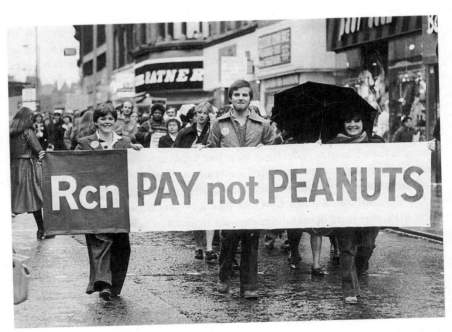

7.3 Pay campaign, 'Pay not Peanuts', 1979.

independent professional body. Affiliation would also solve the bruising question of RCN representation on local union committees. Unusually, Catherine Hall made a personal statement to the RRB that she was in favour of individual liberty, and believed that no-one should be forced to join a trade union; but if the TUC unions managed to exclude the RCN from a closed shop, then the RCN should consider ways of protecting itself. She asked that the RRB give the council discretion in policy.[48] The council took advice from industrial relations experts and from other professional bodies that had already affiliated. The arguments in favour of affiliation seemed strong, for the TUC was a power in the land, and the RCN would be part of it. Conversely, if the RCN was not represented on the TUC, then only the voice of other nursing unions would be heard. The TUC was less dangerous than many members feared, for it could not enforce political affiliation or demand strike action from any member union. Further, as many experts pointed out, the TUC was changing. Its past lay with the old heavy industries, but by this period white-collar workers were beginning to dominate, and several professional bodies had affiliated.[49] The RRB pressed the council to move towards affiliation, and by May 1979, with industrial relations in the health service in a very poor state, the council seemed poised to do so. Several of its members, including a rising figure, Trevor Clay, favoured TUC affiliation as a principle of labour organisation. But at this late stage, two insuperable difficulties arose. The first was the TUC's internal disciplinary measures that were intended to prevent unions from poaching each other's members. If the TUC decreed, members who moved from one union to another might be expelled, but the RCN's charter gave it no powers to expel its members for this reason, even if it wished. The second and probably more significant objection emerged after Catherine Hall reported on her discussions with Len Murray, the general secretary of the TUC. Murray, although personally well disposed towards the RCN, replied candidly when Hall asked whether an application from the RCN would be accepted. Murray believed that the health service unions would probably try to block such a move, and the TUC would defer to the views of these long-standing members. Health unions in Scotland were not expected to oppose affiliation, but it would be impossible for Scottish members to affiliate to the STUC without also being members of the TUC. Catherine Hall knew that RCN members were deeply divided over affiliation. The worst outcome would be to override the wishes of those opposed to affiliation, only to have the RCN's application humiliatingly rejected. After hearing her report, council changed its mind. It submitted the case for and against affiliation in considerable detail to members in the *Nursing Standard*, and the AGM in 1979 voted against it by 3,742 votes to 2,849. The subject was raised again and rejected in 1981. The changing political climate in the 1980s removed this issue from the RCN's agenda, and it has not yet affiliated with the TUC.

Internal affairs and professional development

Rapid changes in the size and composition of its membership, and in the professional work of nurses, led the council to review the structure of the RCN, assisted by Harold Bridger of the Tavistock Institute of Human Relations.[50] A new system came into operation on 1 January 1971. The old titles of Professional Organisation Division and Education Division were scrapped, and the director of education had to report directly to the general secretary rather than the council, in an attempt to improve relations between the educational and professional sides of the College, and to place them under a single executive. The director of education's remit was widened to the whole of the UK, and also to advise council on educational matters. All educational work was brought into a new Institute of Advanced Nursing Education (IANE), with centres in London, Birmingham, Scotland, Northern Ireland and Wales. Jean McFarlane, who took over as Director of Education after Mary Carpenter's retirement in 1968, was the first director of IANE. A UK Education Committee replaced the Education Advisory Board. It had a wide membership of council members, and of both internal and external bodies, including representatives from the Department of Education and Science (DES) and the Department of Health and Social Security.[51] The library also became a direct responsibility of the general secretary. The Department of Education and Science acknowledged its importance in nursing education, and met three-fifths of its expenses.

Until 1967 the RCN council met monthly. This made heavy demands on its members, who were mainly hard-working nurses in senior positions in the NHS, and so monthly meetings were replaced by quarterly ones to discuss major policy issues. After an unsatisfactory experiment with quarterly meetings, the council decided to meet every two months, with monthly meetings by an Executive Committee. The general secretary and a Chief Officers' Committee planned the implementation of policy, made recommendations to council, and monitored the activities of the RCN. Although the Chief Officers' Committee did not have formal executive powers, the RCN's reforms were trying to grapple with the problem of all large trade unions and professional bodies – to vest policy-making in their elected councils, while ensuring efficient executive action through a professional management team. External pressures in the 1960s and 1970s, and the need for rapid reaction to the political situation, inevitably placed considerable responsibility on the general secretary's executive group. As in all such organisations, there was always the potential for friction between the elected and managerial bodies, in this case the RCN council, the RRB, specialist interest groups within the RCN and the permanent staff. Personal relationships helped to prevent divisions, and fortunately for the RCN, during this testing period these relations were usually equable. At council meetings, Catherine Hall's diplomatic opening phrase:

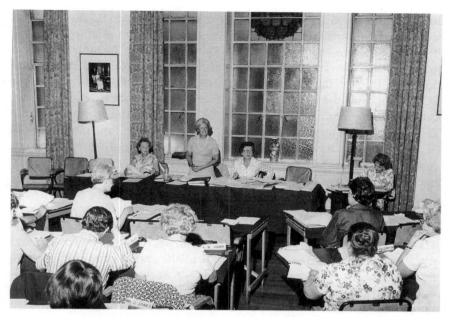

7.4 Council meeting, College of Nursing, London, Sheila Quinn (standing) chairman, 1975.

'Council will be aware that . . .' signalled the carefully balanced relations between general secretary and elected members. The most acrimonious disputes usually occurred at the RRB, but even these had limits. After angry debates over trade union status at the 1976 RRB, many of the younger delegates the following year wore T-shirts with the slogan 'Rcn United', signalling a return to more harmonious discussion.[52]

The new arrangements included a new Professional Nursing Department, with a chief professional nursing officer and a team of nurse officers responsible for the nine specialist sections and specialist groups. Each officer was secretary to a section committee, and was an adviser and consultant in that field. The six area officers, accountable to the chief professional nursing officer, promoted RCN services to local members, recruited new members and ensured effective representation in the workplace. They worked closely with the labour relations staff in dealing with members' employment problems.[53]

In 1972, when the Briggs report was about to be published, and NHS reorganisation was imminent, the council turned its attention to the membership structure, to take account of developments within the profession. Finance was also an important consideration. The RCN's income could be increased only by raising subscriptions or recruiting new members, since subscriptions were its main source of revenue. Given nurses' low pay, raising the cost of subscriptions was always an unattractive option. Catherine Hall observed that it was hardly surprising that the RCN was financially over-strained, since the medical profession had three different bodies to provide the same services in professional advancement, indemnity insurance and workplace representation, and each of these organisations had a higher subscription than the RCN.[54] Nor could the RCN reduce its services without risking loss of members. Once again the branches were said to be moribund, and in May 1973, the Tavistock Institute was asked to assist in a review.[55] A team from the Tavistock's Centre for Career Development and Institutional Change met a representative group of RCN members in an attempt to identify the major issues and to assess what members wanted from the RCN. The Tavistock team, having made a preliminary report, proposed that the membership should be invited to participate actively in evolving a more effective structure.[56]

As the *Nursing Standard* commented, the notion that the RCN headquarters should revolve around the membership and not vice versa was revolutionary.[57] But the council was amenable, and in the spring of 1974 'Operation grassroots' began. Nine regional 'talkabouts' were held, involving over a thousand members. These meetings were to consider the Tavistock report so that representatives could go back to their organisations and continue the discussion about the RCN's future. Teams of staff and council members, together with a member of the Tavistock Institute, attended each talkabout. Margaret Green, the head of the College's Professional Nursing Department, was appointed chairman of all the talkabouts to provide continuity, and she estimated that she travelled 10,000 miles during the whole process.[58] The spring of 1974 was not the best time for this, but despite 'snow in Newcastle, rain almost everywhere, train strikes, no lights, reduced lights, and a day without heat in the University of Edinburgh', all meetings were well attended: 'there were always people waiting to speak . . . and we were always still talking when tea was served at the end of the day'.[59]

Feedback from 'Operation grassroots' was presented to the RRB in Blackpool at the end of March. There was considerable support for continuing all the main functions of the RCN – a professional voice locally and nationally, a forceful approach to labour relations, and a national network for specialist interest groups. There was less agreement about the future educational role of the College, since many felt that this would have to change as departments of nursing developed at the universities and polytechnics. The Tavistock report proposed local centres as the primary point of contact for members. RCN members approved this, for all recognised the need for professional meetings, and welcomed the concept of a local forum for nurses in all fields of practice. Centres would discuss specialist, professional, workplace and social concerns that were currently divided between the sections, specialist groups, stewards and branches.[60] If the new centres were successful, they might also give the RCN an effective presence in the new Area Health Authorities. Having a greater degree of autonomy than the branches, the centres should encourage more member participation.

The strongest message from the grassroots meetings was that more staff were needed in the field, but this had financial implications and so it was decided to redeploy two members of the headquarters' staff from the Professional Nursing Department. These officers were assigned to their local areas, the Midlands and the South East, and besides their usual role of promoting professional activities and giving advice, they piloted the formation of the new centres. The Tavistock concept of centres was philosophical rather than concrete, a centre being wherever a group of RCN members chose to meet, and members were to decide when and where to form them. The first centre was established in September 1974 in Solihull, where members were keen to have one since there were no existing RCN groups. But members were less enthusiastic in areas with flourishing branches and sections. In the South East, where retired members dominated many of the branches, there was considerable resistance to new professional centres.[61] Unlike the branches, the centres were for professional activities, with no provision for the retired member. Also, because the centres usually covered the area of an NHS Area Health Authority, a larger geographical area than a branch, many members were not happy at having to travel further to meetings.[62] The potential membership of a centre included all the RCN members in that area, who would run it and decide what activities to organise. They were to hold regular meetings, to share information from headquarters and the RCN area offices, to promote professional development, and to discuss professional issues for local action or reference upwards.

The changeover from branches to centres proceeded slowly, and by June 1975 there were only seven centres. These were more active than the branches, and the RRB was impatient at the lack of progress. An emergency resolution called for centres to be established throughout the country by 31 March 1976.[63] The Tavistock team had intended that the branches should transform into centres at their own pace, and regretted that the change had been imposed from above. In another break from the Tavistock blueprint, the membership requested a standard constitution for the centres, although a key part of the Tavistock concept had been flexibility to meet local circumstances. In 1981 a follow-up study revealed general disappointment with the centres.[64] Most were balancing their dual role of professional body and trade union along with the sometimes conflicting demands of members and RCN staff, and barely 5 per cent of local members were participating. Few members above the grade of senior nursing officer came to meetings, nor did student and pupil nurses. The idea that all members were equal had not been accepted. RCN officers relied on the centres for feedback on membership opinion, but believed that they were not representative. Some thought that centres could be abolished, since members' needs were met by the specialist associations and societies. But the author of the study concluded that it was unrealistic to expect more than a small proportion of members to participate in the centres. Given that most nurses were married, and 37 per cent of nurses in the NHS worked part-time, centres had to take second place to family and social commitments. Many nurses wanted no more from the RCN than indemnity insurance and to know that they had a professional organisation looking after their interests.

During the grassroots operation, members made plain that they wanted to maintain a specialist structure within the RCN, although they did not agree on what this should be. By 1975 a dual specialist structure was worked out, grouping the membership into three broad functional associations and into numerous specialist societies. The three associations covered nursing management, nursing education and nursing practice. Each association discussed relevant issues in its field, made recommendations to council and formulated resolutions for the RRB. Each elected a national committee, which consisted of voting members of the RRB. Activities were organised regionally and nationally, while locally centres were the focal point. Eventually it was decided that the student body, formerly the Student Nurses' Section, should also become an association, with units in the schools of nursing.

The other part of the structure consisted of specialist societies, and these revealed the increasing complexity and specialisation of nursing practice. At first there were five specialist societies – in geriatrics, occupational health, primary health care and psychiatric nursing, together with the research society. The societies aimed to develop nursing knowledge and standards of care, and each was regarded as the expert body in its own field. The Society of Nursing Research was formed from the Research Discussion Group and included all RCN members engaged in research, regardless of specialisation. During the previous five years, the RCN had set up twelve specialist groups in response to membership requests.[65] These groups represented nursing specialties with small numbers of experts but regarded as professionally significant, such as intensive care nursing and haemodialysis nursing. Under the new structure the specialist groups were called forums, and as the process of specialisation continued their numbers increased. In 1976, when the associations and societies began, seven forums were recognised. Six years later there were twenty-two forums, and by 1990, sixty-five.

The new structure encouraged professional activity. Each association was supported by a professional officer in the Professional Nursing Department at RCN headquarters. Six nurse advisers, based in the six English area offices, assisted the specialist societies and offered expert advice to members in that area.[66] The executive committees of the associations and societies were drawn from nurses at the cutting edge of their field. Through their expertise, energy and enthusiasm the RCN could influence professional policy and contribute to the advancement of nursing practice. The RCN insisted that new specialist societies should include practitioners, teachers and managers, and the first to be recognised was for cancer nursing. At this time, the leading UK nurses in the field were in touch with the American Oncology Nursing Society and a European oncology group that included both doctors and nurses. Drug companies were trying to persuade cancer nurses in the UK to join a nursing society independent of the RCN, but through the skilful negotiations of the professional nursing officer the key people in this specialty became members of the RCN and persuaded the council to establish the new society.[67] In 1984, Societies of Mental Handicap Nursing and of Paediatric Nursing were recognised.

Internal reorganisation did not solve the RCN's financial problems. By the end of the 1960s, inflation added to its annual costs while eating away at income. Between 1968 and 1972 the accounts showed a growing deficit, and council and staff struggled to keep running costs down. They decided not to cut back services, since this would reduce the RCN's attraction for its members.[68] Strict budgetary controls were enforced and staff who left were not replaced. In spite of this, subscriptions had to be increased to £8 in 1971, but this was below the rate of inflation and further increases were necessary in November 1974 to £10.50 and in July 1975 to £15.00. The council knew that raising subscriptions might lead to resignations from the membership. Nurses in the NHS received two pay rises in 1974–75, and a subscription increase in line with inflation (running at 20 per cent) seemed justified. Nevertheless, membership figures dropped from 96,000 in 1972 to 83,000 in 1975. The largest item in the College's budget was salaries, and for most of this period its staff were overworked and underpaid. They were highly committed and prepared to make personal sacrifices; some redundancies were unavoidable, both in London and Edinburgh. The Finance Committee considered making the national boards wholly self-financing from members in their own areas, but rejected this as undermining the RCN's national identity and ability to formulate national policy. The budget of the Labour Relations Department could not be cut, because this service was the main reason for nurses joining the College. Members with employment problems were already criticising the department's standard of service, for they expected instant attention that it could not provide. The Professional Nursing Department in London was the hardest hit, losing eleven staff members within eighteen months. The education staff were least affected because the grant from the Department of Education and Science almost covered the cost of their work. By 1975 the annual deficit was down to £20,500 but there was still an accumulated deficit of over £200,000. The problem was solved mainly by the simple expedient of arranging for members' contributions to be deducted from salary. The RCN's

more forceful approach to pay negotiations, combined with worsening industrial relations in the NHS, and these new financial arrangements, marked a
turning point, and although subscription rates continued to rise, membership
rose too, reaching 150,000 in 1978, 200,000 in 1982, and 250,000 in 1985.[69]

Educational and international activities

In 1965 the director of education, Mary Carpenter, had proposed separate
accommodation for the educational side of the RCN. Space in Henrietta Place
was tight, and the College faced increasing competition from further education colleges in offering post-registration courses to nurses. The Ministry of
Health and regional hospital boards decided where nurses were seconded for
further education, and control of post-registration education was no longer
in the hands of the profession. Mary Carpenter also wanted educational work
to be virtually autonomous from the rest of the College, since the education
staff were wary of the council's control over their work. Her suggestions provoked an internal inquiry into the RCN's multiple responsibilities, and
whether they were impeding one another.[70] Catherine Hall argued that under
the terms of the charter the council must retain control of all College funds
and activities. It could delegate responsibility for education to an academic
board, but could not surrender control. All agreed that the College's dual
responsibility for educational policy and professional work gave it a competi-
tive edge over other educational institutions, but that education could be
administratively and physically separate. Nothing was done until 1969, when
the education staff once again asked the council to launch an appeal for new
student accommodation. The College had 500 students per year, but no adequate facilities for them, and if this continued the College would either have
to rent premises for the students, or cut their numbers. The educationalists
believed that anticipated changes in nurse education following the Briggs
report would reduce the need for post-certificate education, for basic training
would include a specialist element, and further education colleges would
move into the field, freeing the College's limited resources for advanced
courses and experimental work.[71]

   In 1972 the council set up an independent charity, the RCN Development
Trust, aiming to raise three million pounds.[72] There followed a three-year
search for a new home. The RCN intended to raise funds mainly through the
sale of the old headquarters, but after a series of investigations of possible sites
in London and elsewhere, it remained in Henrietta Place.[73] The Development
Trust did not raise any substantial amount, and so the College kept its old
headquarters, and negotiated a large loan to refurbish it.[74] The RCN is still in
its original (though expanded) building in central London, but the debates of
the 1970s over the most cost-effective location continue.

The RCN's financial problems took on an international significance when the College threatened to withdraw from the International Council of Nurses. In April 1975, an extraordinary general meeting passed a resolution on giving notice to the ICN of the RCN's intention to withdraw from membership at the end of that year. The events leading up to this decision were complicated. The RCN had doubts about the role of the ICN, believing that many of its objectives were more appropriate to national nursing associations than to an international body. The ICN aimed to improve nursing standards and influence health policy worldwide but despite its age and its size, its weight in international health politics was small. The RCN believed that the ICN's international advisory role was too ambitious, and that it made unrealistic financial demands on its member associations in order to maintain its staff of nurse advisers. At this time there were seventy-nine national nursing associations in the ICN, paying a per capita levy for each of their members, but few of these associations had enough resources for their national services, and the ICN levy was a burden. The RCN argued that the ICN should cut back its work and reduce its financial demands. The situation was exacerbated when the ICN expanded its definition of a 'nurse' in 1973. Per capita dues were formerly payable only for fully qualified nurses, but were now to include all grades of nurse, including students. The RCN would have to pay for its student and enrolled nurse members, greatly increasing the cost. While the RCN welcomed the inclusion of enrolled nurses in the ICN, it objected in principle to students being regarded as full members of a professional association. The RCN council decided that it could not accept the new charges, and this led to the proposal to withdraw from the ICN.

The ICN's President and Vice-President flew to London, and after discussions with the RCN, issued an agreed statement acknowledging a breakdown in communications, and denying that the ICN had intended to include students in its levy. Although the RCN held its emergency meeting, there was much discussion of the negative effects of withdrawal. The ICN would feel the loss of a substantial member like the RCN keenly, but on the other hand, if the RCN no longer represented UK nurses in the ICN, another nursing association, perhaps a trade union, might take its place.[75] Opinions at the 1975 RRB meeting were divided, but a large majority voted to ask the council to reconsider. For most ordinary members, the ICN probably meant little, but it represented international prestige. After further negotiations, the AGM of the RCN voted to remain in the ICN and to accept an increase of one pound in their subscription to cover the cost of ICN membership. The events of the 1970s were an ironic coda to the RCN's strenuous efforts two decades previously to replace Ethel Bedford Fenwick's National Council of Nurses as the British representatives on the ICN. There were political cross-currents in international nursing at this time that are difficult to interpret, especially as those involved gave different explanations. But behind all these developments, whether in internal reorganisation, physical rebuilding or international representation, lay the problem of supporting an ambitious professional body through the subscriptions of a poorly paid profession.

A voice for nursing: professional life and public policy

The RCN's division into two parts for legal purposes was a genuine reflection of its two main functions: trade union activities, and professional and educational work. Although the former tended to capture the headlines from the 1960s onwards, the RCN was also working steadily for more recognition as an authoritative voice in public policy. The College celebrated its diamond jubilee in 1976 with two royal occasions, a reception in the presence of the Queen at St James' Palace in December 1976, and a visit by the Queen Mother to the London headquarters in June 1977. After sixty years during which it was, for the most part, a small elite professional organisation, it now faced new challenges. It was a hybrid body, a professional union, with a growing membership. But in case anyone feared it was losing its professional ethos, the council chose this point to award the first RCN Fellowships to ten leading nurses. This action was a public statement of the standing of the College as a professional organisation and illustrated how far the nursing profession had moved since the College's silver jubilee in 1941. At that time the council had petitioned for and received the right to award fellowships, but members reacted nervously, believing that the initials FRCN (Fellow of the Royal College of Nursing) would make the College seem pretentious, and the proposal was shelved until a more favourable time. The Fellowships showed greater self-confidence in the profession, and this was reflected also in its growing involvement with public policy.

From its formation, the College had often ruefully compared itself with the British Medical Association. Governments knew that the BMA could be a dangerous opponent, and although the doctors lost several of their political battles, by the mid-twentieth century the Ministry of Health habitually consulted the BMA and the professional associations of medical specialists on many matters of health policy. Decisions on subjects like the nurse's role in the administration of intravenous drugs, or emergency resuscitation, would find their way into nurse training only with the approval of the General Nursing Councils, but the professional bodies often gave early warning of the need for change. Nevertheless, the RCN resented being left out of discussions on day-to-day health policy. In 1963 the College council felt so strongly about this that:

> it was agreed that the Ministry of Health should be asked, in the strongest possible terms, to extend to the College, as the representative body of the nursing profession, the same measure of consultation as it accorded to the BMA.[76]

Consultation with government departments often depended on the warmth (or otherwise) of personal relations between RCN staff and individual ministers. These were strained after Robinson's rejection of the Platt report, but thawed under Crossman, and continued to be more co-operative in the early 1970s. But, because it could not depend on being consulted, the RCN often had to take the initiative on policy decisions or social questions. The press would listen to its views, even if government and the NHS authorities did not invite them. The council received a steady stream of reports from sub-committees, working parties and liaison groups, usually resulting in a publication or a press release on the RCN's stance on NHS administration, nursing practice or wider social questions of the day. The specialised professional groups within the College were essential in this process.

The College had to be ready to respond to official inquiries like the Salmon report, but it was sometimes well ahead of legislation. In 1962 it started to keep a watching brief on the consequences for nurses if Britain joined the European Economic Community (EEC). The RCN knew that a free labour market would require international co-operation over nurse training, entry qualifications for the profession, labour mobility and patient care, and was ready when this happened more than a decade later. In 1972, prior to Britain's entry to the EEC, Tatiana Vergebovsky, the secretary of the RCN's International Department, was appointed Britain's official observer on the EEC Permanent Liaison Committee on Nurses, and the RCN continued to provide a representative when Britain had full membership. The RCN and the British Medical Association worked closely on all matters relating to the health services and the EEC, both organisations having observer status on each others' committees.

As the RCN expanded to include nurses with different types of training, there was always a danger that sectional interests would diverge, and the College could not always formulate policy rapidly in response to changing circumstances. The example most often cited is that of district nurses. After 1948, local authorities had a statutory duty to provide district nurses, but their methods of doing so differed, some continuing to employ Queen's Nurses, who were organised by a voluntary body, others operating their own service under the local Medical Officer of Health. Faced with financial problems and shortages of district nurses, local authorities looked for economical ways of solving the problem, and during the 1950s the Ministry of Health decided on a shorter period of training for district nurses and to employ enrolled nurses in these posts where possible. The RCN has been criticised for its obsession with training an elite group of nurses in the hospitals, and paying scant attention to nurses in the community. District nurses did not work in a controlled environment. They needed considerable social skills, and had to make independent decisions in difficult circumstances, but they were thought to require fewer technical skills than senior hospital nurses.[77] The Salmon reforms gave the nurse administrator some influence in hospital policy, but district nurses had far less influence in the management of community medicine. By the early 1970s, with a major reform of the NHS in prospect, the district nurses' discontent over their loss of status threatened to split the RCN. The council, fearing that district nurses would leave the College, accepted their demand for a separate section, against the strong protests of the Public Health Section.[78] This gave the district nurses an individual voice on the council, and they enlisted the RCN's aid to press successfully for a longer (six-month) period of special training and a new curriculum.

The district nurses' case shows that the RCN did not always foresee problems in its own ranks. Under the RCN constitution, the council was the chief source of policy, and if it failed to understand the needs of its constituent groups, it risked alienating them.[79] On the other hand, the stream of information to the council and the executive, with lengthy reports from the associations and societies, working parties and research groups, permitted rapid response and executive action when necessary. The RCN's excellent publicity and press relations fixed it firmly in the public mind as a body committed to improving nursing standards, not just the economic interests of its members. This was, of course, its intention. The examples that follow show the scope of the RCN's involvement in professional and social issues. They are necessarily selective, and cannot do full justice to the range of investigations carried out in this period. They do, however, reveal some of the RCN's major concerns, including understaffing and violence in the hospitals, the boundaries of nursing responsibility, and social issues such as abortion.

Underlying many of the RCN's public statements was a basic concern about inadequate staffing in the hospitals and the avoidable calamities that resulted. Hospital scandals, usually following press exposure, often began with untrained staff or students being left in sole charge of wards, especially on night duty. This flouted hospital policy, but when there was a shortage of senior staff, some hospitals took a relaxed view of supervision. Student nurses might find themselves in charge of a large ward, with a supervisor theoretically on call, but in reality not always available. This subject recurred with dispiriting frequency in the RRB and in the RCN's correspondence. The RCN could complain to the hospital authorities, with the backing of an indignant press, but the problem still recurs.[80] In the 1960s and 1970s there were several serious and widely reported incidents of cruelty or neglect in psychiatric and geriatric institutions, and the RCN repeatedly pressed the government to provide more funding for these services.[81] The RCN had to provide legal representation for its members in employment tribunals and courts of law. The small number of nursing staff found guilty of criminal behaviour affronted the profession, but the RCN argued that in nearly all cases, the pay and conditions of staff were so poor that nurses with the right training and qualities could not be found for this exacting work. COHSE, with its strong base in the psychiatric hospitals, also blamed bad management and poor environment.[82] At the invitation of the Secretary of State, the RCN and the Royal College of Psychiatrists set up a liaison committee to consider the care of the violent patient.[83] Their report revealed the difficulties of avoiding violent situations where nurses felt unsupported, and were inadequately trained. Violence by, and against, patients was more likely to occur where staff had to cope single-handed, and each hospital needed a clear set of guidelines to forestall and manage violent incidents. The Department of Health was slow to respond, claiming that it was too preoccupied with reorganisation in the NHS, but finally published a circular in 1976 urging hospitals to take note of the management procedures outlined by the Royal Colleges.[84] The RCN returned constantly to this theme in the 1970s and was concerned that in spite of much publicity and several inquiries into individual hospitals, many hospitals still had no clear policy or, if an official policy existed, it was not always heeded.[85]

Nurses were more likely to suffer from violence than to perpetrate it, and in 1971 the annual conference discussed attacks on nurses, especially in casualty wards. Headlines such as 'Junkie hoodlums hold nurses in terror' alarmed the public, but although some hospitals tried to protect their staff, security was left to local discretion.[86] The official circular on violent patients also paid brief attention to this problem, but its directives were vague:

> The handling of patients in a state of temporary intoxication, whether caused by alcohol, drugs or poisons, in accident or emergency departments in such a way that violence can be prevented, or minimised, is a skill which those working in those departments should be enabled to acquire: the experience available in the drug dependence treatment units should, where practicable, be utilised in providing in-service training.[87]

Each hospital had its own way of dealing with such situations, and required regular prodding from the professional associations and the trade unions. Given the expanding number of patients, and the absence of reliable statistics, it is difficult to judge whether violence against nurses was increasing disproportionately, or was the continuance of a very long-standing problem. Extreme cases, such as the murder of a psychiatric nurse at Carstairs Hospital in 1976, caused temporary outrage, and the press would regularly rediscover hospital violence, but the RCN tried to monitor the constant series of minor assaults that many nurses experienced as one of the hazards of their job.[88]

The RCN continued to police the boundary between medical and nursing responsibility. By time-honoured practice, doctors prescribed drugs, pharmacists dispensed them, and nurses administered them. The RCN tried to defend the nurses' territory against carelessness in the other two domains, and in 1965 it investigated bad practice in prescribing and labelling. District nurses produced embarrassing evidence of elderly or confused patients prescribed tablets with no other instruction on the label than 'take as before' or 'take as directed', often involving several bottles of identical pills. Patients were sometimes admitted to hospital bearing collections of unidentified drugs.[89] The College engaged in urgent discussions with the pharmacists' and general practitioners' professional bodies to encourage good practice. In 1971 the focus shifted to drug errors in hospitals, where a hard-pressed doctor might give the nurse a verbal instruction about medication, rather than writing it down. But even with written prescriptions, tests in Sheffield Royal Infirmary showed that staff had trouble in interpreting standard instructions on how to administer drugs. Apart from the perennial problem of medical handwriting, doctors still used Latin abbreviations, but inconsistently, depending on their age and training. On average, doctors understood about eight out of ten written instructions, SRNs seven, and enrolled nurses five.[90]

The RCN was usually circumspect in criticising the medical profession, but many consultants were affronted when in 1971 the RCN sent out a questionnaire to selected members about private patients in NHS wards. In return for their co-operation in establishing the NHS, Bevan had permitted consultants to use NHS facilities for their private patients, a practice which some leading members of the RCN thought open to abuse.[91] Invited by the Labour government's Expenditure Committee to justify this view, the RCN sought evidence from selected hospitals on whether beds were kept empty for private patients and so delayed treatment of NHS patients. Sections of the medical press denounced this as 'spying'. Eighty-four respondents (about half those who received the questionnaire) confirmed that private patients enjoyed better food and more privacy, and did not have to wait long before seeing a consultant, but evidence of actual bed blocking was scanty. Nurses' responses to the questionnaire revealed some antipathy towards private patients, who were seen as demanding and more likely to regard nurses as menials, but some nurses also noted that patients in private rooms probably received less attention than those in the wards.[92] Nurses differed in their views of private medicine, and so in 1979, when the RCN council was negotiating for a discount for its members from a private medical insurance company, it did so 'discreetly'.[93]

In the year of its diamond jubilee, the RCN published two important documents, expressing a growing sense of professional confidence: *What the Rcn Stands For* and *Code of Professional Conduct – A Discussion Document*. Both publications reasserted the RCN's fundamental belief in nursing as an independent profession, and in nurses' responsibility to keep up to date with developments within the profession and their particular sphere of practice.[94] These principles were now set in a modern framework. The first publication covered a range of topics from nursing education to ethical issues such as abortion and euthanasia, while the *Code of Professional Conduct* set out the moral standards that should guide nurses' professional practice.[95] The context for these two publications was the debate about the expanding role of the nurse, since by the early 1970s rapid developments within medical science and technology were propelling nurses into professional situations for which they had not been trained. There were complex boundary issues for general practice nurses, who on one hand might have to take responsibility when the GP was overstretched or on call; or alternatively, might be asked to undertake duties that were more appropriate to a secretary or receptionist. Concern about the legal implications or professional boundaries prompted the DHSS to set up a joint working party with representatives of the nursing and medical professions, 'to identify areas of clinical practice in which the role of nurses is extending in relation to that of doctors' and to determine whether they needed to issue guidance to employers in the NHS. The RCN regretted this narrow approach to the subject, since they would have preferred the working party to consider the principles involved in the development of clinical nursing, rather than drawing up a list of tasks. Some members of the council felt that the RCN should withdraw from the working party, and among these was Charlotte Kratz who believed that the RCN was 'not fulfilling its innovatory and leadership function' if it agreed to these terms.[96] When the working party's report appeared in 1975, Catherine Hall commented that it could be more truthfully entitled 'duties not normally undertaken by nurses, but which in certain circumstances nurses are required to undertake'.[97]

The RCN believed that nursing, like any other profession, needed constantly to upgrade its knowledge and skills, but that these developments should be determined by nurses themselves. The NHS did not recognise advanced clinical nursing, and career progression in nursing still meant moving into management rather than a nursing specialty. In order to advance nursing knowledge and practice the RCN recommended the concept of the clinical nurse specialist and consultant to the Briggs Committee, and, disappointed by the DHSS's narrow view of nursing tasks, returned to the subject again in 1975. In an RCN seminar, leading nurses explored how the role of the clinical nurse specialist could be developed in the United Kingdom. The group, which included a professor of nursing from Toronto and the deputy executive director of the American Nurses Association, drew up a comprehensive case for the clinical nurse specialist and consultant. They discussed the extended role of the nurse and the dangers inherent in nurses taking on tasks previously done by doctors, and accepted that this was inevitable because the boundaries between medical and nursing practice were constantly changing. However, their real concern was to identify and seek recognition for the role of the clinical nurse specialist. These specialists had already emerged in areas such as stoma care nursing (nursing patients with a surgical opening such as a colostomy) and ophthalmic nursing, but the potential of nurse specialists had not been understood. The RCN believed that nursing specialists were improving the quality of care for their patients, and with proper support they could advance nursing knowledge as advisers, practitioners and teachers. The seminar's conclusions were published as *New Horizons in Clinical Nursing*, and with the backing of the RCN council, were presented to the DHSS with a case for further research.[98] The debate surrounding the extended role of the nurse rolled on, since the RCN regarded it as a crucial issue. After consulting all its membership groups, the RCN published *The Extended Clinical Role of the Nurse* in 1979, to stimulate further discussion. It contended that the independent nurse practitioner should have freedom to plan care, though 'care' was a difficult concept to define.[99] The question involved more than professional pride and status, since nurse specialists were in short supply. By early 1978 the waiting list for operations in the NHS was reported to exceed 600,000, one of the main reasons being a shortage of specialist nurses in the operating theatres.[100]

RCN funds for commissioning and publishing research were limited, and, as noted in the previous chapter, a large-scale project on nurses' pay and conditions in the early 1960s lapsed (together with the post of research officer) for financial reasons. From 1966 the College began to publish a series of reports on 'the study of nursing care' at the invitation of the Department of Health. Marjorie Simpson, the RCN's former research officer, had moved to the department as a principal nursing officer responsible for research. Her presence in the department improved communications with the RCN over professional nursing issues. Between 1967 and 1971, the College published fourteen reports on different aspects of nursing practice, though financial problems again interrupted them until in 1974 the Department of Health offered to underwrite them. After this, about four appeared each year.[101] The reports contained valuable guidance on nursing practice, though RCN members were much provoked by one of them. Felicity Stockwell's *The Unpopular Patient* appeared in 1973,[102] causing much press interest, alarm in the *Nursing Times*, and several irate reviews by senior nurses.[103] Stockwell's research, based on a relatively small sample, indicated that nurses were sometimes less than even-handed in their treatment of patients. Nurses might be neglectful, or unkind in small ways, to patients who were surly, disruptive or simply depressed by being in hospital. Cheerful and co-operative patients who cracked jokes with the nurses were likely to receive their best attention. Reviewers either criticised the RCN for associating itself with such unwelcome reflections, or argued that it was hardly worthwhile commissioning research where the results were so predictable. The pamphlet achieved what its author no doubt intended, and promoted some self-reflection in the profession.

For the RCN, one of the most contentious subjects in health policy was abortion, legalised in 1967. Correspondence in the nursing press revealed very deep disagreement in the profession, as in society generally. Contraception had divided nurses in a similar way in the inter-war years, and was still a contested subject in 1960, when the young Claire Rayner's advocacy of it in the *Nursing Times* produced an impassioned response.[104] But by the 1960s the RCN's view was that family planning should be free and an integral part of the NHS. The RCN refused to comment publicly on the 1967 Abortion Act, on the grounds that it was a 'medical matter', but it tried to ensure that hospitals honoured the Act's clause that allowed doctors and nurses to refuse on grounds of conscience to assist in terminating a pregnancy. The RCN also objected to trainee nurses being involved in the procedure. Many nurses, whether or not they approved of the new law, believed that placing abortion cases in general gynaecological wards upset other patients and delayed routine operations. Others did not wish to stigmatise abortion cases by placing them in separate wards. In 1969 the RRB voted overwhelmingly for a review of the Act, with many arguing that abortions should take place in special clinics rather than the general hospitals, to reduce pressure on the wards and allow nurses the freedom of choice. (The Royal College of Obstetricians and Gynaecologists recommended the opposite: that all abortions should take place under the NHS to prevent profiteering by private clinics.) A particularly divisive question was whether the Act effectively permitted abortion on frivolous grounds, for any definition of 'frivolous' was, of course, subjective. The press whipped up anxiety about foreign women flocking to Britain for abortions, and the RCN favoured restricting access by requiring a statutory period of residence. In 1970, theatre nurses at Stepping Hill Hospital in Stockport boycotted abortions, and there was some alarm that the boycott would spread. The RCN was committed to supporting nurses who refused to co-operate, but advised them to give sufficient notice of their intentions.[105]

From 1971 an official committee under a high court judge, Elizabeth Lane, monitored the effects of the Act.[106] The committee, which included two nurses, reported in 1974. Its brief was to investigate abuses or unintended consequences of the Act, not to challenge its basic assumptions about the ethics of abortion. It found fewer abuses than expected, though it recommended reducing the time limit for an abortion from twenty-eight weeks of pregnancy to twenty-four, as a safety measure. In July of the same year, opponents of the Act placed an amending bill before parliament. Since a demand for total repeal was unlikely to succeed, the amendments aimed to control private clinics more tightly, reduce the time limit for a termination from twenty-eight to twenty weeks, and to tighten the conscience clause to permit hospital staff to opt out on ethical as well as religious grounds. Catherine Hall, who had converted to Catholicism in her twenties, was under much personal pressure from members of her faith, though her position required her to remain neutral.[107] The RCN gave evidence to the Lane Committee on the difficulties faced by nurses. In some parts of the country, abortions were performed without undue delay, while in others, a woman would encounter many obstacles. National statistics showed great regional variations in access to the procedure. The law did not allow abortion on demand, but GPs and consultants had to make judgements about a woman's health and environment, and they interpreted the law in different ways. In some hospitals, staff were not permitted to withdraw from the clinical procedure unless they could prove a firm religious commitment. Many RCN members in the hospitals believed that 'frivolous' abortions would block beds for more routine operations.[108]

The RCN took a more conservative view than the Royal College of Midwives or the Association of Health Visitors. After much internal debate the RCN supported the twenty-week limit, but the other two associations opposed this, arguing pragmatically that women who encountered hostile or dilatory GPs would be driven back to illegal abortionists. Nor did they agree with the RCN's view about making access difficult for foreign women. The law was not changed, and the twenty-eight-week limit remained until 1990, when it was reduced to twenty-four weeks. Although more cautious than the community nurses in its approach to abortion, the RCN did demand equality of access across the country, and for better counselling and contraceptive advice for women after a termination.[109] The subject also fell into the problematic area of 'the extended role of the nurse', though in this case, the RCN felt that the Department of Health was forcing nurses to take part in procedures without sufficient legal safeguard. Termination procedures changed rapidly after 1967, and most hospitals favoured the use of prostaglandin, a drug that was introduced into the womb. A doctor inserted the catheter, but instructed a nurse to initiate and monitor the intake of the drug. The RCN questioned the legality of this proceeding, since the Abortion Act permitted only registered medical practitioners to perform an abortion. An anti-abortion group threatened to bring criminal proceedings against nurses who exceeded their responsibility, and the RCN needed legal reassurance that they were protected under the 1967 Act. In 1980 the DHSS tried to resolve the question in a circular confirming that nurses could act as instructed by a doctor, without fear of prosecution. The RCN was not satisfied that the DHSS had the authority to decide this, and took its case to law. *Royal College of Nursing v. the Department of Health and Social Security* went to trial (which found for the DHSS), to appeal (which found for the RCN), and finally to the House of Lords, who declared that the DHSS had not acted unlawfully in instructing nurses to take a more active role in abortion.[110] The case illustrated the RCN's role as boundary keeper. Its long-standing aim was to equip nurses to carry greater responsibilities, but it was always acutely aware of the legal dangers of nurses undertaking unsanctioned work. RCN members saw the question of abortion from both sides, for they were a high-risk group for the procedure. In 1976 nurses accounted for 6.2 per cent of all abortion cases, and were the third largest occupational group among those undergoing repeat abortions.[111]

Overseas nurses

By the 1960s, the NHS was relying heavily on workers from abroad, particularly the Commonwealth, to staff the service at all levels. Movement of nurses to and from Britain was not new, and the Ministry of Health had tried to monitor it, though with much difficulty. Until the late 1950s, the main anxiety was that too many British nurses were emigrating and not enough immigrants arriving to replace them. In 1948, the Australian government had to be persuaded to reduce its demand for British nurses, and in the early 1950s, the number of nurses emigrating to Canada caused alarm.[112] The Board of Trade estimated that 2,616 nurses emigrated in 1959 on the long sea routes, with 1,330 coming in, but this was a minimum figure, since no comprehensive statistics were kept.[113] Nurses continued to arrive from Europe and countries outside the Commonwealth: nearly 1,700 work permits were issued to this group in 1959–60, with Spanish, German, Italian, Dutch and French nurses in the majority.[114] The National Consultative Council on the Recruitment of Nurses and Midwives monitored the movement of nurses as best it could. The council was a large body, with representatives from national and local government, nursing organisations, the NHS and the TUC. Florence Udell, then chief nursing officer at the Colonial Office, reported to the council in 1960 that NHS hospitals were still accepting overseas women for nurse training without screening them effectively, and that some had been rejected for training in their own countries.[115] The council believed that most Commonwealth nurses who trained in Britain would not return home, and was anxious that British hospitals accept only the most suitable applicants. Some trainees were sponsored by their own governments, who were irritated when British hospitals tried to persuade them to stay after qualifying. The RCN's reaction to this situation was complex. It had strong international ties through the International Council of Nurses, hosted many students from overseas in its advanced training courses, and some of its most distinguished members were foreign born.[116] Any publicly voiced anxieties about overseas nurses were on linguistic rather than racial grounds, and did not apply to the largest group of immigrants in the 1960s, who were English-speakers from the Caribbean. Nevertheless, the growing number of overseas nurses in the NHS was a bleak reminder that the profession in Britain was not attractive to domestic recruits. The RCN welcomed overseas nurses as potential members; but their presence was a reflection on the perennial problems of British nursing: low pay and poor working conditions.

Before the Commonwealth Immigrants Act of 1962, Commonwealth citizens could enter Britain and work without restriction. The Act made entry far more difficult, and immediately produced bureaucratic wrangling, since certain immigrants were permitted to stay indefinitely if they had desirable skills, while others had temporary employment vouchers that lapsed if they changed or lost their approved employment. Bona fide students were admitted, but while those who qualified for the register were allowed to stay, pupil nurses were on more doubtful ground, since the Home Office did not consider that an enrolled nurse was 'qualified'.[117] While enrolled nurses worked for the NHS, their work vouchers were extended, but if they left that employment, they lost the right to remain. NHS managers, who employed overseas staff in all sections of the service, were alarmed at the possible loss of labour. Private nursing agencies were also concerned, since they had many overseas nurses on their books, some having trained abroad and others in Britain as pupil nurses. Although technically self-employed, these nurses were in fact working for the NHS, which relied heavily on agency services, especially in London. Asked by the agencies to intervene, the RCN approached the Ministry of Labour, but received a negative response.[118] Although the Act was not intended to exclude nurses, the Ministry refused to accept enrolled nurses and ancillary staff employed through the agencies. The RCN was alarmed lest the restrictions on immigration precipitate a crisis in the hospitals, and Monica Baly wrote to the Ministry of Health to inquire how many 'non-British' staff were employed in the NHS. Internal communications within the Ministry were blunt: 'There is no information whatsoever on foreign nurses employed in the N.H.S.' There was a single attempt at the end of 1961 to calculate the number of overseas nursing students and pupils in preparation for the Act, and this information was used in a bland reply to Baly's letter. Less than 15 per cent of this group came from the Commonwealth, and:

> It has, of course, long been the case that numbers of girls from the Commonwealth come here for training and so take back to their own countries the high standards of nursing learned here; this is a very desirable situation and one which will, we hope, continue.[119]

Ten years later, the proportion of overseas-born trainees had risen to nearly 30 per cent.[120] But if the statistical methods of bureaucracy lacked rigour on this subject, the RCN's were also deficient, and no information on the numbers of overseas-born nurses in the RCN has yet come to light. Because so many Commonwealth immigrants were relegated to less skilled posts, it is likely that their representation in the RCN was relatively low compared with their presence in the trade unions. COHSE, after some racial tension in the 1950s, made more effort to recruit immigrant workers in the 1960s.[121]

British hospitals relied on a steady stream of overseas students, but did not always treat them fairly. Many came for what they believed was a high quality training that would be recognised internationally, but before they could train for the register, they had to pass a GNC proficiency test. This took place shortly after they arrived in Britain, and if they failed, they would be given the shorter apprenticeship of an enrolled nurse, although the SEN qualification was not recognised outside Britain. Stanley Holder, chairman of the RRB, stated forcefully that, 'It is sheer hypocrisy to tell students that they will be trained as nurses, when what we mean is that they are needed as labour'.[122] Private agencies were accused of bringing trainee nurses into the country, and placing them on SEN courses.[123] The Student Nurses' Section of the RCN employed its own overseas student officer, Frank Rice, to look after these students' interests and to ensure that they understood the terms on which they were being trained and employed. He visited many training schools, and recalled that administrators who were not keen to invite scrutiny often tried to fob him off by missing appointments, or passing him on to junior staff who could not answer his questions.[124]

RCN members from overseas remember that they were often bewildered and ill informed. One student from Mauritius had the necessary O-levels, and was accepted for training in England after an interview with a matron in Mauritius. She started work in a large asylum the day after she arrived in Britain, having made her way to the hospital with some difficulty, and without any directions from her employer. She began work as a nursing assistant, but prompted by a student from Guyana, had to ask to be put on a training course, since the matron made no mention of training. Her spoken English was fluent, but she was offered no help in improving her written English. She had trouble with her examinations for personal reasons, and at first settled for the roll rather than the register. The RCN's base in the psychiatric hospitals was less firm than in the general hospitals, and she joined COHSE as a student. Membership of the RCN came later when she became an SRN.[125]

Race Relations Acts were passed in 1965 and 1968 to prevent discrimination against immigrants. Enoch Powell, the former Minister of Health who had encouraged the immigration of nurses from the Commonwealth, made his anti-immigration 'Rivers of Blood' speech in April 1968. The numerous supportive letters he received revealed a deep vein of prejudice in British society, and it would be unrealistic to pretend that all nurses were exempt from it.[126] But the founders of the RCN had seen nurses as an international community, and the College had long welcomed overseas students into its educational courses. The many pictures in the early nursing journals of British nurses presiding over training schools of the empire and even further afield can be read in two ways. They certainly carried an imperialist message about the benefits of a 'superior' British training, but the trainees were always presented

as studious professionals, accepted into the sisterhood by virtue of their training and their British-style uniforms. The small group of overseas nurses
among RCN members interviewed for this book certainly encountered occasional racist prejudice, though mainly from patients rather than fellow nurses.
Crotchety seniors feature regularly in the reminiscences of British nurses, and
it is difficult to separate racism from personal temperament. Overseas nurses
experienced more prejudice from the public, especially in areas with a large
immigrant community: by 1969, 72 per cent of trainee nurses in one
Metropolitan hospital board were from overseas.[127] But, unlike overseas
doctors, the nurses had trained in Britain, and seem to have attracted less
hostility.[128] At the 1972 RCN annual professional conference there were unfavourable comments about the standards of Commonwealth doctors, but
members made no comment on Commonwealth nurses; rather, they worried
about a possible influx of non-English speaking nurses when Britain joined
the EEC in 1973. The *Nursing Times* was rather defensive about the conference
discussion: 'There was little chauvinism, but there was real apprehension
grounded in deep thought'.[129]

The RCN tried to assist overseas nurses with information and advice. It
produced an information leaflet for arrivals, and in 1965 its Public Health
Section organised a conference on 'Our part in integration' in Leicester, for
public health nurses, social workers and schoolteachers. In 1974, with the aid
of the Gatsby Charitable Foundation, it set up a special project (CHANNEL)
to provide a more welcoming reception and welfare service for incoming
nurses, regardless of whether or not they joined the RCN.[130] CHANNEL also
assisted overseas nurses at the end of their training, when they were likely to
fall into the bureaucratic black hole of the Department of Employment. The
RCN was particularly anxious to prevent overseas nurses from unwarily
embarking on the wrong course of training, since this not only restricted their
opportunities when they returned home, but they might be denied permission
to stay in Britain after their two-year training for the roll. It also complained
to the Ministry of Health that hospitals admitted students from abroad without
an interview, or employed untrustworthy interviewers in the students' home
countries. This was a problem that pre-dated the Commonwealth Immigration
Act, and the Ministry, at the RCN's request, issued lists of reputable interviewers in each country to the hospitals recruiting students from overseas.
Interviewers, however, were not always reliable, and concentrated on trying to
screen out grossly unsuitable candidates rather than assessing whether the
students were adequately prepared for training in Britain. Some students
arrived speaking little English, and a few were in poor health. Those who could
not cope with the training courses because of language difficulties were effectively being recruited as ancillary staff, although they did not know this, and
the RCN contended that such practice amounted to false pretences. Briggs also

recommended effective screening of applicants from abroad, and the need for mandatory orientation courses for them, but his suggestions were not followed up.[131] There was a further problem with nurses who had already trained overseas, but whose qualifications were not recognised by the GNC. They were welcome in the hospitals, because they could be paid less than their qualifications merited. The RCN wanted the GNC to offer them practical and theoretical examinations to regularise their position. The GNC refused, mainly on grounds of cost, since nearly 4,000 trained nurses entered the country in 1974.[132] The RCN also battled with the Department of Employment over work permits for overseas students who passed their examinations and wished to stay in Britain. They had the full backing of the Department of Health, whose main priority was the labour needs of the NHS. Student nurses from overseas had visas that expired when they finished their studies, but they could not be employed by a hospital until they had received their examination results and been registered by the GNC. This could take months, during which time the nurses were threatened with deportation for having overstayed their visas.[133]

By the early 1970s, the nursing shortage was again acute, and regular NHS advertisements appeared in the press urging school leavers and others to consider nursing as a profession. Apart from the difficulty of domestic recruitment, many British nurses emigrated after American and Australian recruiting bodies came on widely publicised 'trawling' expeditions, offering attractive salaries. But by the later 1970s, with unemployment rising rapidly, there were more domestic recruits for nursing, and the Department of Employment (formerly the Ministry of Labour) was less disposed to allow qualified students from overseas to remain in the country, even though their labour had been essential to the NHS while they trained. A study by Susan Walsh, commissioned by the RCN and published in 1980, showed that little had changed. Students were still being placed on courses that did not qualify them for nursing in their own countries, and the process of gaining an employment voucher was still extraordinarily complicated. No-one kept an adequate record of the number or subsequent careers of overseas trainees. The researcher concluded grimly that the system showed a considerable moral turpitude on the part of the Home Office and the Department of Employment, who accepted overseas students without giving them adequate guidance, used them as cheap labour and then ejected them.[134] Her recommendations were essentially those that the RCN had been putting forward for some twenty years: to stop recruiting for the roll, since other countries did not recognise the qualification; to recruit overseas nurses through a central clearing system rather than the individual hospital training schools; and to offer these students independent counselling and career guidance.

Overseas trainees were caught between the Department of Health, always ready to welcome cheap labour into the NHS, and the Department of

Employment and the Home Office, who policed immigration policy in accordance with fluctuating labour demand, under increasing pressure from popular anti-immigration sentiment. In the early 1980s the Commission for Racial Equality reported that racism was rife in the NHS, and that nurses from ethnic minorities were less likely to be promoted or to reach the upper levels of their profession. They were still concentrated in geriatric and mental hospitals, in low status jobs and unpopular fields of nursing.[135] Similar criticisms were still being made in 1996.[136]

In 1979, Briggs finally arrived, though several years of negotiation among interest groups in the profession had chipped away at the unitary structure envisaged in his report. The Queen's speech in 1978 promised a Nurses, Midwives and Health Visitors Bill, and this passed through parliament with little controversy, to become law in 1979.[137] The new UK Central Council for Nursing, Midwifery and Health Visiting, which replaced the GNCs, was responsible for planning new patterns of nurse education, though regional and specialised groups had separate boards or standing committees. The length and content of training courses would have to conform to EEC directives, but this was already planned for. The RCN had a direct input into the new system, for Catherine Hall, who was due to retire as general secretary in 1982, became interim chairman of the UK Central Council for Nurses, Midwives and Health Visitors during its foundation period, a part-time task that challenged even her redoubtable energies. The processes of change begun by Briggs in 1972 were still being painfully worked out in the 1980s, as will be discussed in the next chapter. Although histories such as this never fall neatly into periods, the end of the 1970s seems in retrospect to form a natural divide. In 1979, the RCN was moving into its new role as a trade union, though constrained by its constitution and professional traditions. The Nurses Act promised new directions in nurse education. Catherine Hall's imminent retirement gave cause for reflection on the great changes in the composition and activity in the RCN during her lengthy tenure as general secretary. For much of her time in office, the RCN had to deal with a rapid succession of government ministers against a background of political and economic instability. Nursing was rarely high on the political agenda, as the sluggish response to Briggs revealed.

Conclusion

The turbulent industrial relations of the 1970s forced the RCN to become a trade union, not because of any change of heart by its leadership, but by force of circumstances. The labour policies of Conservative and Labour governments, although differing greatly in their attitude to the unions, both wanted to place union activity in a firm legal framework. If the RCN had rejected unionism, and remained as a professional body, it would have lost its authority to speak for nurses in the workplace. Many of its members, particularly the nursing students, were, in any case, trying to push it into a more radical position. Its difficult relations with other health services unions were not resolved by its new status: rather, they resented it as a direct competitor that was not willing to join the workplace disruption of that difficult period. The change of status was more than a legal manoeuvre: it led to major local reorganisation of the RCN, and a more efficient system of workplace representatives. The RCN shared the problems of all large unions in trying to attract members with different interests, and it made further efforts to accommodate specialist interests in the profession, and to foster nursing research.

Since the time of the Horder investigations, the RCN had been active in trying to influence nursing policy, both in wider issues like nurse training, and in everyday practice. From 1970 to 1972 it participated in Asa Briggs' major report on nurse training, but political instability and economic chaos made this a particularly unfavourable time for major change. The profession was never unanimous on this crucial issue, but the RCN had dropped its older stance of opposing practical training that was not under the control of ward sisters, and it welcomed Briggs' proposal to set a basic educational standard for nursing recruits. The standard of women's education had risen since the war, and social change made possible the long-standing desire of the College founders to present nursing as an educated profession. But this desire still ran counter to the health service's demand for cheap labour, which was being increasingly met by overseas nurses. With Catherine Hall as general secretary, the RCN had proved adaptable to changing conditions, as its healthy membership figures showed, and it needed to maintain this momentum. At the 1977 conference, during the debate on TUC affiliation, June Clark made a prescient comment: that there was no guarantee that the TUC would remain a major force in politics.[138] The Nurses Act had barely passed through parliament when a general election brought the Conservatives under Margaret Thatcher into power, which they retained for nearly two decades. The RCN, like other trade unions, now had to work within a programme of radical change.

Notes

1 RCNA T30, interview with Dame Kathleen Raven, 1988.
2 Briggs report, p. v.
3 In all, twenty people served on the committee, but one nursing member left the committee early for personal reasons, and was replaced.
4 It published its own evidence in *Rcn Evidence to the Committee on Nursing* (London: RCN, 1971).
5 For the details of governments' slow progress with the Briggs report, see Webster, *Health Services Since the War. Vol. 2*, pp. 686–92.

6 For a full account of the Briggs recommendations, and their consequences, see Celia Davies and Abigail Beach, *Interpreting Professional Self-regulation. A History of the United Kingdom Central Council for Nursing, Midwifery and Health Visiting* (London and New York: Routledge, 2000), pp. 3–39.

7 National Board for Prices and Incomes, *Report No. 60. Pay of Nurses and Midwives in the National Health Service*, p. 8.

8 RCNA pamphlet collection, *Rcn Comment on the Report of the Committee on Nursing* (London: RCN, 1973), pp. 1–2.

9 For a detailed analysis, see Robert Taylor, *The Trade Union Question in British Politics: Government and the Unions Since 1945* (Oxford: Blackwell, 1993), pp. 177–93.

10 RCN/5/2/10, Catherine Hall to E. Caines [DHSS], 16 Dec. 1970.

11 RCN/5/2/10, notes by the Labour Relations Department on counsel's opinion on the Industrial Relations Bill.

12 CM 27 Jan. 1971, pp. 2–6.

13 RCN/17/4/3, press cuttings, *NM* 23 March 1971.

14 RCN/17/4/3, press cuttings, *Sunday Times* 31 Oct. 1971.

15 RCN/5/2/10, *Sunday Times* 3 Jan. 1971.

16 *Report of a Committee of Inquiry into the Regulation of the Medical Profession* Cmnd 6018 (London: HMSO, 1975).

17 For progress, see CM 1974, appendix, RCN/74/8, Labour Relations Report.

18 Below Grade 7.

19 RCNA T297, interview with James P. Smith, 2006.

20 CM 24 July 1975 p. 136.

21 Carpenter, *Working for Health*, p. 348.

22 RCN/17/4/5, press cuttings, *NT* 5 April 1973.

23 Taylor, *Trade Union Question*, p. 234.

24 Barbara Castle, *The Castle Diaries 1974–76* (London: Weidenfeld and Nicolson, 1980), p. 88.

25 Castle, *Diaries*, p. 101. The 'mass resignation threat' is described in the following interviews: RCNA T274, Margaret Green, 2005, T283, Val Harvey, 2006.

26 RCN/17/4/6, press cuttings, *Evening News* 14 May 1974.

27 Carpenter, *Working for Health*, p. 73.

28 Hart, *Behind the Mask*, pp. 130–3.

29 RCN/17/4/6, press cuttings, *Daily Telegraph* 13 May 1974.

30 See Christopher Hart, *Nurses and Politics: the Impact of Power and Practice* (Basingstoke: Palgrave Macmillan, 2004), chapter 4, for an excellent analysis of the 'angels' image.

31 RCN/17/4/6, press cuttings, *Daily Express* 1 May 1974.

32 RCN/17/4/8, press cuttings, *Daily Mail* 1 June 1974.

33 The report did not cover Northern Ireland.

34 Department of Health and Social Security, *Report of the Committee of Inquiry into the Pay and Related Conditions of Service of Nurses and Midwives*, Chairman: The Rt. Hon. The Earl of Halsbury, FRS [Halsbury report] (London: HMSO, 1974), p. 12.

35 Halsbury report, paras 39, 53. The Clegg report subsequently explained that hospitals, which avoided the higher costs of overtime pay as far as possible, tended to resort to time off in lieu when they asked nurses to work outside their normal shifts.

36 Unions had to meet certain conditions regarding their constitutions and the transparency of their financial practices, but most were already conforming to these.

37 CM 22 July 1976, p. 442.

38 CM 25 Nov. 1976, p. 420; RCNA T283, interview with Val Harvey, 2006.

39 AR 1977–78, p. 7.

40 Although this was the most publicised incident it was not the only one. A former nurse recalls similar action in Aberdeen Royal Infirmary, after a senior nurse persuaded the consultants to join her in defying management (personal information).

41 See RCN/17/4/11, press cuttings for Feb. 1977 for numerous examples.

42 RCN/17/4/11, press cuttings, Eastern Daily Press 6 June 1978 and 9 June 1978.

43 RCN/17/4/11, Bucks Examiner 20 Oct. 1978.

44 For a detailed account of these negotiations, see Webster, Health Services Since the War. Vol. 2, pp. 712–14.

45 RCN/17/4/12, press cuttings, The Guardian 19 Jan. 1979.

46 RCN/17/4/12, press cuttings, The Scotsman 7 March 1979.

47 RCN/5/2/10, contains a detailed account of the RCN processes over affiliation.

48 RCN/25/1, RRB minutes 1977, pp. 36–7.

49 Other professional bodies that affiliated at this time were the First Division Civil Servants, the National Association of Schoolmasters and the Association of University Teachers. The Health Visitors' Association was a long-standing member.

50 Bridger was programme director, Career Development and Institutional Change at the Tavistock.

51 The Board comprised council members, and representatives of the sections, the national boards, the IANE London, current students and the association for former students. It had external representatives from the General Nursing Council, the Joint Board of Clinical Nursing Studies, the Council for the Education and Training of Health Visitors and the Departments of Education and Science, and of Health and Social Security.

52 NT 19 May 1977, p. 717.

53 The area officers were based in Bath (Western Area); Darlington (North Eastern and North Western); Birmingham (Midlands); and in Headquarters London (South Eastern and Eastern).

54 RCN/4/1965/2, report of a special group set up to consider the future development of the RCN. Most doctors subscribed to the BMA, the Medical Defence Union, and a professional association in their own area of medicine.

55 RCNA T274, interview with Margaret Green, 2005.

56 RCN pamphlet collection, Tavistock Institute of Human Relations, An Exploratory Study of the Rcn Membership Structure (London: RCN, 1973).

57 NS leader, 'Operation grassroots', Jan./Feb. 1974.

58 RCNA T274, interview with Margaret Green, 2005.

59 RCN/3/42/4, speech by Margaret Green to RRB, 1974.

60 Bridget Ramsay, *Expectations and Disappointments: a Perspective on Reorganisation in the Royal College of Nursing* (London: RCN, 1981), p. 15.

61 RCN/3/42/4, Steering Committee on reorganisation of the membership structure, 1974–76, and RCNA T28, interview with Margaret Lee, 2006.

62 One officer remembered being told in no uncertain terms by members in the North West that they would not travel to Lancaster for a meeting. RCNA T304, interview with Moureen White, 2006.

63 By this date there were seventy-two centres. There had been 214 branches in 1973.

64 Ramsay, *Expectations and Disappointments*.

65 Before the change to associations and societies in 1975 there were ten sections – the former Public Health Section had become Community Health in 1971; District Nurses (1972); Enrolled Nurses; Nurse Administrators; Occupational Health; Private Nurses; Psychiatric Nurses (1966); Student; Tutor; Ward and Departmental Nurses. The twelve specialist groups were accident and emergency nursing; clinical teachers; community health administrators; district nurse administrators and tutors; health education; intensive therapy nursing; nursing agencies administrators; public health tutors; registered homes administrators; research discussion; top management; university health.

66 The nurse adviser for the Society for Primary Health Care Nursing was based in the South Eastern area office at the RCN headquarters, the nurse adviser for the Society of Geriatric Nursing and Society of Nursing Research in the Western area office; the nurse adviser for the Society of Occupational Health Nursing in the North Western area office; the nurse adviser for the Society of Psychiatric Nursing in the Midland area office; the nurse adviser for Overseas Students in the Central Southern area office at the RCN headquarters; and, the nurse adviser for Specialist Entities in the North Eastern area office. *Rcn Members Handbook* (Royal College of Nursing of the United Kingdom, 1977).

67 RCNA T304, interview with Moureen White. The key people involved in the formation of the RCN Oncology Nursing Society in 1978 were Richard Wells, Robert Tiffany, Norman Beasley and Gill Hill. The society changed its name to the RCN Cancer Nursing Society in 1991.

68 CM 15 March 1973, p. 112.

69 Basic subscription rate increases: 1975 £15; 1976 £18; 1977 £23; 1978 £27; 1979 £30; 1980 £36; 1981 £40; 1984 £45; 1987 £50; 1989 £55; 1990 £65; 1991 £75.

70 RCN/4/1965/2, report of meeting of special group set up by the Chairman's Committee to consider the future development of RCN, 1965–6.

71 CM Jan. 1969, pp. 49–54.

72 Although independent, the Development Trust was tied closely to the RCN through the appointment of the trustees. These were the president, the chairman of council, the chairman of the Finance Committee, the Marchioness of Lothian (a vice-president of RCN), the Duke of Atholl (Lord Cowdray's nephew), Lord Rosenheim (a vice-president of RCN and president of the Royal College of Physicians), Sir Brian Windeyer (vice-chancellor of London University) and Brian Salmon.

73 CM 27 July 1977, pp. 180–1; 22 Sept. 1977, p. 280.

74 CM 24 Nov. 1977, p. 375.

75 CM 21 March 1975, p. 65.

76 CM 21 Feb. 1963, p. 49.

77 For a critical approach to the RCN stemming from experience of that period, see Rosemary White, 'Political regulators in British nursing', and Jean B. McIntosh, 'District nursing: a case of political marginality', in Rosemary White (ed.), *Political Issues in Nursing: Past, Present and Future* (Chichester: John Wiley, 1985), vol. 1, pp. 31–3 and pp. 55–7. For an alternative view, see Dingwall et al., *Introduction to the Social History of Nursing*, pp. 210–13.

78 CM March 1971, p. 30; July 1971 p. 374; May 1972, p. 213.

79 In 1976 regional, area and district nursing officers requested permission to set up their own society within the RCN, but this was discouraged at first until they threatened to go to NALGO; the RADNO Group was established in June 1977. In 1984 the group voted to become a forum of the RCN Association of Nursing Management. In 1986 it became the Forum for Chief Nurses in Health Authorities.

80 'NHS leaving students in sole charge of patients', *The Guardian* 17 April 2007. Similar complaints had been made of the former voluntary hospitals.

81 For example, Farleigh Hospital where a number of male staff received gaol sentences, *NM* 16 April 1971.

82 Hart, *Behind the Mask*, pp. 120–1.

83 CM 18 May 1972, Report of the Psychiatric Committee, 'The care of the violent patient', pp. 144–53.

84 RCN/5/2/100. DHSS HC(76)11, 'The management of violent, or potentially violent, hospital patients', 10 March 1976.

85 Rcn Society of Psychiatric Nursing, *Seclusion and Restraint in Hospitals and Units for the Mentally Disordered* (London: RCN, 1979).

86 RCN/17/4/3, press cuttings, *Daily Sketch* 24 March 1971.

87 RCN/5/2/100. DHSS HC(76)11, 'The management of violent, or potentially violent, hospital patients', 10 March 1976.

88 A patient and a policeman also died in this incident. For press alarm at violence against nurses, see RCN/17/4/11, press cuttings, *Liverpool Daily Post* 22 March 1977 and *The Sun* 7 April 1977. For similar accounts in later years, see RCN/17/4/21/6, press cuttings, *London Standard* 30 Dec. 1985, and 'Attack alarms for nurses and a crackdown on dirty wards', *The Guardian* 26 Sept. 2007, p. 10.

89 RCN/17/5, press release, Oct. 1965.

90 RCN/17/4/3, press cuttings, *Medical News* 1 Oct. 1971.

91 RCN/17/4/3, press cuttings, *NT* 19 Aug. 1971.

92 *The Times* 25 March 1971, p. 2.

93 CM 26 Feb. 1979, pp. 22–3.

94 *What the Rcn Stands For* (London: RCN, 1976), p. 3.

95 *Rcn Code of Professional Conduct – A Discussion Document* (London: RCN, 1976).

96 CM 19 Sept. 1974, p. 381.

97 CM 21 Mar. 1975, p. 60.

98 *New Horizons in Clinical Nursing* (London: RCN, 1975).

99 *The Extended Clinical Role of the Nurse* (London: RCN, 1979), p. 3. In the 1980s the RCN continued to promote the development of the clinical nurse specialist through its work on standards of care. See chapter 8.

100 RCN/17/4/ 11, press cuttings, *The Observer* 12 Feb. 1978.

101 H. Marjorie Simpson, 'The Royal College of Nursing of the United Kingdom 1916– 1976: role and action in a changing health service', *Nursing Mirror* (2 Dec. 1976), 39–41.

102 Felicity Stockwell, *The Unpopular Patient (Study of Nursing Care Project, Series 1, No.2.)* (London: Rcn, 1972).

103 RCN/17/4/5, press cuttings, *NT* 22 March 1973.

104 *NT* 25 March 1960, p. 394.

105 RCN/17/4/2, press cuttings, *Daily Telegraph* 18 June 1970.

106 For the workings of this committee, see Ashley Wivel, 'Abortion policy and politics on the Lane Committee of Enquiry, 1971–1974', *Social History of Medicine* 11: 1 (1998), 109–35.

107 RCN/15/1/3/4, miscellaneous correspondence on the Abortion Act.

108 For an analysis of the report, see J. Temkin, 'The Lane Committee report on the Abortion Act', *Modern Law Review* 37: 6 (1974), 657–63.

109 RCN/15/1/3/1, Abortion Act 1967.

110 *The Times* 1 Aug. 1980, p. 4; 7 Nov. 1980, p. 14; 6 Feb. 1981, p. 9. Also, RCNA T287, interview with Margaret Lee, 2006.

111 Colin Brewer, 'Why nurses?', *NT* 9 Dec. 1976, p. 1909.

112 TNA MH 55/2197, A. M. Reisner to M. M. Wilkins, 11 March 1948; memo by M. G. Lawson, 11 May 1956.

113 TNA MH 55/2197, 'Passenger Movement Department of the Board of Trade, estimates by migration by long sea routes of nursing profession'. Numbers leaving the country included overseas-born as well as British-born nurses, and students as well as qualified nurses.

114 TNA MH 55/2197, Ministry of Labour. Permits issued for nursing from 1 April 1959 to 31 March 1960. It was not known how many of those who acquired permits actually worked as nurses, and the Ministry estimated that about a third were not taken up.

115 TNA MH 55/2197, National Consultative Council on the Recruitment of Nurses and Midwives, minutes, 26 Oct. 1960, p. 3.

116 For example, Annie Altschul, Lisbeth Hockey and Charlotte Kratz.

117 The debate on SEN status is rehearsed exhaustively in TNA HO 344/208.

118 CM 17 May 1962, pp. 231–2.

119 TNA MH55/2197, M. M. Perry to M. E. Baly, 1 Aug. 1962.

120 TNA MH 165/243, evidence to the Halsbury Committee by the management side of the Nurses and Midwives Council, p. 9. This figure fell to 24.6 per cent in 1972, including 19.2 per cent from the Commonwealth.

121 Carpenter, *Working for Health*, p. 285.

122 RCN/17/4/3, press cuttings, *Times Educational Supplement* 30 April 1971.

123 RCN/17/4/3, press cuttings, *The Guardian* 6 May 1971.

124 RCNA, T329, interview with Frank Rice, 2007.

125 RCNA T311, interview (anonymised), 2007.

126 Penny Starns, *March of the Matrons*, pp. 89–93, argues that racist attitudes inherited from the military were carried over into the nursing hierarchy, but does not offer much evidence. For a 1990s study offering evidence of discrimination against ethnic minority nurses, see Sharon Beishon, Satnam Virdee and Ann Hagell, *Nursing in a Multi-ethnic NHS* (London: Policy Studies Institute, 1996).

127 RCN/17/5/11, press release, Aug. 1973.

128 TNA MH 149/1671, this file contains many racist complaints about Commonwealth doctors, but very few about nurses. This is, admittedly, negative evidence.

129 RCN/17/4/4, press cuttings, *NT* 30 March 1972.

130 Centre of Help and Advice for Newcomers to Nursing Education and Life in the UK.

131 Briggs report, p. 213.

132 CM 19 Sept. 1974, pp. 407–8.

133 CM 13 Sept. 1979, pp. 435–7.

134 Susan Walsh, *Overseas Nurses: Training for a Caring Profession? A Study Identifying the Needs of, Resources Available to, and the Employment Expectations of Overseas Nurses Whilst Training in the NHS* (London: RCN, 1980).

135 RCN/17/4/20/1, press cuttings, *The Guardian* 7 Jan. 1984.

136 Beishon et al., *Nursing in a Multi-ethnic NHS*.

137 See Margaret Green, 'Nursing education – "Reports are not self-executive"', in Baly, *Nursing and Social Change*, pp. 295–310.

138 RCN/25/1, RRB minutes, 1977, p. 38.

8

Nurses, managers and politicians

One of the Callaghan government's last efforts to restore calm in the public services was to set up a Standing Commission on Pay Comparability, chaired by Professor Hugh Clegg. The commission, established in March 1979, investigated pay in various occupations by analysing their duties and comparing them to similar groups in both the public and the private sectors. Like Briggs, Clegg began his work under a Labour government, and presented his report to a Conservative one. As ever, it was difficult to compare nursing with other occupations, and Clegg called in business consultants to work through the complex activities of nurses, analysing a small sample to find out how they spent their time. The consultants used a ready-made system of analysis based on the 'know-how, problem-solving and accountability' of each worker, and claimed thirty years' experience of collecting empirical data.[1] Whether this took into account long-standing gender prejudices was not mentioned in the report. The RCN was anxious lest nurses be compared once again with the average of non-manual female workers, because many of these, having few O-levels and no special training, were confined to junior posts. Nurses, the RCN argued, were highly trained, and should not be disadvantaged because their work was traditionally seen as female; rather, they should be compared with other professions, such as teachers, though teachers worked significantly shorter hours and had longer holidays. In 1978, male primary school teachers earned an average of £99 per week compared with an average of £54 for female registered and enrolled nurses.[2]

The Clegg report was a curious mixture of formal managerial rhetoric and pragmatism. It decided that ward sisters and staff nurses, highly experienced and working long shifts, were underpaid in comparison with other professional groups. The commission recommended a substantial rise for them, and assumed that their weekly working hours would soon be cut from forty to thirty-seven. Nurse administrators, working shorter hours and with higher salaries, were seen as adequately paid in comparison with junior management elsewhere, and many received no pay rise. Nurse tutors caused a problem.

They too had shorter working hours than staff nurses, and it was difficult to justify a substantial raise for them by Clegg's criteria. Should they be regarded as nurses, or compared with teachers in further education? Practical issues determined the outcome. Like psychiatric and geriatric nurses, nurse tutors were in short supply, so Clegg proposed a substantial pay rise to attract recruits. The average recommended increase was 19 per cent, but most of the benefits were for staff nurses, who received 23 per cent, against 17 per cent for nurse tutors. Senior administrators, area and district nursing officers had no rise at all.[3]

The RCN council was dismayed by the Clegg report, particularly because it threatened to divide the profession. The *Nursing Times* was inundated with passionate complaints from nurse administrators, who felt that their position after years of struggle had been completely undermined, while staff nurses were reasonably content with the offer. Many pointed out that the report assumed a shorter working week, but that hospital management had not yet agreed this. Catherine Hall had to deal with many aggrieved letters from members of the RCN complaining of discrimination. She was in a difficult position, as both staff and management sides of the Whitley Council had agreed to accept the report if the government did so, and it was not certain whether the Conservative government would honour any of its predecessors' industrial relations commitments. The government made plain that it had little interest in comparability discussions, and rapidly discarded the Standing Committee. If the RCN objected too strongly to Clegg's proposals, it might receive a worse offer. The pay settlement favoured nurses in the wards rather than nurse managers, and the RCN had been arguing for some years that staff nurses had been left behind, with few career incentives. The settlement also assumed a shorter working week for hospital nurses, another of the RCN's goals. Hence the council accepted the Clegg report as the best that could be achieved under the circumstances. Catherine Hall's standard reply to complaints stated: 'I have to advise you that, unacceptable though the recommendations are, it is neither possible nor practical to reject the report'.[4] The council had to fend off a formal motion from the Derby centre of no confidence in the RCN's negotiators. Derby also demanded that the council repudiate the Whitley Council as a method of pay bargaining.[5]

One of the main priorities of the Thatcher governments was to attack inflation through a tight control of the money supply. Whether their tactics amounted to 'monetarism' as defined by economists, caused much debate then and later, but they certainly led to much discussion on how to cut 'wasteful' expenditure in the public services. The government's response to Clegg was an early indication of their tactics towards public spending. They accepted the report, together with Clegg's separate recommendations for ambulance staff and ancillary NHS workers – again divisive, with a 10 per cent raise for the first group and 22 per cent for the second. But for all NHS workers the message was the same: the government would meet only part of the cost of their pay increases, and the rest would have to be covered by local health authorities through 'efficiency savings'. Health authorities had already been asked to make £23.4 million savings, and an additional £3.4 million was demanded to demonstrate 'improvements' in working practice among ancillary staff. For nurses, too, the amount offered by the government fell short of the agreed pay rise.[6] Since productivity was almost impossible to measure for nursing staff, and difficult enough for most workers in the NHS, health authorities looked desperately for ways of saving money. To employers faced with the long-term problems of rising health care costs and growing demand from an ageing population, cutting staff seemed the easiest option.

The RCN was also affected by the government's second priority: to curb the power of the trade unions. Elected in a landslide vote after the 'winter of discontent', in the following years the government passed a number of measures that restricted strike action, laid unions open to civil action for damages, and virtually abolished the closed shop.[7] Rising unemployment made the task easier, and Margaret Thatcher succeeded where Edward Heath had failed. The last major confrontation with the health service unions, before these restrictions began to bite, came in 1982. After the Clegg report, some NHS workers received more substantial pay rises than others, but low pay among ancillary staff was still a serious problem. About 400,000 health workers earned considerably less than the government's own poverty line of £82 a week for a married person with two children, and the government's offer in late 1981 of a 6.4 per cent rise for nurses and 4 per cent for other workers was not accepted.[8] In December the RCN launched a pay campaign under the slogan 'Bridge that gap', which proved one of the longest and most bitter of its kind. The government made no pretence of equality of sacrifice in the public sector. Although there was a nominal ceiling of 4 per cent, selected unions, including the police and fire service, received much higher awards. The health service unions, who had become very unpopular in 1979 because of disruption to the hospital services, prepared for a series of one-day strikes from 18 May 1982, though with firmer control of their members' actions, and they promised not to impede the emergency services. This did not prevent the *Daily Mail* from accusing them of waging a 'war . . . against the sick'.[9] The RCN, which did not take part in the strikes, balloted its own members over the government's offer, and Norman Fowler, the Secretary of State for Social Services, refused to respond to the other unions until after the RCN ballot.

Early in June, RCN members rejected the government's offer by 41,297 votes to 20,457, with about a third of members voting. The government responded by raising its offer to 7.5 per cent. In a plain attempt to divide the unions, Fowler met with a RCN delegation on 22 June and persuaded them to accept

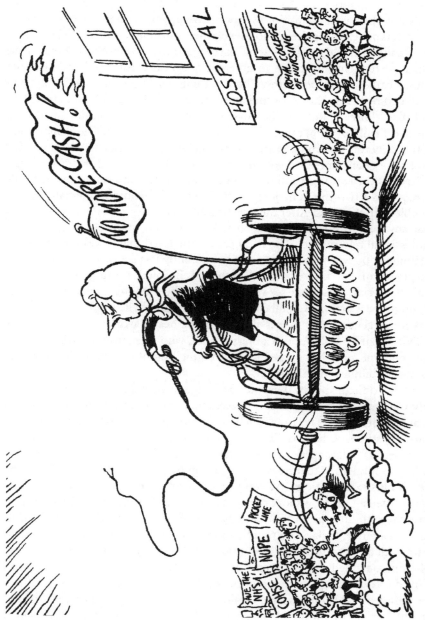

8.1 The *Guardian* cartoonist Les Gibbard comments on the relationship between Mrs Thatcher and the health service unions, February 1988.

this, while keeping the other union representatives waiting for four hours before presenting them with a lower offer.[10] Itself divided, the council agreed by a narrow majority to advise members to accept, but in a second ballot an even larger majority rejected the offer, and half the membership voted. Many RCN members were in mutinous mood, not only over their pay, but also over the effects of health service economies on their working conditions. Meanwhile, thousands of health workers took part in a fourth twenty-four-hour strike aimed at reducing hospitals to emergency services only, and several other unions came out in sympathy. The RCN council knew that two resolutions would come before the AGM that autumn: that the RCN affiliate to the TUC, and that it discard Rule 12, the no-strike policy.[11] Both resolutions had been rejected firmly in 1979, but support for them was growing. The constitution of the RCN was becoming more democratic. In 1982 the charter was amended to allow student nurses to vote in ballots and elections, and they were likely to have a much stronger influence on the outcome. A motion to discard Rule 12 required a two-thirds majority, but if successful would immediately cause trouble with the GNC. After the 1979 health service disputes, the GNC decided that any nurse who put patients at risk by striking could be disciplined for professional misconduct. The RCN council believed that it was impossible to distinguish between emergencies and apparently less serious cases. Action by hospital workers immediately lengthened hospital waiting lists and put patients at risk, so any nurses who withdrew their labour might be in danger of disciplinary action. Several council members also believed that government was more generous to nurses than to other health workers because of the RCN's no-strike policy, but Catherine Hall, who was strongly committed to the policy, nevertheless argued that the council should be prepared to change tactics if members demanded it.

At this difficult point, there was a change of management in the RCN. In July Catherine Hall retired. Her successor, Trevor Clay, had been appointed deputy general secretary in 1979. The appointment of a male general secretary caused a stir, especially as Clay's background differed so markedly from his predecessors'. Clay, aged forty-six, was the son of a wheelwright, eldest of a family so numerous that he was brought up by a paternal aunt. He failed the eleven plus examination, and went to a secondary modern school, which he left at fifteen. During a short period as a trainee shoe salesman, he went into hospital with an injured foot, and as a result of this experience, decided to become a nurse.[12] Clay rose rapidly in the nursing profession, at a time when it was still fairly unusual for men to be accepted for general training; indeed, when he qualified in 1957, men were still excluded from the RCN. He soon moved into nursing administration, and by 1974 he was area nursing officer for Camden and Islington Area Health Authority. His nursing career was successful in spite of continual struggle against debilitating emphysema, which

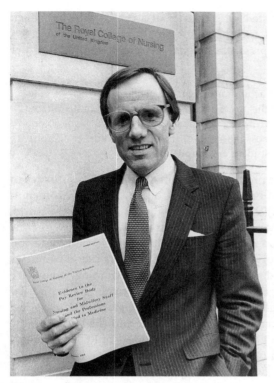

8.2 Trevor Clay, general secretary 1982–89.

he knew would shorten his life. Clay was an excellent communicator who made a powerful impression at public meetings, and he was adept at dealing with politicians and the press. Like his predecessors, he was unmarried, and devoted his life to his work. Catherine Hall had presided over the transformation of the RCN into a trade union. She had not desired this outcome, but accepted it pragmatically when political pressures made it inevitable. Clay was an enthusiastic union man, but was at one with Catherine Hall in their belief that the RCN must achieve its ends without resorting to strikes. For Clay, this was making a virtue of necessity, since he knew that public sector workers had little economic leverage over government. He emphasised the importance of favourable publicity for their cause. 'They have virtually nothing but the balance sheet of public opinion'.[13]

Catherine Hall was sorry to leave the RCN at such a difficult time, but was already working part-time in setting up the UKCC, which was replacing the General Nursing Councils. It is appropriate to pause the story of the RCN to comment on the career of Dame Catherine, as she soon became. Her managerial role in the RCN lasted for a quarter of a century, during which time the College's nature and membership went through many changes. Among many tributes in the press, the *Sunday Telegraph* summarised her work:

> it is very much because of her achievements that the college – which 25 years ago represented the elite end of the profession, the 'ladies' who went into nursing subsidised by their parents – is now a formidable body grown from 30,000 members to 200,000 (out of a possible 375,000) including the former National Council for Nurses, and male, student and pupil nurses.[14]

Catherine Hall deserves a more prominent place in British labour history than she has received. As a leader of one of the largest organisations of women in the country, and one of the largest professional bodies of nurses in the world, her contribution has been underestimated. This is probably because she fits no accepted pattern: she is too conservative for labour historians, and too conventional for feminist historians. She belonged to a generation of nurses without higher education and with little management training, who were forced to renounce family if they wanted a career, though she supported adjustments in professional life to meet the needs of married nurses. She resembled the commanding matrons of former times, and she had the same alarming effect on the younger generation in the corridors of RCN headquarters as an old-style matron on unwary probationers. Christine Hancock, her successor but one, recalled the awe that she inspired, 'I always called her Dame Catherine and she always told me to "call me Mary" but I never really could'.[15] Catherine Hall dealt patiently but firmly with politicians who did not take nurses seriously, with doctors who wanted to keep nurses in their place, with the sometimes fractious sectional interests in the RCN, with a sentimental press that could easily become hostile, with severe critics in the health service unions, with traditionalists among older RCN members, and militants among the young. The RCN's no-strike policy, in which she passionately believed, won her few friends in the other unions, but RCN members in her day overwhelmingly supported it. Yet she also made a strong impression on politicians. Barbara Castle recalled a confrontation, with the tall general secretary towering over her and threatening, 'if you do *that*, Secretary of State, I can guarantee that you will not have a single nurse left in the NHS'.[16] Although her tactics did not please all members, expressions of respect from the nursing profession on her retirement were numerous and sincere.

While the health service unions continued a series of short strikes, the RCN mustered once more to lobby MPs, organise marches, and put its case to the public. Public opinion, if the press views are an accurate representation, stayed solidly behind the nurses because of the no-strike policy. Even *The Sun*, normally a warm supporter of the Prime Minister, chided the government for failing to take care of the 'angels': 'GIVE NURSES THEIR RISE, MAGGIE!' Like Trevor Clay, *The Sun* was acutely sensitive to public opinion, and having found from a poll of its readers that eight out of ten supported the nurses, it prudently stayed on their side.[17] The dispute rumbled on into the autumn, with neither side making any progress. Norman Fowler was criticised for inaction, especially since he took his August holiday at a particularly fraught time. Once again, waiting lists rose, hospitals were without clean laundry or hot meals, and in some cases patients were asked to provide their own sheets. Kenneth Clarke, the Minister for Health, was frequently photographed dodging pickets when he visited NHS hospitals. Acquiring a certain reputation for pouring oil on conflagrations, Clarke announced that the army was standing by in case the emergency services were unable to cope; this had to be hastily corrected by Fowler, who stated the army would take over only ambulance work.[18] Margaret Thatcher went into hospital for a varicose vein operation, but, unlike David Ennals in similar circumstances, opted for a private hospital, a decision that created its own problems. When she emerged, uncharacteristically clad in a trouser suit to cover her bandages, she was spared press comments on her relationship with NHS nurses, but provoked allegations that the NHS was 'not safe' in Tory hands. The TUC involved itself in industrial action for the first time since the general strike of 1926, by co-ordinating a day of strikes and protests in support of the health workers on 22 September.[19] This was now a dangerous tactic, as new legislation allowed legal action with heavy damages against unions taking part in sympathy strikes, and some employers were already taking advantage of it. The TUC and the health service unions were in a difficult position. Their action was making little headway, but attempts to widen it might produce a humiliating public defeat in the courts.

By the time the Cabinet met after the parliamentary recess, Fowler's colleagues were exasperated by his handling of the dispute. Critics as disparate as Edward Heath and Paul McCartney (son of a midwife) publicly attacked the government's stance. The government was preparing for confrontation with more powerful unions, and as the events of the next few years showed, was prepared to take tough and calculated action against them, culminating in the breaking of the miners' strike in 1984. But a fight with nurses was counter-productive. The public was distressed by the disruption in hospitals, but did not turn against nurses, and the RCN's no-strike policy was popular. Inside sources leaked to the press that several Cabinet members felt that this was 'the wrong battle against the wrong people at the wrong time'.[20] The government then decided to conciliate the RCN, in an attempt to drive a further wedge between professionals and other health service workers. In November they offered a staggered increase for nurses averaging 12 per cent, and promised to replace the Nurses and Midwives Whitley Council with an independent Pay Review Body (PRB). They were apparently willing to return to the principle of pay comparability for nurses and other professional groups in the NHS, such as physiotherapists and radiographers. From 1984, decisions on nurses' pay would be in the hands of this body. The RCN had long desired such a measure, and its members accepted the new offer. At almost the same time, the AGM by a large majority rejected the motions to discard Rule 12 and to affiliate with the TUC.[21] The other health service unions continued an inconclusive series of actions until December, and had to settle for the original offer, which was lower than the nurses'. They were not given a review body, and, as privatisation began to spread in the NHS, were pushed towards local rather than national pay agreements.

The RCN's desire for a new method of arbitration stemmed from growing disillusion with the Whitley Councils, where union and management representatives met, first in their own group, and then collectively, to thrash out pay agreements. The government had only two representatives on this body, but they nevertheless had the ultimate authority, since the management side had no power to award pay increases higher than the government of the day would allow. The notion of an independent body was seductive to an aspiring professional organisation. There were already a few models, including those introduced by Labour governments in the 1970s for doctors and dentists, who had previously negotiated directly with government without going through a Whitley Council. But for the RCN council, a major advantage of the pay review system was that they would no longer have to negotiate alongside other unions. The health service unions resented the RCN's numerical superiority on the staff side of the Whitley Council, and there were frequent internal arguments, both about representation and over tactics to be employed. Pay Review Bodies heard evidence from unions and management separately, and then met in camera to decide the outcome. At first, Fowler and Clarke hoped to divide the unions further by permitting only nursing unions that had not taken part in industrial action to come under the PRB, but it was impossible to divide nursing in this fashion, and so all the relevant unions were allowed to present their case.[22] The RCN was unhappy about auxiliary nurses being included in the PRB's remit, and argued that it undermined what should be a principal aim of the NHS: to employ only fully trained nurses by the end of the century, but it was overruled on this.[23]

The Review Body for Nursing Staff, Midwives, Health Visitors and Professions Allied to Medicine was established in 1983, chaired by Sir John Hedley Greenborough, a former director of Shell UK, and former chairman of the Confederation of British Industry. Bodies of this type were supposedly independent of government – though they were firmly instructed by government on its current financial priorities – and have been variously seen as too close to government policy or, conversely, as prone to 'go native' and empathise with their clients.[24] They dealt with occupations in the public sector, such as the armed forces, the judiciary and the police, for whom normal union tactics were thought inappropriate. They had no power to impose their wishes, but were likely to embarrass government by protesting or resigning if their recommendations were not honoured. Greenborough made it plain that the PRB would make its own decisions, and that it was then up to government to find the means of implementing them. One indication of the importance of the new PRB for nurses and midwives was that Kenneth Clarke personally presented evidence at its meetings, rather than leaving it to civil servants. In such a system, compromises were inevitable. Ironically, after much discussion over the PRB's foundation, its first recommendations for nurses in 1984 offered an average rise of 8 per cent for qualified nurses and 7 per cent for auxiliaries, and pleased no-one. Kenneth Clarke indicated that any increase over 3 per cent must be met by the health authorities, while the RCN was dissatisfied at the amount offered and mounted another pay campaign under the title 'Don't squeeze the nurses'.[25] The PRB dealt only with pay, not terms of service or working conditions; and against some opposition from the nursing unions, in 1984 the government disbanded the Whitley Council and replaced it with a Nursing and Midwifery Staffs Negotiating Council. Its job was to grapple with the extremely complex problem of pay grading and comparability for nurses in the NHS.

The PRB took evidence on nurses' pay and responsibilities, and offered variable pay rises to different grades of nurse. Its recommendations were usually above the government's target and above the level of inflation, but nurses were still trying to bridge the historical gap between their salaries and comparable professions. As usual, a major problem was their large numbers – over half a million nurses, auxiliaries, midwives and health visitors were employed by the NHS in 1983, and even a modest pay demand was very costly.[26] The system relied heavily on unqualified staff – a fifth were students and nearly a quarter were auxiliaries. The government honoured the commitment to lower nurses' working hours, which averaged thirty-seven and a half hours per week, but this exacerbated the problem in the hospitals, where shorter hours for trained nurses meant employing more unqualified ones. Although the government did not reject the PRB's decisions, it found ways to circumvent them, such as delaying the payment of an award, and insisting that most of the finance come from efficiency savings in the NHS. Efficiency savings meant fewer posts for qualified nurses. Recently qualified nurses had more difficulty finding jobs, and unemployment in the profession, as in the nation, continued to rise.

The Griffiths report

The whole question of nurses' pay, however, could not be divorced from what was happening in the NHS as a result of the government's drive for efficient and economical management, as defined in its own terms. The government looked to businesspeople for advice, assuming that market forces produced better management in the private sector. Accordingly, in 1983 it appointed Roy Griffiths, a managing director of Sainsbury's, the supermarket chain, to lead a small team to advise on NHS management and cost effectiveness. Other members of his team came from enterprises such as British Telecom and United Biscuits. Griffiths reported in October, urging the government not to delay in imposing a new system of management on the NHS. For too long, he maintained, the NHS had relied on 'consensus management' that produced sluggish administration; there were no incentives for efficiency or penalties for poor service; budgets were too centralised and poorly audited; and authority was too widely spread. Clinical staff were barely mentioned in the report, and nurses appeared only in a phrase that attracted much attention: 'if Florence Nightingale were carrying her lamp through the corridors of the NHS today she would almost certainly be searching for the people in charge'.[27] The Griffiths report, a twenty-four-page typed letter to Norman Fowler, had more immediate impact on the NHS than many of the lengthy and exhaustive reports of previous commissions of inquiry. Fowler began to implement it in the following year, replacing regional and hospital management teams with general managers. The NHS itself was to be under the general direction of a manager appointed from outside the service, while local management posts were open to internal and external competition. The aim was to emphasise the strategic virtues of general management over the (allegedly) narrow views of specialists. Griffiths was 'quite deliberately anti-professional'.[28]

The medical and nursing professions reacted sharply to the Griffiths report, arguing that it undermined clinical responsibility in the hospitals. They were not convinced that consensus management had failed, nor that the NHS was unduly expensive compared with health systems in other countries.[29] The implications for the RCN were profound, since Griffiths threatened to undo the work of decades and remove nurses from any influence on management. The power of the medical profession meant that the reforms had a different effect on nurses and doctors, and although the district medical officer post survived, the chief nursing officer post was abolished.[30]

The Thatcher government produced a measure of unity in the health services unions, since all felt equally threatened. Trevor Clay cultivated good relations with the other unions, and met informally with their leaders. He also tried to keep on amicable terms with the Department of Health and Social Services, and was on first-name terms with Norman Fowler, a familiarity unthinkable in Catherine Hall's day. But Griffiths drove another wedge between the government and the RCN. Kenneth Clarke once more managed to stoke the flames by commenting urbanely on the Jimmy Young radio show that many hospital wards were overmanned.[31] This produced a furious response from the unions, but Mr Clarke demonstrated to his own satisfaction that nursing shifts sometimes overlapped by as much as four hours, a needless luxury, he considered. The nurses retorted that this was uncommon, and that overlapping shifts were necessary to ensure smooth running of the wards and make time for training students, but they were wrong-footed on this matter.[32] Clay urged Fowler to ensure that nurses were represented in senior management, since the post of chief nursing officer would be absorbed under the new arrangements. Fowler was emollient, replying that

> In practice so far as nursing is concerned we would expect that authorities will need a nursing adviser at a senior management level whose main responsibility is the provision and quality of nursing advice to the authority. The officer may of course carry out other duties in support of the general manager.[33]

Fowler also promised Clay that new management structures would not be approved unless they included a 'single identifiable source' of professional advice, and, in response to many similar protests from doctors about their own loss of power, Barney Hayhoe, who had replaced Kenneth Clarke as Minister for Health, wrote to all regional health authorities suggesting that the 'co-operation' of clinicians should be sought in the new system. Hayhoe added, however, that the government did not wish to be 'prescriptive' in implementing the Griffiths report, which meant that the authorities were at liberty to ignore this advice.[34]

The RCN closely monitored the appointment of general managers, and, like the British Medical Association, was increasingly dissatisfied with the new system. By January 1986, of the 138 District Health Authorities in England and Wales whose new management systems were approved by the Department of Health, twenty-eight had no chief nursing officer post and no nurse member of the management team; nine authorities had a chief nursing officer who was advisory only, and not part of day-to-day management; while forty-six had a nursing officer directly responsible to management, but also in charge of nurse education, a division of duties that the RCN thought undesirable. Even worse, five authorities had 'hybrid posts with new titles such as "quality assurance manager"', in which the officer in charge of nursing services had other duties, such as management of the ambulances, or even of public relations.[35] Technically, 'matron' had disappeared from the hospitals after the Salmon reforms, but Griffiths seemed to signal the end of the authoritative (and sometimes authoritarian) nurse of the kind who had founded the RCN. Griffiths' reforms were not just about efficiency, they were a moral crusade; the traditional management structure was swept away and large numbers of senior nurse managers were removed or resigned.[36] The discontent of the RCN in England was worsened because Scotland successfully resisted some of the more extreme elements of the new system. The Scottish Home and

Health Department required that each management team include a senior nurse, not as an adviser, but as professional head of the nurses in that area.[37] If Mrs Thatcher had managed to divide the RCN in accepting the Clegg report, her championing of Griffiths reunited it. Invited to attend the RCN's annual formal dinner, the Prime Minister took the opportunity to express her views in a long political speech, which her hearers received in a hostile spirit. The RCN president, Sheila Quinn, whose work for the International Council of Nurses had required considerable diplomatic skills, pondered her response, and told herself, 'You weren't elected to be polite in these circumstances'.[38] In her reply she said that the RCN did not agree with Griffiths' recommendations, 'but the decision was made and as nurses we are committed to making it work because it directly affects our patients'.[39]

Griffiths saw patient, or 'customer', satisfaction as a high priority, but this often conflicted with economical management. The government seized enthusiastically on his suggestion that in-house NHS services should compete with private suppliers. Replacing cleaners, kitchen staff and other ancillary workers on the NHS payroll with contract staff would save money, though the unions saw this as yet another attempt to reduce their influence, since hourly-paid contract staff had few employment rights and were less likely to be unionised. By 1984, NHS planning included selling off hospital residences for nurses and junior doctors, for the government argued that the recent salary rises would enable students to find more agreeable private accommodation. Only first-year students would be accommodated. The RCN fought this decision, and managed to prevent wholesale evictions, but the slow process of selling off continued.[40] The disposal of nurses' homes ended a system that was often an extension of the disciplinarian regimes of the hospital, and nurses had long complained about poor accommodation. Nevertheless, many nurses, especially in expensive cities like London, found that their pay would hardly stretch to rented accommodation, let alone a mortgage.

The RCN mounted a vigorous publicity campaign, mainly against the Griffiths report, but also against other economies in the health service. Even before the report appeared, the RCN was planning a 'Nurse Alert' strategy to draw attention to the effects of government policy. Nurses were asked to inform the RCN of any problems in their local hospitals arising from the new system. *Nurse Alert: the Effects of Financial and Manpower Cuts in the NHS* was published in March 1984, and received much attention from the national and local press. A series of publications made the RCN point. *Feeling Better, Getting Better. Why the Nursing Voice Must Be Heard* appeared in 1986. It argued that the government had taken economical management in the NHS to an extreme that even the managing director of Sainsbury's, Roy Griffiths, had not intended, and that 'any supermarket which pursues its profit margins so relentlessly would soon go bust'.[41] The RCN's £250,000 advertising campaign asked, 'Why is Britain's nursing being run by people who don't know their *coccyx* from their *humerus*', and added:

> we wish the Health Authorities shared our view that accountants and adminis-
> trators don't know the best bed for a severe burns case, or how many night staff
> are needed to run a busy intensive care unit. We accept that a professional
> administrator should run a hospital. But we passionately believe that only nurses
> can run nursing.

A second advertisement, targeting cuts in nursing staff, ran the dramatic heading: 'You're in hospital. It's dark. You're all alone, surrounded by strangers. You're worried in case something happens. And you're the nurse'.[42] District nurses reported that they were struggling to cope with patients who were being discharged from hospital prematurely in order to cut costs and reduce the waiting lists. Trevor Clay attacked the new management in a *Times* article entitled, 'Why matron is sorely missed'. He described decisions by hospital managers that included expecting two hospitals to share a defibrillator, and trying to cut back on nursing staff at night and weekends to avoid paying overtime rates.[43] Margaret Thatcher's successor accepted 'clinical directorates' in the hospitals in order to avoid some of these problems, though Clay had dismissed such moves as cynical, noting that in the Griffiths report, 'The doctors were deemed important only in so far as they could be nudged into managerial positions and thereby be best placed to control expenditure by other doctors'.[44] Although the RCN's campaign probably had more effect on individual hospital practices than on the NHS as a whole, it did convince many of the public that the absence of matron, representing nursing author-ity, was responsible for many of the continuing problems in the hospitals, from inadequate cleaning services to the spread in later decades of diseases caused by drug-resistant bacteria. The new managers had their own griev-ances, and saw the medical and nursing professions as obstructive in charac-teristic ways. In the hospitals, medical specialists were too important to be overridden, and this, managers alleged, prevented radical change. Conversely, nurses, lacking education, seemed too subservient and hierarchical, unwilling to make decisions for themselves, and capable of slowing the wheels of prog-ress simply through indecision.[45] It seemed that the traditional view of the nurses' role in the hospital hierarchy had left them unfitted to deal with the new managerial world.

The RCN's attitude to another political issue did not please the govern-ment. In 1983 the RCN and the BMA produced separate responses to the government's publicity on how the emergency services would cope in the case of nuclear war.[46] Their view was that even with a limited explosion in one area, few nurses would be left to deal with the casualties, and 'the skills and training of any surviving nurses would be rendered virtually irrelevant'.

The nurse on the left established British nursing standards. The nurse on the right is being forced to compromise them.

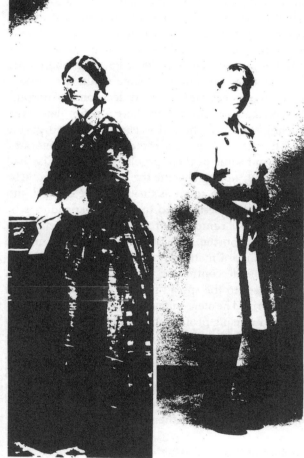

Over a century ago, Florence Nightingale brought to nursing a degree of professionalism, commitment and care that has been its hallmark ever since.

As a result, thousands of little children grew up wanting to be nurses.

Today, many of the children who did become nurses are wishing they hadn't.

Because since the Griffiths Report, nurses are increasingly being treated like children.

The Griffiths Report recommended major changes in the way that the National Health Service is run. Chief among them is the idea that it can be made more cost-effective by employing managers from the business world.

WHO PAYS?

We would argue that in many places, cost-cutting is being carried out at the patients' expense.

Because, whilst we agree that administrators can run hospitals, we don't believe that they can run nursing.

More and more Health Authorities are appointing executives: at the same time, they are depriving nurses of any meaningful management role.

The results could be frightening.

Imagine a hospital where the nurses have no say at all in the choice of beds or other equipment. Where nursing staff can advise on patient care, but can't take any decisions. Where a matter of life and death can become a matter of pounds and pence. A hospital where the patients' spokesman has lost her voice.

Now stop imagining.

Because this is what's starting to happen in Health Authorities throughout the country.

As the protector of nursing standards, the Royal College of Nursing is appalled.

THERE MUST BE A BETTER WAY.

We want to see a director of nursing appointed in every health unit in Britain.

Someone with the power and the nursing experience to make health care more effective.

Whilst the administrator concentrates on making it more cost-efficient.

We think that Miss Nightingale would agree with us. If you do too, please add your name to our petition by sending us the coupon.

And, if you're as worried as we are, please write to your Member of Parliament now (the address is the House of Commons, Westminster, London, SW1A 0AA).

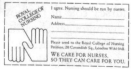

ROYAL COLLEGE OF NURSING

I agree. Nursing should be run by nurses.

Name_____

Address_____

Please send to the Royal College of Nursing Petition, 20 Cavendish Sq., London W1M 0AB

WE CARE FOR NURSES,
SO THEY CAN CARE FOR YOU.

8.3 RCN newspaper advertisement criticising the effects of the Griffiths reforms, 1986.

Transport of casualties would be impossible, and radioactive fallout would prevent any outside movement. Few dressings and drugs would have survived, and these would be rapidly used up. The Home Office, they contended, had an unrealistic expectation that the population would receive enough warning to take shelter in protective buildings. The RCN statement confirmed the worst fears of many of the public, and received a great deal of press coverage.

In the dispiriting atmosphere of efficiency savings and privatisation, the RCN's battles were mainly to ensure that nurses were graded appropriately for the work they were doing. The Pay Review Body did not end disputes over pay settlements. Hospital management had to honour national awards, but tried to achieve savings by other means, such as grading systems that were unfavourable to staff, or reducing special payments that were locally determined. In January 1987, health service union nurses in Manchester took industrial action over cuts in their special duty payments for night work and overtime, and, as similar actions began to spread, it looked as though another major labour dispute was about to break out in the NHS.[47]

The pay and management disputes of the mid-1980s meant that Trevor Clay had a high public profile from the moment he became general secretary. The 'Nurse Alert' campaign was also successful in keeping the RCN in a favourable public light, and Clay reinforced this by commissioning MORI polls on the image of nurses in British society. Not surprisingly, 78 per cent (including a majority of Conservative voters) thought that nurses should be paid more, and that their pay ought to be comparable to the police or fire services. Asked whether they approved of the RCN's no-strike policy, the MORI sample was 45 per cent in favour and 32 per cent against, with a higher proportion of trade unionists, predictably, being against it.[48] The results were perhaps not as overwhelmingly in favour of the RCN's policy as expected, but the polls reaffirmed a high public support for nursing which was useful in the 'balance sheet of public opinion' that Clay was anxious to monitor. More worryingly for the government, the RCN's poll confirmed that 63 per cent of respondents did not think that the NHS was safe in the Conservatives' hands, including 32 per cent of Conservative voters. Clay's approach to nursing questions was distinctly political, as he indicated in his personal manifesto, *Nurses: Power and Politics* in 1987. Nurses, he maintained, could not ignore their part in fighting for resources in the NHS. 'The route lies through organising as a profession and as a trade union, by recognising that the public control of the national health service gives us the opportunity to bring public pressure on government and employers alike'.[49]

Clay had only two more years as General Secretary but they were to be the most political of his career and to radicalise the RCN in an unprecedented way. The issue was clinical grading, a process which aimed to restructure nurses' pay and provide nurses who stayed in the clinical field with a career structure which rewarded their knowledge and skills. A new nine point grading scale had been agreed and was introduced in 1988 linked to the nurses' pay award. Four per cent would be paid immediately, the remainder after each nurse's job had been assessed. The government was optimistic that the whole exercise would be completed within a year.

On their side, nurses were optimistic that they would get a fair grading. Both sides were disappointed. Cash limits were imposed by the Treasury so the health authorities and boards had to adopt a mechanistic approach of deciding how many nurses at each grade they could afford. Nurses' disappointment was inevitable, since they had welcomed the clinical grading structure as a recognition of their skills and experience. Instead it was widely used to downgrade their jobs. They reacted angrily and the RCN and the other health unions had difficulty managing the strength of feeling and spontaneous outbursts, which included strikes and demonstrations around the country. A survey of RCN branches showed that members were disillusioned with the grading process and believed that the NHS management would cheat them of their financial reward. The RCN responded with a 'Fair Grades for Nurses' campaign, launched at a mass meeting in London but there was growing pressure on the RCN to call an extraordinary meeting to discuss strike action. Clay resisted this pressure but did agree to a ballot of members on Rule 12 and, although there was much criticism of the wording of the ballot papers, the membership voted against strike action and to retain Rule 12. The other health unions, particularly COHSE, publicly accused Clay of being on the side of the government.[50] COHSE's nurse members were mainly enrolled nurses and nursing auxiliaries, groups which had been particularly badly treated in the grading process, and they were demanding tough action. The RCN's campaign was based on keeping the issue in the public's attention and supporting the appeals of individual nurses throughout the country. A special training programme to assist stewards was set up, and extra staff were taken on to deal with the accumulating appeals. By the end of the year they had fought and won over 20,000 appeals. While a number of dissenting members left the RCN and joined COHSE, the RCN appeared to have got the mood right, for recruitment figures grew by 14,000 during the year.

Clinical grading continued to dominate the work of stewards and officers for the next five years and by the time the last case was settled it was estimated that 120,000 appeals had been heard. Although the Thatcher government had to back down and make an extra £138 million available, the whole process damaged the relationship between the profession and their employers.[51] The position was not improved by the publication of a White Paper in 1989 proposing that health authorities might become self-governing trusts. This carried with it the possibility that salaries might be locally rather than nationally determined. The RCN's history began in a period when nurses' salaries were entirely at the discretion of local employers, and the RCN, like other unions, had no wish to return to this.

The reform of nursing education

While the Griffiths reforms were sweeping away the traditional nurse managers, an equally fundamental reform of nurse education was being debated. In many ways, the Griffiths report revived long-standing concerns over the nature of nurses' education, since the new managers complained that lack of education was at the root of nurses' problems in the NHS. In January 1981 the RCN council received an ultimatum from the RCN Association of Nursing Education, that if the council did not act to improve their salaries and working conditions, nurse teachers would take their grievances elsewhere – presumably to a trade union.[52] This crisis was another example of the long-running grievances of nurse tutors, but the final straw for them was the Clegg report on pay comparability. Clegg had overridden his consultants' recommendation that tutors receive no pay increase because their hours were shorter than clinical nurses', but their pay rise was lower than the average, and seemed to confirm that they were held in low regard. Nurse teachers had been in short supply since the Second World War, and despite many attempts to improve their position, grievances identified in the 1950s were still apparent in 1980. Their teaching qualifications were not given weight in their salaries, making recruitment and retention difficult and leading to excessively high tutor–student ratios. But the main cause was a pervasive low morale among nurse teachers due to the continuing subordination of nursing education to the needs of the service. This diminished the status of nurse education, and caused many tutors to leave teaching after a couple of years. Following the Clegg report, the frustration and anger of nurse teachers was channelled into the report *To Teach or Not to Teach?* by the RCN Association of Nursing Education. This was presented to council in January 1981 with the teachers' ultimatum calling for 'urgent and drastic' measures:

> Since the 1950s nurse teachers have waited for their just reward. We have waited for Platt, for Salmon, for Prices and Incomes Board, for reorganisation, for Halsbury, for Briggs, for Clegg. Thirty years is a long time to wait.[53]

The general secretary managed to dissipate their anger by persuading council to agree to the Association of Nursing Education Advisory Group taking on an advisory role to the RCN Labour Relations Committee, so that they would be more closely involved in preparing their salary claim and the subsequent negotiations.[54] But the sense of crisis within this section of the profession remained.[55]

The RCN had pleaded for the reform of nursing education after the Platt report over a decade previously, but the government had not supported it. A move towards reform was made with the passing of the Nurses, Midwives and Health Visitors Act of 1979. This Act dissolved six statutory bodies including the old General Nursing Councils and Central Midwives' Boards for Scotland, England and Wales, and replaced them with one large council representing the wider nursing profession for the first time.[56] The new statutory body, the United Kingdom Central Council for Nurses, Midwives and Health Visitors, was responsible for setting the standards for the education, registration and discipline of these three professional groups.[57] Transfer of functions to the UKCC was slow while a shadow council and working groups planned the structure and working practices that would be needed. The working group which was considering the reform of pre-registration education issued two preliminary consultation documents in 1982 but these caused more anxiety than useful discussion among the profession and the shadow council decided to wait until the elected council took office before proceeding.[58] Meanwhile, a flurry of working parties appeared elsewhere, spurred on by *To Teach or Not to Teach*. One, involving the RCN, the GNC and the DHSS, considered the recruitment and retention of nurse teachers. A Scottish group, chaired by the chief nurse, Margaret Auld, proposed reorganisation of post-registration education.[59] The DHSS also funded an RCN working party to investigate the educational needs of nurse teachers.[60] The RCN had long advocated that nursing students be treated like students in higher education, and not regarded as part of the NHS labour force, but the UKCC's early consultation papers rejected this, and the RCN Association of Nursing Education demanded fundamental reform.[61] Trevor Clay, dismayed by the lack of co-ordinated action, and fearing that the cause might once again be lost, urged the RCN council to produce a comprehensive plan for nursing education for the next century.[62]

The RCN's Commission on Nursing Education began its work in March 1984, chaired by Dr Harry Judge, Director of the Department of Educational Studies at the University of Oxford. The commission had twenty members, mainly from the field of nurse education. They worked quickly and presented their report to the RCN council in April 1985.[63] The Judge report rejected the apprenticeship model of nurse training and recommended moving nurse education from the health service into mainstream higher education. Schools of nursing would be transferred to polytechnics, colleges of higher education, and in some cases universities, alongside comparable disciplines and professions. Nursing students would be supernumerary in the hospitals, although they would make a contribution to the nursing service. Judge proposed an integrated three-year course for all nursing students comprising a common foundation programme followed by a choice of specialisation and leading to a single basic qualification, a diploma in Nursing Studies. This structure had some affinities with Briggs – indeed, Asa Briggs had recommended Harry Judge for the task – but it placed more emphasis on nursing education outside the hospitals.[64] The RCN and the Association of Nursing Students welcomed the report enthusiastically. This marked a final movement away from the principles of the RCN's early years, when the matrons on its council refused to contemplate any loss of authority over probationers.

Shortly after the appearance of the Judge report, the English National Board published alternative proposals for the future of nurse education.[65] The publication of these two reports put pressure on the UKCC to set out its future strategy, and it decided to engage in widespread consultation with the profession.[66] The proceedings were as open as possible, with a series of discussion papers and roadshow meetings throughout the country to encourage feedback. The UKCC's plans were published in May 1986 as *Project 2000: a New Preparation for Practice*.[67] This inspirational title, usually shortened to 'P2000' by those involved, was to become synonymous with nursing education over the next fifteen years, even though it was not implemented in full. *Project 2000* proposed fundamental reforms but was less visionary than the Judge report. The two reports shared several recommendations: a common foundation programme with a greater emphasis on health rather than illness, followed by specialisation, the end of enrolled nurse training, and mandatory graduate qualifications for nurse teachers.[68] The UKCC accepted that student nurses should be supernumerary labour, not part of the establishment, but their education would remain in hospital training schools, where they would make a contribution to the nursing service. Instead of transferring nursing education into higher education, closer links between the schools of nursing and higher education institutions were recommended, with joint professional and academic validation for nursing programmes. During the consultation process serious concerns were raised in the profession about the labour and financial implications of student status, and this had contributed to the compromise.

Although it was not happy with all aspects of *Project 2000*, particularly the approach to higher education, the RCN accepted that nurses should present a united front to the government, and welcomed the report. The overwhelming response from the RCN membership was one of enthusiasm and impatience for the reforms.[69] There was unanimous support for phasing out enrolled nurse training, but the wisdom of replacing enrolled nurses with 'nursing aides', unqualified support workers, was questioned. The example of other countries, such as Finland, where nursing education had successfully moved into higher education was cited. But the *Project 2000* compromise was made not only because of fears over the cost of losing student labour, but because many felt that nursing was not yet ready to move into higher education, and that the educational gap between schools of nursing and institutions of higher education must be narrowed. This was the view of Margaret Green, the RCN director of education, who sat on the Judge commission and chaired the UKCC committee that produced *Project 2000*. She also believed that the RCN, by proposing radical change, had enabled reformist members of the *Project 2000* committee to move their conservative colleagues a little closer to higher education for nurses.[70] Celia Davies has written that conservative forces in the profession had contributed to the slow progress in educational reform over the years, and that whenever radical changes were proposed the profession opted for a series of small concessions that did not challenge the basic assumption of hospital organisation: that trainee nurses would provide a large proportion of nursing labour.[71] Clay knew this, and was anxious to precipitate the RCN council into different ways of thinking.

The RCN regarded *Project 2000* as an important step towards reform and the council pledged to make nursing education its first priority for the next ten years.[72] The council had accepted Judge's argument that removing student nurses from the NHS payroll was fundamental to the whole reform, and that this could only be achieved when nursing education was moved into higher education. The UKCC's compromise, with shared responsibility between the training schools and higher education, would not give future nurses an education equal to that of related professions. Trevor Clay feared that once again conservative forces within the profession had triumphed, and that it had chosen the gradualist approach rather than a major overhaul. Although Clay had left school as early as possible, he later took a Masters course at Brunel University, which, he argued, had transformed his life. He firmly supported college education for nurses, and denied charges of elitism:

> [Higher education] would simply be giving to those same kind of young people who opt for nursing at the moment a better chance to learn the skills of their chosen profession, a less stressful environment and a more useful qualification at the end of it. It would be the same people, except that we would want to train fewer of them because the drop-out rate would have declined.[73]

The publication of *Project 2000* was followed by a lengthy consultation period during which the UKCC held discussions with the DHSS, the nursing profession and the doctors. The latter were not enthusiastic, and the BMA was concerned about the blurring of professional boundaries.[74] Nor did the trade unions welcome *Project 2000*, since most of their nurse members were enrolled nurses who inevitably saw the phasing out of enrolled nurse training as an attempt to create an elitist profession.[75] At the end of the consultation period the final proposals were presented to the Ministers. Consultation with the health authorities then began, during which significant changes were made to the *Project 2000* package. The original P2000 report included a vision for the future of nursing practice in which nursing care would be directed and delivered by a team of registered nurses, specialists and generalists, prepared through a common foundation programme and grounded in health rather than illness.[76] But as the impact of the proposed changes in nursing education on the hospitals' services began to be calculated, the benefits of a better educated and more satisfied nursing workforce were overlooked. The cost of replacing student nurses in the nursing service was the biggest obstacle, for students provided a quarter of the NHS labour force and three quarters of direct care in hospital wards.[77] When in May 1988 the government finally announced that it accepted *Project 2000* in principle, it was referring to the educational reforms. It rejected the UKCC's vision of a nursing workforce of 64 to 70 per cent qualified nurses as unrealistic.[78] Further concessions were necessary: the contribution of student nurses to the nursing service had been agreed at approximately 20 per cent of their three years' training, while the phasing out of enrolled nurse training was postponed for five years and it would be linked to the introduction of support workers with a shorter training and less responsibility.[79] The new P2000 training schemes would be introduced gradually when funds were available and the move to a graduate teaching staff was also postponed.[80] By the mid-1990s changes within the structure of the NHS and the higher education sector overtook the *Project 2000* reforms and accelerated the transfer of nursing education into higher education. This was a cornerstone of the RCN's Judge report but not part of the P2000 report. Once again nurse education policy became the by-product of government priorities in other areas.[81]

The educational work of the RCN in the 1980s

The Institute of Advanced Nursing Education began the 1980s by moving from the original College headquarters in Henrietta Place into new accommodation in the refurbished Cowdray Club at 20 Cavendish Square. During this decade there was more emphasis on academic content, and where possible certificate courses were upgraded to diplomas, and diplomas to degrees. The number of full-time students declined and part-time students increased, and by the middle of the decade accommodation was again insufficient.[82] At the same time the Department of Education and Science reduced its grant, and the RCN had to contribute a greater proportion of the funding for its educational work. The internal structure of the IANE's work was reorganised in 1983 with the setting up of a curriculum development group for each course and the appointment of an Academic and Administrative Affairs Committee to replace the Committee on Education and Training. The Board of Education continued in its role of determining the educational role of the College.

By 1989 the work of the IANE presented a complex picture of degree and diploma programmes in association with four universities, and the long struggle for higher education for nurses was finally resulting in a major shift in nurse education. The first degree programmes, a BSc in nursing studies, and a BA in nursing education, were offered in collaboration with the University of Manchester in 1987, and achieved one of the early aims of the College. Subsequently a BSc in nursing studies was offered with the University of London and a multi-disciplinary degree in occupational health with the University of Surrey. The diploma courses were run with the University of London, the University of Surrey and the City University, and included a diploma in occupational health nursing (the former certificate course), a diploma in community mental health nursing, and a diploma in therapeutic community practice. A new diploma in international health services management replaced the former certificate course for overseas nurses in 1986, in response to demand from foreign governments. The RCN remained the leading educational body in occupational health nursing. There were over thirty centres around the country offering the RCN courses at different levels, and a distance-learning course began in conjunction with the Health and Safety Executive for nurses working in isolated areas. By 1990 the RCN had developed a diploma and a degree course in occupational health, but the most significant achievement was central recognition of these qualifications, which would appear in a nurse's entry in the statutory register. After a period of joint approval with the RCN, the statutory bodies, the English National Board, the Welsh National Board, the National Board for Scotland and the National Board for Northern Ireland, took over responsibility for the certificate in 1988. The international reputation of the RCN in the field brought requests from overseas governments for advice about setting up and validating courses. In the University of Ibadan in Nigeria, a member of the RCN Institute staff actually ran the course for the first two years until a suitably qualified nurse was available.[83]

In addition to the degree and diploma work the IANE continued to offer courses leading to RCN certificates, to approve and validate external centres for these courses, and to develop short courses in specialist subjects. The types of course offered reveal the expanding social role of nursing. They included in-flight nursing, working with ethnic minorities, and adolescent risk taking, particularly solvent abuse. In developing these courses the IANE staff worked with the experts in the field both from the RCN's professional staff and from other organisations, as in the case of the nurse practitioners' course. Nurse practitioners were becoming more common, as changes in NHS funding for general practice encouraged many doctors to give up single-handed practices and join in group practice clinics, where highly trained nurses could take over many of the doctors' former tasks. The RCN Community Nursing Association was concerned at the lack of appropriate training for nurse practitioners, and following a resolution at Congress in 1987, the RCN set up a curriculum development group. They invited representatives of the Health Visitors'

Association and the District Nursing Association to join them. It took two years to agree a definition of the nurse practitioner's role on which to base the course curriculum. Over twenty interested parties were consulted.[84] The course began in September 1990.

The RCN also worked closely with government and the UKCC to deal with new problems. During the 1980s, medicine internationally had to respond to the growing threat to public health from HIV. The government, at first reluctant to act, sponsored an effective publicity campaign, 'Don't Die of Ignorance'. Ignorance among nurses as well as the public led to a few well-publicised cases of nurses refusing to treat AIDS patients for fear of infection. The *News of the World* ran excitable stories of community nurses refusing to enter the homes of two dying patients, and of porters at a Liverpool hospital unwilling to move victims' bodies. A pathologist allegedly refused to perform an autopsy.[85] The College issued best-selling guidelines on nursing patients with AIDS, and made two public statements on the subject, the first emphasising the responsibility of each health authority to plan for the treatment and support of patients, the second asserting the professional responsibility of nurses to care for AIDS sufferers. The RCN warned that nurses who would not assist on moral or religious grounds, or through unjustified fear of infection, could be contravening the code of professional conduct.[86] The IANE staff worked at the request of the statutory bodies to develop the first course on AIDS nursing. This short course, funded by the DHSS, proved very popular, but overstretched the RCN's ability to take all the applicants. It had a twelve-month waiting list for several years.

The RCN was more frequently asked to validate courses run by other bodies. The University of Aberdeen Institute of Environmental and Occupational Medicine wanted validation for their offshore occupational health course for health workers on the oil rigs. Candidates for the course were registered general nurses, enrolled nurses and ex-Service medical attendants. There were some reservations about awarding RCN accreditation to students who were not nurses, but an exception was made.[87] Other requests for validation came from BUPA, for a health screening course, and the Royal Marsden Hospital, London, for a course in nursing patients with breast cancer. The RCN would have preferred the latter course to be validated by the statutory body but the English National Board had decided not to validate the course and the RCN, considering that such a course was needed, gave approval. At the end of the decade the RCN council decided to review the future educational role of the College once more. During the 1980s there were considerable changes in both nursing and general education, the profession's needs had changed and *Project 2000* was contemplating new structures for nursing. In 1987 the government announced major changes in funding for higher education, which would affect the work of the IANE. In future it would be recognised as an institution of higher education and would receive its grant from the Polytechnic and College Funding Council instead of the Department of Education and Science. The director of education was optimistic that this would mean increased funding, but there was doubt over the future of the non-advanced courses that the IANE provided.[88] The new grant would cover only advanced courses, and the RCN would have to fund non-certificate work. Previously, all the IANE's courses were classified as advanced by the DES because they were post-registration. A small committee of council carried out the review and concluded that the educational work of the College had never been more necessary. The IANE's role should be expanded within the RCN, which should fund educational work that fell outside higher education. This was the basic in-service work that responded to the profession's needs in short courses, workshops and seminars, held all over the country. The IANE would continue to provide a comprehensive range of higher education courses from certificates through to higher degrees, develop its degree programme and in the long term move towards offering Masters degrees. It should be accredited by a university but remain physically within the RCN, and independent of other institutions.

The new funding arrangements, to be applied from 1990, affected the work of the Birmingham Education Centre. The centre specialised in short clinical care courses, such as its very successful and innovatory course on infection control nursing, but these courses did not qualify for the Polytechnic and College Funding Council grants. Like most RCN courses, they were not an integral part of nurse education, but were regarded as useful additional skills, often paid for out of nurses' own pockets. During the 1980s nurses found it increasingly difficult to get secondment for courses of this type, and the changes taking place in post-basic education put the centre's future in doubt. It closed in 1991 after thirty-eight years of pioneering post-registration nursing education in the Midlands.

Internal affairs

The Professional Nursing Department had been set up in the early 1970s to provide a service to members in the practice of their profession and to ensure that the professional viewpoint of nurses was put forward nationally. With the appointment of David Rye as director of professional activities in 1977 the department began a period that some considered the best time for the RCN.[89] The introduction of new specialist associations and societies created the conditions that allowed the College's professional work to flourish. The department had a team of professional officers and nurse advisers whose task was to assist members in the practice of their profession. They were experts in their field and worked closely with the active members in the associations, societies and forums.[90] This kept the professional staff in touch with each field of practice and enabled the RCN to respond quickly to DHSS initiatives and to produce detailed evidence on any aspect of health care. The combination of innovative thinkers on the staff and professionals in the field produced an impressive range of publications in the 1980s and gave the RCN considerable influence in the formulation of professional policy. The department's growing influence was reflected in its change of name in 1987 to the Department of Nursing Policy and Practice.

The department's brief was to maintain and improve standards of professional practice, and as the economic and political climate of the NHS changed in the 1980s this subject became even more important. The RCN had always been concerned to monitor standards of nursing care. In the 1960s it embarked on a 'study of nursing care' project, funded by the Ministry of Health.[91] The economic problems of the 1970s created considerable anxiety about deteriorating standards of care, and the RCN began to take the lead in defining and monitoring nursing standards. This drew it further into the political arena. Well before the 'Nurse Alert' campaign of the 1980s, RCN members, particularly clinical nurses, reported a range of problems resulting from financial cutbacks that made their work difficult and raised fears that patients were not receiving the best attention.[92] In response the RCN collected evidence, particularly about the problems in wards where the number of beds was being reduced while the throughput of patients was increasing. A deputation to the Secretary of State in 1974 confirmed that the government shared their concerns, especially over standards in geriatric care. They invited the RCN and the British Geriatrics' Society to draw up guidelines for improving nursing care of the elderly in hospital and funded a pilot study to test their recommendations.[93] The RCN also collaborated with the Royal College of Psychiatry and the British Psychological Society to produce guidelines for patient care in this field. As the cutbacks continued members asked the RCN for help in dealing with local crises and the general secretary cautioned that the issue should be treated as a professional rather than labour relations issue.[94]

In 1975 Barbara Castle tried to find a method of distributing NHS capital and revenue in a more egalitarian way.[95] This led to reduced funding for hospitals in the London area, and the Thames region was one of the worst hit. The RCN conducted a survey in that region to assess how far standards were being eroded. Its report drew attention to the dangerously low staffing levels, with a rise in the number of unfilled vacancies and a reduction in student recruitment. So serious was the threat to standards of care that it might be necessary to close units or wards and concentrate resources, in order to protect patients and staff.[96] Sheila Quinn chaired a committee, which included a representative of the DHSS, to provide guidance to nurses on acceptable standards of nursing care, and it published two reports. The committee believed that the profession as a whole had to agree on acceptable standards, and all nurses should examine critically the care they gave their patients. In an attempt to define professionally acceptable standards, the first report raised three questions: what is nursing, what is good nursing care, and can nursing care be measured? In answering the first of these, the long-standing problem of nursing boundaries arose. The nurses' dilemma was in knowing where, in the patient's interest, they should concentrate their activity. If they took on more tasks delegated from others, basic nursing might be neglected or given to those less competent to do it. In clinical nursing, the ward sister was crucial in maintaining nursing standards, and the importance of this general role increased as specialisation expanded.[97] In deciding what constituted 'good nursing care' the committee drew on research from the USA, which described the 'nursing process' and defined 'good nursing' as a continuous and dynamic pattern of assessment, planning, action and review.[98] In measuring quality, the report recommended studying what nurses did, how they did it, and the effect on patients. This required performance indicators to be developed for each of these areas.

Inevitably the committee found the subject more complex than they expected, as the title of the second report, *Towards Standards*, indicated. It argued that in aiming for agreed professional standards, every nurse needed to understand the basic distinction between medicine and nursing. It outlined a philosophy of nursing where the patient was central and the nurse was the patient's advocate, and this approach to patient-centred care was distinct from medicine or any other discipline. Many doctors, and some nurses, still regarded nursing as a collection of tasks or procedures requiring a certain amount of skill, but which were initiated by, and under the direction of, doctors.[99] The professionally accountable nurse understood that a nursing view of a patient's needs might differ from, or even conflict with, those of medicine, but that both must work in partnership. Accountability was the basis of professional standards, and clinical nurses must be accountable for their conduct. This would provide a basis for professional practice and raise the standards of nursing.[100] In the climate of the 1980s, standards of care were tested when staff shortages tempted nurses to depersonalise patients, who might receive the minimum of care necessary for basic comfort. The publication of each report was followed by a series of successful conferences and seminars, and it was clear that nurses accepted the challenge of examining their standards critically.

In 1983 the Griffiths report ended consensus management in the NHS, and the new general managers, often with backgrounds in hospital administration, accountancy or industrial management, introduced a fast-track approach to care. The turnover of patients became the yardstick of efficiency and the quality of care, being hard to measure, was not a priority. In this context the

RCN's work on standards of care became highly significant, and the council decided to develop it further, as a matter of urgency, for use in nurses' day-to-day practice. A Standards of Care Project was set up and Alison Kitson appointed as a project co-ordinator in 1985. At first there was no clear view of how the project should proceed, but through David Rye, Kitson connected with the innovators of the emerging clinical practice movement. These included Sue Pembrey and Alan Pearson who pioneered a nurse-led unit at the Radcliffe Infirmary in Oxford, and Helen Kendall in West Berkshire who was applying quality assurance methods to nursing.[101] They wanted to empower clinical nurses to take control of patient care, and this linked with the RCN's aim to assist nurses in evaluating their own work. The Standards of Care team spent three years on a new theoretical framework for quality assurance, building on existing fieldwork.[102] They co-operated with members from each specialist professional group to establish a series of guidelines for good practice and national standards, and in 1989 published the first six of these, on standards of care in rheumatic disease nursing, health visiting, family planning nursing, district nursing, orthopaedic nursing and nursing management. A teaching package for setting, monitoring and evaluating standards of care for ward and community staff was produced in 1990. Known as the *Dynamic Standard Setting System*, or DySSSy, the workbook offered theory and methodology for quality patient care. News of the system spread through workshops and it became a run-away success, requiring a team of facilitators to work with nurses across the country.[103] Within a year, twenty-four health authorities were using it in England and Wales, all the health authorities in Scotland had expressed an interest, and it was being applied in at least sixty other locations.[104] Two successful international conferences in London advertised DySSSy, which was beginning to be adopted by groups of nurses in Europe. Sheila Quinn was a member of the World Health Organization European Region working group on standards of care at this time, and introduced Kitson to the group as a technical expert. In this way DySSSy spread to Europe where it was particularly popular in the Scandinavian countries.[105]

The overwhelming success of the RCN system surprised even its authors, for it seemed to capture the imagination of clinical nurses and became a major catalyst for change. Part of its success was that it empowered nurses to set their own achievable clinical standards. The DHSS welcomed the RCN's work on quality, and agreed to fund research into the evaluation of DySSSy – it may be surmised that they hoped that nurse-led wards might reduce expenditure on the more expensive medical staff. This evaluation was transferred from the RCN headquarters to Oxford to become part of the Institute of Nursing. This new venture, led by Sue Pembrey, was funded by the Regional and District Health Authorities and the Sainsbury's Trust, with the professional support of the RCN. The Institute of Nursing, in the Radcliffe Infirmary, gave nursing an independent university unit after the demise of the Radcliffe's nurse-led wards due to lack of support from the medical profession.[106] The new institute flourished. It was the first practice development and research unit, and influenced the introduction of nursing audit and then clinical audit. Kitson became director of the Institute of Nursing in 1992, and the RCN's standards of care project became the Dynamic Quality Improvement Programme, with a UK and European quality assurance network, assisting nurses and other health care professionals to audit their own standards.

In 1982 the College also achieved its ambition to establish a research unit, first contemplated over twenty years earlier, when problems of cost and finding suitably qualified staff prevented it. Nevertheless, the College sponsored thirty monographs in the 'Study of Nursing Care' project during the 1970s. After the DHSS refused to continue underwriting the research series the RCN decided to set up a research unit with funds collected by the Appeals Committee in the 1970s.[107] A director was appointed in February 1982. Located in the Professional Nursing Department, the Daphne Heald Research Unit was named in honour of Lady Heald who had been a vice-president of the College and chair of the Appeals Committee since 1950. It aimed to establish links between nursing research and nursing practice.[108] The first research project evaluated the contribution to patient care made by different groups of clinical nurse specialists, focusing on the care of patients with stomas, and then on the care of diabetic patients. The unit's staff worked closely with the adviser to the RCN Research Society and in 1984 the council agreed to fund the core staff, rather than relying on external sources.[109] By 1990 the unit had a staff of six and new research projects included the effects of early discharge after surgery on patients, their carers and the community nursing and GP services; the care received by elderly people; and the nursing and care of HIV and AIDS patients.

At this time the RCN library was going through a rapid transformation. Several factors combined to change it from a quiet professional library serving a small part of the membership and a mature student body, to a crowded place that could barely cope with the demands of busy members and part-time students with many commitments. The RCN's membership was expanding, its profile changing, and many more nurses were taking post-registration education. Growing demand for further education also increased the number of members using the library's services, for the libraries in their hospitals and local educational institutions had inadequate resources for nursing studies. By the 1980s the RCN library had a stock of over 25,000 volumes, was taking over 200 journals, and was building up a collection of nursing research.[110] During the 1970s it started to publish a monthly bibliography of new books to keep the profession informed of new developments. The bibliography grew into an essential reference tool before being replaced by electronic databases in the 1990s. At its peak the nursing bibliography had over 500 subscribing libraries in the UK and overseas.[111] Over the years the RCN library has built up its reputation to earn the title the Library of Nursing and is now the major library for nursing literature in the United Kingdom.

In 1983, after twenty years in post, Lt. Col. Douglas de Cent, the director of the Press and Public Relations Department retired. He held office for almost the entire period that Catherine Hall was general secretary and they worked closely together. During his time the department established an effective relationship with the media, providing comments, press releases, interviews and briefings and measured its success each year by the number of column inches devoted to the RCN in the national and provincial press. Although the department was small, with a staff of three (increased to five by 1977), they supplemented their limited resources through a network of 200 honorary public relations officers based in the RCN branches. This gave the RCN a local voice and these officers, who received training in public relations work, could call on the professional expertise of the headquarters' staff when required. The department also produced and distributed to branches, stewards and membership groups, newssheets and promotional material, all of which carried the corporate image of the RCN (circulation just under 5,000). During 1982 the RCN's pay campaign took up much of the department's time, achieving a record of 25,000 column inches in the press, 50 per cent more than the previous year. The department deplored the occasion for these extra inches, but true to their PR brief, were pleased at the effective publicity. The campaign presented an ideal opportunity to introduce the new general secretary, Trevor Clay, whose skills as a communicator quickly made him a favourite of the media, and established him as the spokesman for the nursing profession. Clay's goal was to take nursing into politics, and he achieved this through his skilful use of the media and by setting up a parliamentary office within the RCN. The first parliamentary liaison officer, Neil Stewart, was appointed in 1984, and from this point the political activities of the RCN increased significantly, including systematic lobbying of MPs and external organisations, monitoring government health proposals, and attendance at political party conferences.

One of Clay's first duties as deputy general secretary in 1979 was to chair the working group on communications, and their fractious meetings influenced his ideas on how the RCN should manage its public image. In 1983 De Cent was replaced by Alison Dunn, the editor of *Nursing Times* since 1975. During her editorship, the journal was re-branded and became the market leader. With the appointment of Dunn the Press and Public Relations Department moved to centre stage. Previously it had operated on a very constrained budget and by 1980 was having difficulty meeting the expectations of members and staff. The total public relations budget, exclusive of the *Nursing Standard*, was approximately £14,000, which was the equivalent of a single one-minute advertising spot on television at peak time.[112] The *Nursing Standard* had suffered extensively over the years from lack of finance, resulting in the use of poorer quality paper and a restriction on the use of artwork and photographs. In contrast, under Clay the department was placed alongside the Professional Nursing Department and the Labour Relations Department in the allocation of financial resources. This fitted the managerial approach of the 1980s. The Thatcher government encouraged the spread of business practices in the public sector, with a strong emphasis on advertising and public relations. The RCN's new interest in this side of its activities mirrored the practices of many other organisations, both public and private.

The new general secretary wanted a total re-branding of the RCN, including a new address and a new logo. The refurbishment of the headquarters' building was finally completed in 1983 and its address became the decidedly aristocratic 20 Cavendish Square, the former entrance to the Cowdray Club. The old entrance at Henrietta Place was reserved for deliveries. The RCN's logo dated back to 1963, when 'Rcn' was a symbol of the merger of the College of Nursing and the National Council of Nurses. In 1973 it had turned into RCN, and its origins were largely forgotten. For the new logo, Dunn commissioned David Hillman who made his name designing magazines like *Nova* in the 1960s and had redesigned the masthead of the *Nursing Times*. His linked hands symbol for the RCN pleased Trevor Clay. It was adopted in 1984 and, with a few amendments, has been in use ever since. The old coat of arms was seen occasionally after 1984 but during the 1990s it fell out of use. In 1987 Clay attended the American National League of Nursing convention and was impressed by the professional presentation of the event. In future the RCN's Congress auditorium would mirror this stylish appearance, moving away from the traditional trade union congress model to a modern image of a powerful political party.[113]

With Clay behind it the Press and Public Relations Department expanded. It now comprised three sections, one for producing the *Nursing Standard*, one for public relations and the third for marketing. The last function, which included organising RCN conferences and exhibitions, had previously been contracted out, but was brought in-house by Dunn, and within a few years had become so profitable that there was concern that it would affect the RCN's charitable status. In the autumn of 1984, two new quarterly journals were launched, *Lampada* for full members, and *Tradimus* for student members. These did not satisfy the expectations of members and in 1987, Scutari Projects Limited was set up as an independent company to combine the publishing and marketing sides of the RCN and to avoid problems over charitable status.[114] Dunn became managing director of the new company and moved

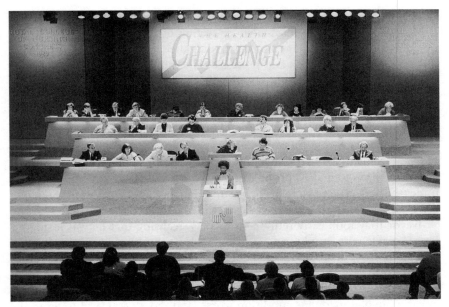

8.4 New look Congress, Glasgow, 1989. The new RCN logo appears on the podium.

to Harrow with the journalist and marketing staff. The remaining staff, under their new director, Neil Stewart, took on the work of promoting the RCN and providing the free publications together with publicity material, and public relations support to the branches, membership groups and staff. The growing parliamentary work, which now had a staff of three, was integrated into the department.

The marketing side of the new company continued to prosper, as did the new book publishing wing, but the success of Scutari was tied to the launch of the *Nursing Standard* as a weekly glossy journal and this was not a success. Although the *Nursing Standard* was redesigned and re-launched, sections of the membership were still critical of it. Extensive market research tried to establish what type of journal would attract nurses, and the design and tone of the new *Nursing Standard* was based on this. Described as a 'popularist' style, it contained short news items and easy-to-read clinical pieces. The first three issues were mailed to the entire membership, but thereafter only RCN activists received it free, and other members had to pay, either by subscription or from newsstands. The *Nursing Standard* aimed to challenge the monopoly of the *Nursing Times*, which had recently taken over the *Nursing Mirror*, its main rival. To compete with the *Nursing Times*, the *Nursing Standard* had to present itself as an independent journal, and so it no longer carried official

RCN news, with free advertisements for RCN events and meetings. This was a mistake, and efforts to reach a wider section of the profession by reducing the journal's serious content also misfired. It alienated its potential readership – the educators, specialists and professionally minded nurses, who perceived it as lightweight, and it could not change the habits of advertising agencies who continued to support the *Nursing Times*. Much public relations work was required to overcome reader's hostility. The editorial style was changed to a more authoritative tone, and the *Nursing Standard* was re-launched in September 1989 with a more academic appearance. Parts of Scutari Projects Ltd were immediately profitable but it was a decade later before the *Nursing Standard* began to make a profit. The company was brought in-house in 1995, under the next general secretary, Christine Hancock, and the *Nursing Standard* did eventually eclipse *Nursing Times* as the market leader.

Trevor Clay took early retirement in 1989, realising that he was losing his long struggle with emphysema. During his time in office, RCN membership rose from around 200,000 to 280,000. He died in 1994, after an active retirement in journalism and in promoting his 'Breathe Easy' campaign, to assist emphysema sufferers. Although never a heavy smoker, he knew that smoking in early life had made his condition worse, and did a great deal to wean the nursing profession from cigarettes. His two predecessors belonged to a generation where smoking was adopted by many professional women as a sign of their independence. Under Clay, the RCN took a firm anti-smoking stance. Christine Hancock became general secretary in September 1989. She trained at King's College Hospital, and had trained as a midwife and worked in mental health. In addition, she was a graduate of the London School of Economics, the first general secretary with an undergraduate degree. She had been chief executive to Waltham Forest Health Authority, one of the relatively few nurses to survive the managerial changes of the 1980s and remain in a position of authority.

Christine Hancock presided over one of the most significant shifts in the RCN's view of its role and its membership. By the 1980s, the RCN was determined to move students out of the hospital training schools, but its old ambition for a fully qualified nursing staff remained unfulfilled. The RCN's views prevailed in that nursing students were increasingly removed from basic duties and spent more time in the classroom; but as trained nurses' salaries rose, so the service became more reliant on a cadre of trained nurses supervising teams of unqualified helpers, known at various times as nursing assistants, nursing auxiliaries, nursing aides, and latterly as care assistants. Ironically, the structure came to resemble that of the old poor law hospitals, where a small number of trained nurses supervised a larger body of untrained staff, rather than the voluntary hospitals, which expected probationers and junior nurses to undertake unskilled nursing tasks and domestic labour. The governments

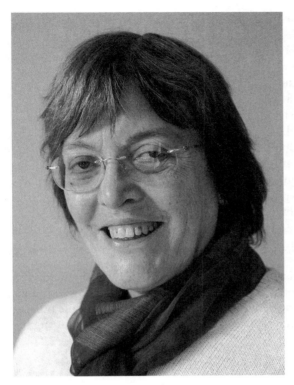

8.5 Christine Hancock, general secretary, 1989–2001.

of the 1980s made it plain that the price of higher education in nursing was the employment of more support workers, and *Project 2000* acknowledged them as an important part of the health system. This presented a challenge for the RCN, and the 1987 RRB in Glasgow passed a resolution (though with many abstaining) calling on the council 'to consider the implications of not incorporating the helper grade in the structure of the RCN'.[115] Kenneth Clarke reinforced the message in a speech to the RCN Congress in 1989, stressing the importance of care assistants to the health service, though acknowledging that they would need to be directed by trained nurses, and the government promised short but specialised training programmes for them.

The council tested members' views by moving an amendment to the College's charter to admit 'support workers' (as defined by the RCN) to a separate grade of membership. Support workers were important, not only in the hospitals, but in the growing number of nursing homes for the elderly. The council set out a careful set of arguments on both sides. They acknowledged that care workers were an essential part of the health team, and that they were already included in the decisions of the Pay Review Board. Arguments against included reluctance to antagonise other unions, and the possibility that the RCN's work would become unbalanced, with more emphasis on trade union activity and less on professional work. Further, offering support workers fewer benefits for a lower subscription might be creating a 'bogus' membership.[116] Those in favour of a separate membership for support workers noted that the RCN's Royal Charter clearly referred to nurses on the register, and that a major revision would be necessary to include those who were not. The 1989 AGM accepted the resolution but it was over a decade before membership was offered to health care assistants. The field of vocational qualifications was constantly changing and when in 2001 the RCN first widened its membership criteria to include this group of workers, it restricted access to those with a National Vocational Qualification level 3 or above. A very small number of this group joined the RCN and in the following years the membership criteria was further extended to embrace almost all levels of health care support workers.[117]

Was Arthur Stanley a visionary or a realist when in 1916 he envisaged a College of Nursing that would embrace all hard-working nursing assistants, regardless of the length of their training? They were as essential to the nursing service at the end of the twentieth century as the VADs had been during the First World War.

Conclusion

Under the Conservative governments of the 1980s, the RCN's fortunes were mixed, with turbulence in its employment negotiations for nurses, but a more rapid movement towards many of its goals in nurse education. Unflagging public support for nurses helped to maintain it in years when the trade union movement was in bitter conflict with the government. The government was not slow to exploit the RCN's no-strike policy, using this as a reason to reward nurses in preference to other health service unions. But the government's reforms in the structure of the NHS had the paradoxical effect of driving the RCN closer to the traditional unions, as all resented the effects of economies in the NHS and the changes towards a more localised, managerial system as a result of the Griffiths report.

Changes of leadership in the RCN also prepared it for a more managerial world in its own internal arrangements. The RCN's effective handling of public relations, where it had developed much expertise in earlier decades, gave weight to its objections to changes in hospital management and their effects on patient care. Campaigns such as 'Nurse Alert' did not endear it to the government, nor did they restore senior nurses to an authoritative position in the hospitals, but they made a considerable impression on the public and resulted in significant local changes. The founders of the RCN believed that trained nurses should be regarded as professionals, with an important place in the health services. They also believed that nurse management should be under the control of nurses themselves. To many, Griffiths constituted a setback to nurses in management, though in such a decentralised system, wide variations in local structures were possible. It was surely no coincidence that much of the RCN's most valuable research in this period concentrated on redefining the role of nurses, while defending their traditional values. Patient care and quality management in nursing were at the heart of these investigations – areas where the nurse's territory had to be defended.

In nurse training, there was a decisive shift towards college-based courses. This was possible only in a society where a much larger proportion of women were reaching this standard. The combination of basic training and specialist courses, where the college rather than the hospital set the student's agenda, had featured in several earlier investigations into nursing education, and the RCN itself had finally dropped its long-standing attachment to a hospital-dominated training system. In an earlier period, when secondary education for women was not compulsory, the founders of the RCN generally believed that further education would be confined to a small group of nursing leaders; and they had not foreseen that it would become a possibility for all trained nurses. But the economic costs of such a move were high, and the price of a professional education was the employment of growing numbers of care assistants, and a wider division between trained and untrained workers in the hospitals.

Notes

1 Standing Commission on Pay Comparability, *Report No. 3, Nurses and Midwives*, Chairman: Professor H. A. Clegg [Clegg report] Cmnd 7795 (London: HMSO, 1980), p. 30.

2 RCN/5/2/70, 'A summary of the evidence submitted by the staff side of the Nurses and Midwives Whitley Council', p. 2.

3 Clegg report, pp. 48–50. The zero pay rises, affecting a small minority, did not affect the average.

4 RCN/5/2/70, draft of Catherine Hall's standard letter.

5 CM 10 April 1980, pp. 183 ff; RCN/2/1980/183.

6 RCN/5/2/70, DHSS statement, 25 Sept. 1979.

7 For an overview, see Alastair J. Reid, *United We Stand: a History of Britain's Trade Unions* (London: Allen Lane, 2004), pp. 396–410.

8 *The Times* 17 May 1982, p. 2.

9 RCN/17/7/6, press cuttings, *Daily Mail* 4 June 1982.

10 RCN/17/7/6, press cuttings, *Financial Times* 21 Sept. 1982.

11 CM 11 March 1982, RCN/2/1982/185.

12 Monica E. Baly, 'Clay, Trevor (1936–1994)', *Oxford Dictionary of National Biography*, on-line edn, Oxford University Press, www.oxforddnb.com/view/article/54813, accessed Mar. 2008.

13 Trevor Clay, in association with Alison Dunn and Neil Stewart, *Nurses: Power and Politics* (London: Heinemann Nursing, 1987), p. 128.

14 RCN/17/4/16, press cuttings, *Sunday Telegraph* 11 July 1982.

15 RCNA T301, interview with Christine Hancock, 2006, transcript p. 3.

16 As told by Barbara Castle to Christine Hancock. RCNA T301, interview with Christine Hancock, 2006, transcript p. 3.

17 RCN/17/7/16, press cuttings, *The Sun* 16 Aug. 1982.

18 RCN/17/7/16, press cuttings, *The Times* 25 Aug. 1982, p. 1; 26 Aug. 1982, p. 1.

19 Carpenter, *Working for Health*, pp. 378–80.

20 RCN/17/4/17/1, press cuttings, *Daily Mail* 8 Sept. 1982.

21 *AR* 1982–83, pp. 4, 17. Members not attending the AGM could vote by proxy on these issues.

22 For a general account and debate on the formation of PRBs, see Geoff White, 'The Pay Review Body system: its development and impact', *Historical Studies in Industrial Relations* 9 (Spring, 2000), 71–97; Frank Burchill, 'The Pay Review Body system: a comment and a consequence', *Historical Studies in Industrial Relations* 10 (autumn 2000), 141–57.

23 RCN/17/4/19/2, press cuttings, *The Guardian* 7 April 1983.

24 RCN/5/2/55, minutes of working party to consider the Rcn input into the joint Rcn/TUC discussions on industrial relations in the NHS, 1980–81.

25 RCN/28/11/AB/1985, 'Please don't squeeze the nurses'.

26 Review Body for Nursing Staff, Midwives, Health Visitors and Professions Allied to Medicine, *First Report on Nursing Staff, Midwives and Health Visitors*, Cmnd 9258 (London: HMSO, 1984), p. 3. The figures refer to full-time equivalents.

27 Department of Health and Social Security, *NHS Management Inquiry Report* [Griffiths report] (London: DHSS, 1983).

28 Philip Strong and Jane Robinson, *The NHS – Under New Management* (Milton Keynes and Philadelphia: Open University Press, 1990), p. 24.

29 RCN/5/6/14, RCN, *Comment on the National Health Service Management Inquiry* (Jan. 1984).

30 Philip Strong and Jane Robinson, *New Model Management: Griffiths and the NHS*. Nursing Policy Studies 3 (University of Warwick: Nursing Policy Studies Centre, 1988), p. 38.

31 RCN/17/4/19/4, press cuttings, *The Sun* 13 Sept. 1983.

32 Clay, *Nurses: Power and Politics*, pp. 95–8.

33 RCN/5/6/14, T. Clay to N. Fowler, 15 Nov. 1984; N. Fowler to T. Clay, 16 Nov. 1984.

34 RCN/5/6/14, N. Fowler to T. Clay, 16 July 1985; circular from Barney Hayhoe to all Regional Health Authority chairmen, 20 Nov. 1985.

35 RCN/5/6/14, ms. 'RCN briefing', Jan. 1986, pp. 2–3.

36 Strong and Robinson, *New Model Management*, pp. 15, 54. Also, Jane Robinson, Phil Strong, and Ruth Elkan, *Griffiths and the Nurses: a National Survey of CNAs*, Nursing Policy Studies 4 (University of Warwick: Nursing Policy Studies Centre, 1989).

37 *AR* 1986–87, p. 3.
38 Sheila Quinn, *A Dame Abroad* (Stanhope: Memoir Club, 2004), p. 148.
39 *Nursing Standard* (381), 24 Jan. 1985, p. 1.
40 *AR* 1986–87, p. 1.
41 *Feeling Better, Getting Better. Why the Nursing Voice Must be Heard* (London: RCN, 1986), p. 4.
42 RCN/17/9 for a collection of posters and advertising for this campaign.
43 RCN/17/4/21/6, press cuttings, *The Times* 13 Jan. 1986.
44 Clay et al., *Nurses: Power and Politics*, p. 57.
45 Strong and Robinson, *The NHS*, pp. 31–48.
46 RCN/17/4/19/4, press cuttings, *The Guardian* 30 Sept. 1930, and Royal College of Nursing of the United Kingdom, *Nuclear War, Civil Defence Planning, the Implications for Nursing, Report of an Rcn Working Party* (London: Royal College of Nursing, 1983).
47 *AR* 1987–88, Jan. report, n.p.
48 RCN/28 MORI, 'Public attitudes towards nurses' pay' and 'Public attitudes towards trade unions. Research study conducted for the Royal College of Nursing', 1985.
49 Clay et al., *Nurses: Power and Politics*, p. 3.
50 Chris Hart, *Behind the Mask: Nurses, Their Unions and Nursing Policy* (London: Baillière Tindall, 1994), pp. 223.
51 Chris Hart, *Nurses and Politics: The Impact of Power and Practice* (Basingstoke: Palgrave Macmillan, 2004), pp. 74–84.
52 CM, Jan. 1981, pp. 17–20 and for background 13 March 1980, pp. 129–32.
53 *To Teach or Not to Teach? That Is the Question* (London: Royal College of Nursing Association of Nursing Education, 1981), pp. 4–5.
54 CM, 8 Jan. 1981 pp. 17–20 and 9 Nov. 1981 pp. 453–95.
55 For an overview of nursing education from 1950 see Weir, *Educating Nurses in Scotland*.
56 Also dissolved were the Northern Ireland Council for Nurses and Midwives and the Council for the Education and Training of Health Visitors and three non-statutory bodies, the Panel of Assessors for District Nurse Training, the Joint Board of Clinical Nursing Studies, and in Scotland the Committee for Clinical Nursing Studies.
57 The UKCC was supported by four national boards, the English National Board, the National Board for Scotland, the Welsh National Board, and the National Board for Northern Ireland. For a thorough account of the work of the UKCC and the reform of nursing education see, Davies and Beach, *Interpreting Professional Self-Regulation*.
58 United Kingdom Central Council for Nursing, Midwifery and Health Visiting, Working Group 3 Consultation Paper, *Education and Training: the Development of Nurse Education*, 1982; and *Education and Training: Report to the UKCC Following Consultation with the Professions*, 1982.
59 *Continuing Education for the Nursing Profession in Scotland. Report of a Working Party on Continuing Professional Development for Nurses, Midwives and Health Visitors* (Edinburgh: HMSO, 1981).

60 *The Preparation and Education of Nurse Teachers* (London: RCN, 1983).

61 *Report of the Working Group on Education and Training, 1984, Recommendations for Nursing Education Through the Next Decade* (London: RCN, 1984).

62 CM Nov. 1983, pp. 866–7.

63 *The Education of Nurses: a New Dispensation*, Commission on Nursing Education [Judge report] (London: Royal College of Nursing of the United Kingdom, 1985). The commission funded two pieces of research, one on the workforce implications of supernumerary status by the Institute of Manpower Studies, and one on the relative costs of nurse training in the NHS and higher education by the Centre for Health Economics, University of York.

64 RCNA T285, interview with David Rye, 2006.

65 The English National Board for Nurses, Midwives and Health Visitors, *Professional Education/Training Courses*, consultation paper, 1985.

66 Davies and Beach, *Interpreting Professional Self-Regulation*, p. 77.

67 *Project 2000: a New Preparation for Practice* (London: United Kingdom Central Council for Nursing, Midwifery and Health Visiting, 1986).

68 Five branch programmes were proposed, adult nursing, children's nursing, mentally ill, mentally handicapped and midwifery. In the final structure there were four branch programmes, adult nursing, children's nursing, mental health and mental handicap nursing.

69 *Comments on the UKCC's Project 2000 Proposals*, report on local and national RCN membership entity consultation (London: RCN, 1986).

70 RCNA, T274, interview with Margaret Green, 2005.

71 Celia Davies, 'A constant casualty: nurse education in Britain and the USA to 1939', in Celia Davies (ed.), *Rewriting Nursing History* (London: Croom Helm, 1980), p. 122 fn, 33.

72 *AR* 1986–87, p. 1.

73 Clay, *Nurses: Power and Politics*, p. 76.

74 Davies and Beach, *Interpreting Professional Self-Regulation*, p. 94, fn 31.

75 Ibid., pp. 80 and 86.

76 Davies, *Gender and the Professional Predicament in Nursing*, p. 107–27.

77 Celia Davies, 'Nurse odyssey 2000', and Tom Jones, 'Speculating on the "futures" market', *Health Service Journal* (24 July 1986), 986–7.

78 Davies, *Gender and the Professional Predicament*, p. 119.

79 Health care support courses were offered in colleges of further education from the early 1990s, these courses were three or four months in length, see Weir, *Educating Nurses in Scotland*, pp. 55–8.

80 The first *Project 2000* courses began in England in 1989, in Northern Ireland in 1990, in Wales in 1991 and in Scotland in 1992.

81 John Humphreys, 'English nurse education and the reform of the National Health Service', *Journal of Education Policy* 11:6 (1996), 655–79.

82 Full-time students numbered 137 in 1983 and 82 in 1989; part-time students numbered 163 in 1983 and 436 in 1989. Whole-time equivalent totals were 300 in 1983, 518 in 1989. These figures did not include those attending short and special courses where the numbers were slightly less, 1,000 in 1983, 700 in 1989.

83 B. M. Slaney, *Nursing at Work: the Direction and Development of Occupational Health Nursing 1947–1984* (Bushey: B. M. Stanley, 2000), pp. 110–11.

84 This was a two-year part-time course leading to an RCN diploma. RCN/7/2A/3/5–6, Board of Education minutes, 27 June 1988 p. 7; 24 Oct. 1988, p. 4; 26 June 1989, p. 10; 23 Oct. 1989, p. 7; 26 Feb. 1990, p. 8. See June 1989 for paper on agreed role definition.

85 RCN/17/4/20/1, press cuttings, *News of the World* 8 Jan. 1984.

86 *AR* 1986–87, p. 5.

87 RCN/7/2A/3/4, Board of Education minutes, 20 Oct. 1986, p. 6.

88 The RCN successfully negotiated an increase in its final grant from DES, receiving £750,000, an increase of £200,000 over the previous year. This was because for many years the grant was below the usual rate, for it was not calculated according to the formula used by the National Advisory Board for Higher Education for similar colleges and institutions.

89 RCNA T302, interview with June Clark, 2006.

90 They supported four associations, Education, Management, Practice and Students; and seven societies, Occupational Health, Geriatric Nursing, Psychiatric Nursing, Oncology, Primary Health Care, Mental Handicap and Paediatric Nursing; and two research groups, the Research Society and the Daphne Heald Research Unit. By 1990 the number of specialist membership groups had reached sixty-three.

91 The first report sets out the background to the project. Jean K. McFarlane, *The Proper Study of the Nurse* (London: RCN, 1970).

92 CM 14 March 1974, pp. 69–70 and 128–36.

93 British Geriatrics Society and Royal College of Nursing, *Improving Geriatric Care in Hospital: a Handbook of Guidelines* (London: RCN, 1975).

94 CM 23 Feb. 1978, p. 60.

95 She employed a Resource Allocation Working Party for this.

96 An Assessment of the State of Nursing in the NHS (London: Royal College of Nursing, 1978).

97 *Standards of Nursing Care: a Discussion Document* (London: RCN, 1980), pp. 4–7.

98 Ibid., p. 9, and RCNA T302, interview with June Clark, 2006.

99 *Towards Standards: a Discussion Document, the Second Report of the Rcn Working Committee on Standards of Nursing Care* (London: RCN, 1981), p. 4.

100 Ibid., pp. 8–9.

101 For further details on innovations in clinical practice of this time, see RCNA T316, interview with Alison Kitson, 2007, and RCNA T318, interview with Alan Pearson, 2008.

102 *RCN Standards of Care Project, A Framework for Quality, a Patient-centred Approach to Quality Assurance in Health Care* (London: Scutari Press, 1989).

103 Royal College of Nursing, *Quality Patient Care: the Dynamic Standard Setting System* (London: RCN, 1990).

104 CM March 1990, Report on Standards of Care Project, pp. 262–7.

105 RCNA T316, interview with Alison Kitson, 2007.

106 RCNA T339, interview with Sue Pembrey, 2007.

107 £250,000 was assigned to the establishment of the Research and Development Unit in 1980, CM 8 May 1980, p. 229.
108 CM 12 March 1981, pp. 112–18, also RCN diary, 1987.
109 CM 15 Nov. 1984, pp. 832–9.
110 The Steinberg Collection of Nursing Research, a collection of theses relating to nursing.
111 Four volumes of the Nursing Bibliography were published as cumulative editions between 1968 and 1986, *A Bibliography of Nursing Literature, 1859–1960; 1961–1970; 1971–1975;* and *1976–1980* (London: The Library Association).
112 RCN/4/1980/1, 'The future development of the Rcn – a Review', p. 16.
113 RCNA T308, interview with Brian French, 2006.
114 Scutari Projects Ltd was wholly owned by the College.
115 CM June 1989, p. 293.
116 CM June 1989, pp. 295–301.
117 As associate members they pay a reduced subscription rate, they have voting rights but cannot stand for council or president.

Conclusion

The history of the RCN's first ninety years shows how far it has changed since a group of hospital matrons met to plan a professional association for nurses. Its strategies continue to alter, as do its size and the social and ethnic composition of its membership. But it still adheres to the principles of its founders, that a College of Nursing should support the professional advancement of nursing, and improve the working lives of nurses.

These two principles have not always fitted together easily as the RCN pursued its role as both professional association and trade union. It wished to defend the professional status of nurses, but began as a very exclusive body, believing that only long and rigorous nurse training would define nursing as a profession rather than a craft. As late as the 1950s the RCN hoped that the NHS would come to employ only fully trained and registered nurses, but NHS economics made this desire unrealistic. As the educational standards of trained nurses rose, so employers tried to reduce costs by dividing nursing tasks into numerous grades based on skill, and paying them accordingly. The RCN altered its membership rules to take account of these divisions in nursing, but there are still problems in defining a 'nurse'. Many hospital patients probably see health care assistants as the 'nurses' chiefly responsible for their general comfort; and these assistants are now responsible for tasks that would have fallen to trained nurses or nursing students well into the twentieth century. The answer to the question posed in the Wood report, 'what is the proper task of the nurse', therefore remains open, given the wide range of groups described as 'nurses'. For these reasons, nursing has been described as one of the 'insecure' professions, less able to defend itself through its scarcity value than professions such as medicine.[1]

The RCN's membership currently stands at around 327,000 nurses working in the UK, and 34,500 students.[2] As ever, it is difficult to calculate what proportion of all nurses this represents. In 2007 there were 660,502 registered nurses working in the UK.[3] NHS annual average employment figures for 2005 were 404,161 full-time and part-time qualified nurses, and 376,219 support staff, including health care assistants and other clinical support workers.[4] The NHS figures do not include nurses in the private sector, though agency nurses are still vital in supporting the system. These figures suggest that around 50 per cent of nurses on the nursing register are members of the RCN, though the register does not indicate how many nurses are working part-time, and perhaps less likely to keep up their RCN subscriptions.

Until late in the twentieth century, nursing students were included in NHS nursing statistics, since they were an integral part of ward labour. The founding matrons of the RCN did not want to give up their control over the management of probationers, but the RCN gradually shifted its position on this subject in response to changes in women's education and the growth of other possible careers for them. None of the women who founded the RCN had much formal schooling, and none had attended university. Like Florence Nightingale, they tended to see nursing skills as something quite distinct from passing examinations, but they also appreciated that as other opportunities for women expanded, nursing would have to compete for recruits. Educationalists in the RCN argued that moving the early years of nurse training into colleges and universities, already the practice in the USA, would reduce wastage among trainees, maintain the reputation of British nursing abroad, and keep nurses abreast of new developments in medicine. But the RCN was not united over this, for some believed that too much time spent in the classroom devalued traditional nursing skills and deterred less academic candidates.[5] Genuine concerns about the appropriate balance between theory and practice were frequently muddied by spokespeople from the medical profession who argued that nursing was a trade best learned at the bedside, and blamed the RCN for encouraging nurses to waste time on study. The crude gender bias in early statements on this subject, which echo even now, has made impartial assessment of nurse training difficult, and the debate has not ended. For a long time the RCN argued that students dropped out of training because classes were poorly organised, and education was sidelined because students provided cheap ward labour. Moving nurse training into higher education has not solved the problem. The student attrition rate from university courses is certainly lower than in the old hospital-based training schools; and the official wastage figure for England is 16 per cent; though for Scotland it is 26 per cent.[6] The RCN believes that the English figures are a considerable underestimate, because returns from individual universities give variant figures, which may be as high as 24 per cent. Nurse training, with its combination of theory and practice, is arduous, and many aspiring nurses may prefer to move into less skilled posts for the sake of an immediate salary, as they did in the past.

Although the RCN offered membership to certain grades of health care assistant from the beginning of the 1990s, members in this group number only

3,600. This section of NHS staff relies heavily on workers born overseas or from ethnic minorities, and if they join a union, it will probably be the general public sector union UNISON, which claims 1.3 million members. In 1993 the RCN's old rivals COHSE, NUPE and NALGO amalgamated to form UNISON, regrouping in reaction to the Thatcher government's industrial relations policies, as did several other general workers' unions. But, with part-time and casual work common among health care assistants, many belong to no union. Although the rise of more powerful general managers in the NHS hospitals did not seriously undermine national pay bargaining, it allowed management to develop a variety of employment practices.[7] Care workers employed by private agencies or in private nursing homes are often isolated, and difficult to organise, while their low and sometimes erratic pay makes membership an expensive proposition for them.[8]

As we have seen, the RCN tried to pursue its second aim of improving the working lives of nurses while specifically rejecting trade unionism. Union tactics were believed to be incompatible with the professional ideal, while the social class of the early leaders of the RCN also made unionism unpalatable. The RCN held to this position for fifty years, and abandoned it only when forced to do so by the political currents of the 1970s. But by this time the views, and the social and gender mix of its members were also changing. Well-publicised pay campaigns from the 1960s revealed a growing militancy among members, especially the nursing students, and the RCN leadership needed to be flexible in the face of competition from the health service unions. The pragmatic response of its leaders to these challenges maintained the popularity of the RCN among registered nurses, and greatly increased its membership.

As a trade union, the RCN has been distinctive because of its long antipathy to industrial action by nurses. From the 1960s, this policy came under severe strain as the RCN and the health service unions shared the fate of most public sector workers, and their wages were usually the first victim of government economies. The RCN's refusal to join the NHS unions in their more disruptive pay campaigns led to much animosity and competition for members. Other unions contended that the RCN undermined the bargaining strength of nurses in the NHS. Yet the health workers who did strike often experienced bruising defeats. Nurses retained a positive public image because they refused to take part in disruption to the health services, and RCN leaders believed that this image was their most powerful weapon in negotiating with government. The opposing points of view may be tested if the RCN ever decides to instruct its members to strike. In 1979, the GNC declared that nurses who put patients at risk through a strike or other action 'would have a case to answer on the score of professional misconduct'. But the Code of Professional Conduct drawn up by the GNC's successor, the UKCC, contained no such warning.[9]

Rule 12 of the RCN constitution forbade members to withdraw their service, and a two-thirds majority at a general meeting was necessary to amend the rule. After a particularly unsatisfactory decision from the Pay Review Body in 1995, an emergency meeting of the College council finally broke with the policy of nine decades, and requested Congress delegates to allow it to amend Rule 12. Congress backed them by 488 votes to three. The council then put the following resolution to a ballot:

> It is a fundamental principle of the College that its members shall not act in any way which is detrimental to the well being or interests of their patients or clients. Without prejudice to this fundamental principle, the council is empowered to authorise action by members of the College in furtherance of an industrial dispute and to make regulations governing the procedure to be followed.

Nearly 100,000 nurses balloted in favour of the resolution, a majority of 94.7 per cent; though following another tradition of the RCN, less than half the membership voted.[10] Although the RCN Council has considered applications from branches to initiate industrial action ballots and has agreed such ballots, the members have not yet taken industrial action.

The changing views of the RCN, on both educational issues and industrial relations, have inevitably been shaped by its distinctive character as an organisation composed largely of women. Only one in ten RCN members is male, and this proportion is consistent with the gender balance of all registered nurses in the UK. The most striking difference between nursing in 1916 and nursing today is that women with family responsibilities are now the largest group; and nurses under thirty are only 10 per cent of the total.[11] The founding matrons of the RCN sought the patronage of influential males, who also remained on its governing body until the Second World War. It was paradoxical that a professional body that excluded men from membership nevertheless relied on male support, not least in financial matters. This alienated more militantly feminist nursing organisations, but the RCN's pragmatism won it political acceptance and gave it a secure foundation. But gender issues continued to affect virtually all of its work, particularly in education, pay and power.

The RCN hoped that nursing would draw in women from the 'officer class', which in practical terms meant women with a secondary education, and its early membership rules assumed that women could afford to wait until they were eighteen before starting nurse training. This was a luxury that many could not afford, and the health services had to employ men and women whose education had ended at fourteen. The RCN's aims were unrealistic in this context, and more than thirty years passed before the coming of compulsory secondary education made the original ideal feasible. The continual lag in nurses' pay is also part of a wider problem, for, in spite of equal pay legislation, the average wage for women is still lower than that of men. Critics of the RCN have argued that its non-militant tactics have contributed to nurses' relatively weak position in the workplace, but inequalities in pay have affected women in most occupations, regardless of their union affiliation. It is unlikely that the RCN alone would be able to effect the change in social attitudes necessary to alter this position. Similar gender questions also arise with the subject of nurses and health service management. As Catherine Hall perceptively noted, the dual responsibilities of married nurses hindered managerial ambitions, and left the way open for a disproportionate number of men in higher administrative positions in the health services (including in the RCN itself). Again, this reflects the general position of women in Britain, for they have moved into many occupations, but are not well represented at the upper levels of management. Many RCN members have little time for activism, although they now see nursing as a long-term career rather than a short break before marriage.

Since the RCN in its earlier days spoke largely for the elite of nurses from the voluntary hospitals, its problems have often been blamed on its attachment to the Nightingale legacy. Florence Nightingale was praised, or condemned, for having presented nursing as a selfless vocation, whose practitioners saw their pay as less important than their social duty. In fact, Florence Nightingale insisted that nurses should be properly paid for their work, but her image was too closely associated with discipline and self-sacrifice. During each RCN pay campaign since the 1960s, the press has asserted that nurses have finally flung aside the Nightingale mantle – though apparently they pick it up again between campaigns. This is part of the paradoxical image of the RCN; for according to union-minded historians, the RCN was for too long restrained and ladylike in its dealings with authority, yet at the same time senior nurses were criticised for their strong and authoritarian ways. The middle-class ideals and outright social snobbery of early RCN leaders are difficult to dispute, but the vocational ideal may have been as much a response to difficult circumstances as the cause of them. Nurses in Britain, whether in the hospitals or in the community, have nearly always worked in systems with constrained resources, and the vocational ideal has been a way of maintaining a service in spite of this.

The RCN has achieved the ambition of its founders in that most career-minded nurses and nursing students become members. As a union, it has rivals, but there is no comparable professional body for all nurses. While union activities and lively Congress debates capture media attention, the everyday professional work of the RCN is the enduring experience for many of its members. The authors, none of whom is eligible for membership of the College, did much of their research in the College archives in its Edinburgh headquarters. In this building, as in its other centres, the constant hum from conferences, seminars and study groups, and the (somewhat) quieter clusters of students in the library, are part of a history of activity that goes back to its founding days. Its notice boards carry news of meetings, courses, social activities and welfare services. Sarah Swift and Arthur Stanley might be perturbed by the less starched dress of today's nurses, but they would recognise the professional atmosphere of the institution that they created.

Notes

1 See Chris Nottingham, 'The rise of the insecure professionals', *International Review of Social History* 52: 3 (2007), 445–75 for a wider analysis.
2 Figures provided by the RCN for Feb. 2008. A further 32,000 members are retired nurses, associate members, members overseas, etc.
3 Nursing and Midwifery Council, *Statistical Analysis of the Register*, 1 April 2006 to 31 March 2007, p. 5, www.nmc-uk.org/aFrameDisplay.aspx?DocumentID=3600, accessed 31 March 2008.
4 www.ic.nhs.uk/statistics-and-data-collections, accessed 27 March 2008. These figures do not include students.
5 Davies, *Gender and the Professional Predicament in Nursing*, ch. 6.
6 *NS* 22: 31, 9 April 2008, pp. 12–15. The higher Scottish rate is attributed to the longer course, four years rather than three.
7 Stephen Bach, 'Health sector reform and human resource management; Britain in comparative perspective', *International Journal of Human Resource Management* 11: 5 (2000), 932–3.
8 Stephen Bach 'International migration of health workers: labour and social issues', International Labour Office, Geneva (2003), p. 19 http://medact.org/content/health/docments, accessed 27 March 2008.
9 CM April 1995, p. 217.
10 CM July 1995, p. 462.
11 Nursing and Midwifery Council, *Statistical Analysis of the Register*, 2006, p. 5.

Appendix 1 timechart

[Royal] College of Nursing	Date	Related events
College of Nursing Ltd founded	1916	
Mary S. Rundle, secretary		
Standing Committees set up		
Scottish Board established in Edinburgh		
Irish Board established in Dublin	1917	
Nation's Fund for Nurses provides endowment for College	1919	Nurses Registration Acts Dr Addison, Minister of Health General Nursing Council established
Badge introduced	1920	
Quarterly College *Bulletin* published		
Endowment fund set up for a chair of nursing		
	1921	Cowdrays purchase 20 Cavendish Square for the College
Sister Tutor's Section established	1922	Irish Free State founded
Public Health Section established	1923	
Student Nurses' Association formed by College as a separate body	1925	
Decision to close Irish Board of the College: focus shifts to Committee for Northern Ireland in Belfast		
Opening of College of Nursing building in Henrietta Place	1926	
Queen Mary becomes official patron		
Nursing Times becomes the official journal of the College of Nursing	1927	
Royal Charter granted to the College, but title of 'Royal' not permitted	1928	Federated Superannuation Scheme for Nurses and Hospital Officers established
College of Nursing Ltd becomes College of Nursing		
	1931	Report of the *Lancet* Commission on Nursing
Frances Goodall appointed secretary	1933	
Indemnity insurance established	1936	
George VI grants the title 'Royal' to College	1939	Report of the Interdepartmental Committee on Nursing Services (Athlone)
College badge redesigned		
Private Nurses Section established		
War Emergency Committee established for duration of war		

Nursing Reconstruction Committee   1941   Nurses Salaries Committee
(Horder) established   (Rushcliffe) set up
Society of Registered Male Nurses and
Association of Sick Children's Nurses
affiliate to the College
First use of the title 'general secretary'   1942   Beveridge Report on Social
First report of Horder Committee, on   Insurance and Allied Services
Assistant Nurses
Second and third reports of Horder   1943   Nurses Act establishes roll of state
Committee, on education and training,   enrolled assistant nurses
and on recruitment
Princess Elizabeth becomes president of   1944   Education Act expands secondary
the Student Nurses' Association   education and improves access to
higher education
1945   Aneurin Bevan becomes Minister of
Health
1945–49
1946   Report of the Royal Commission on
Equal Pay
1947   Report of the Working Party on the
recruitment and training of nurses
(Wood)
1948   NHS Act (England and Wales)
National Association of State Enrolled   1949   Whitley Councils of the NHS set up
Nurses (NASEN) affiliates to the College   to arbitrate on pay
Ward and Departmental Sisters Section   Nurses Act (England and Wales)
established   NHS Act (Scotland)
Third report of Horder Committee, on
social and economic conditions of the
nurse
Society of Mental Nurses affiliates to the   1951
College
Occupational Health Section established   1952
Association of British Paediatric Nurses   1953   Nuffield Provincial Hospitals Trust
affiliates to the College   publishes *The Work of Nurses in*
Queen Elizabeth II becomes patron   *Hospital Wards*
following death of Queen Mary
Birmingham Education Centre
established
Catherine Hall appointed general secretary   1957
1959   GNC incorporates the
supplementary registers into the
general register
Membership opens to all registered   1960
nurses including men
Nurse Administrator's Section established
Information officer appointed   1961
Reform of Nursing Education Committee
(Platt) appointed

RCN launches first highly publicised pay campaign	1962	
Welsh Board established		
RCN amalgamates with the National Council of Nurses: becomes Royal College of Nursing and the National Council of Nurses of the UK (Rcn)	1963	
Queen Mother, patron of NCN is joint patron of Rcn		
International Department established		
Report of Platt Committee	1964	
Northern Irish Committee becomes a Board		
	1966	Report of the Committee on Senior Nursing Staff Structure (Salmon)
Branches Standing Committee becomes the Royal College of Nursing Representative Body (RRB)	1967	
First meeting of the RRB		
Computerised membership records begin		
Nursing Times returns to independent status		
Membership opened to student nurses	1968	Joint Board of Clinical Nursing Studies established
Princess Margaret patron of SNA, becomes joint patron of RCN		
Nursing Standard begins as bi-monthly publication, free to members		
Student Nurses' Section established		
Welfare Advisory Service established	1969	
Raise the Roof campaign		
NASEN amalgamates with RCN	1970	The Committee on Nursing (Briggs)
Enrolled Nurses' Section established		
Education Department becomes the Institute of Advanced Nursing Education (IANE)	1971	Industrial Relations Act UK enters EEC
Professional Nursing Department established		
District Nurses' Section established	1972	Report of the Committee on Nursing (Briggs)
Membership re-organisation begins, following review by Tavistock Institute	1973	NHS Act (consensus management introduced)
Local Centres established		
Stewards scheme established		

Threat of withdrawal from ICN	1974	Barbara Castle becomes Secretary of State for Social Services*
		Report of Committee of Inquiry into the Pay and Related Conditions of Service of Nurses and Midwives (Halsbury)
		Trade Union and Industrial Relations Act
		EEC Directives on Nursing
Membership Centres re-organised to match NHS boundaries	1976	PCN Permanent Committee of Nurses in Liaison with the EEC established
RCN registered as a trade union		
First Fellowships (FRCN) awarded		
CHANNEL set up		
New title, Royal College of Nursing of the UK (RCN)		
	1977	Royal Commission on the NHS set up (Briggs)
	1978	David Ennals becomes Secretary of State for Social Services
Nursing Standard becomes a weekly journal	1979	Nurses Midwives and Health Visitors Act; replaces GNCs with UKCC and National Boards
Records Department moves to Cardiff		Margaret Thatcher Prime Minister 1979–90
AGM amendment to charter giving students limited voting rights		
Trevor Clay becomes deputy general secretary		
Motion to discard Rule 12 (right to strike) rejected at AGM	1980	Report of Standing Commission on Pay Comparability, *Report No. 3, Nurses and Midwives* (Clegg)
Catharine Hall becomes first chair of the UKCC		
Bridge that Gap pay campaign	1981	Norman Fowler becomes Secretary of State for Social Services*
Membership re-organisation		
Trevor Clay appointed general secretary	1982	TUC backs industrial action by Health Service Unions
	1983	Pay Review Body established
	1984	NHS Management Inquiry Report (Griffiths)
Commission on Nursing Education (Judge)	1985	Review of Community Nursing (Cumberledge)
	1986	Nurse Practitioner and Nurse Prescribing introduced
	1987	UKCC publishes Project 2000
	1988	Clinical grading introduced
		Kenneth Clarke becomes Secretary of State for Health*
Christine Hancock appointed general secretary	1989	

*Minister of Health to 1968; Secretary of State for Social Services to 1988; Secretary of State for Health to date.

Appendix 2 RCN membership, 1916–2007 (000s)

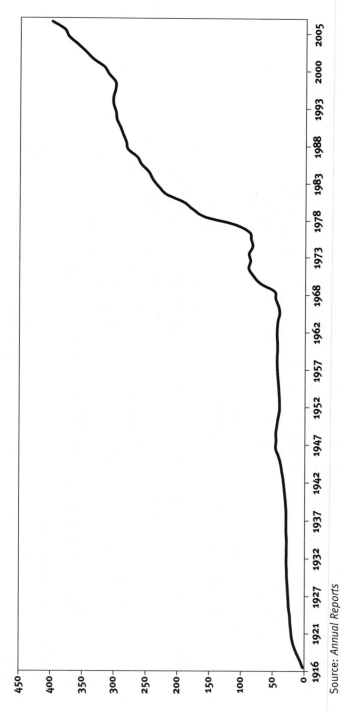

Source: *Annual Reports*

Appendix 3 Structure of the College, 1932–49

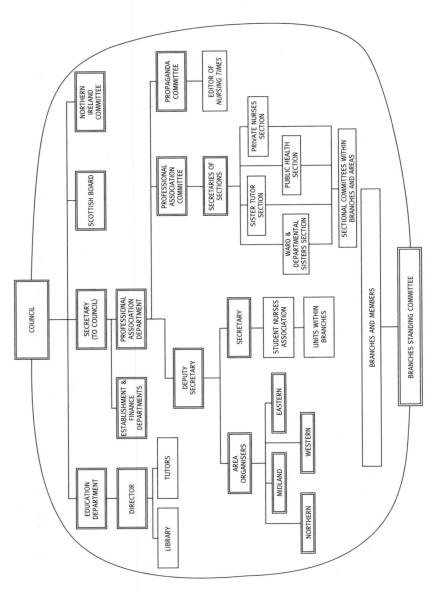

Appendix 4 Structure of the College, 1950–70

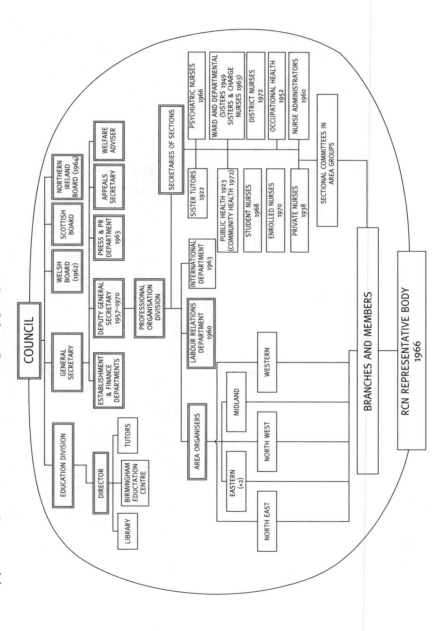

COUNCIL

EDUCATION DIVISION
- DIRECTOR
  - LIBRARY
  - BIRMINGHAM EDUCTATION CENTRE
  - TUTORS

GENERAL SECRETARY
- ESTABLISHMENT & FINANCE DEPARTMENTS

DEPUTY GENERAL SECRETARY 1957–1970
- PRESS & PR DEPARTMENT 1963
- PROFESSIONAL ORGANISATION DIVISION
  - LABOUR RELATIONS DEPARTMENT 1960
  - INTERNATIONAL DEPARTMENT 1963
  - SECRETARIES OF SECTIONS

WELSH BOARD (1962)

SCOTTISH BOARD

NORTHERN IRELAND BOARD (1964)
- APPEALS SECRETARY
- WELFARE ADVISER

AREA ORGANISERS
- NORTH EAST
- EASTERN (×2)
- NORTH WEST
- MIDLAND
- WESTERN

SECRETARIES OF SECTIONS
- SISTER TUTORS 1922
- PSYCHIATRIC NURSES 1966
- WARD AND DEPARTMENTAL (SISTERS 1949 SISTERS & CHARGE NURSES 1963)
- PUBLIC HEALTH 1923 (COMMUNITY HEALTH 1972)
- DISTRICT NURSES 1972
- STUDENT NURSES 1968
- OCCUPATIONAL HEALTH 1952
- ENROLLED NURSES 1970
- PRIVATE NURSES 1938
- NURSE ADMINISTRATORS 1960

SECTIONAL COMMITTEES IN AREA GROUPS

BRANCHES AND MEMBERS

RCN REPRESENTATIVE BODY 1966

Appendix 5 Structure of the College, 1970–77

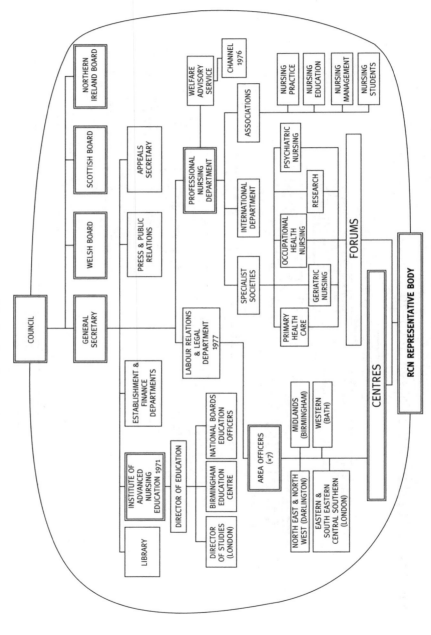

COUNCIL

NORTHERN IRELAND BOARD

SCOTTISH BOARD

WELSH BOARD

GENERAL SECRETARY

PRESS & PUBLIC RELATIONS

APPEALS SECRETARY

PROFESSIONAL NURSING DEPARTMENT

WELFARE ADVISORY SERVICE

CHANNEL 1976

ASSOCIATIONS

NURSING PRACTICE

NURSING EDUCATION

NURSING MANAGEMENT

NURSING STUDENTS

INTERNATIONAL DEPARTMENT

SPECIALIST SOCIETIES

PSYCHIATRIC NURSING

RESEARCH

OCCUPATIONAL HEALTH NURSING

GERIATRIC NURSING

PRIMARY HEALTH CARE

FORUMS

LABOUR RELATIONS & LEGAL DEPARTMENT 1977

ESTABLISHMENT & FINANCE DEPARTMENTS

INSTITUTE OF ADVANCED NURSING EDUCATION 1971

LIBRARY

DIRECTOR OF EDUCATION

NATIONAL BOARDS EDUCATION OFFICERS

BIRMINGHAM EDUCATION CENTRE

DIRECTOR OF STUDIES (LONDON)

AREA OFFICERS (x7)

MIDLANDS (BIRMINGHAM)

WESTERN (BATH)

NORTH EAST & NORTH WEST (DARLINGTON)

EASTERN & SOUTH EASTERN CENTRAL SOUTHERN (LONDON)

CENTRES

RCN REPRESENTATIVE BODY

Select bibliography

Manuscript sources

Modern Records Centre, University of Warwick: NALGO papers.
The National Archives, London: nursing material in the Ministry of Health (MH) and
    Ministry of Labour (LAB) series.
Royal College of Nursing Archives, Edinburgh.
Wellcome Library, Archives and Manuscripts, London: Health Visitors' Association
    papers.

Unpublished theses

Beaumont, Catriona, 'Women's citizenship: a study of non-feminist women's societies
    and the women's movement in England, 1928–1950', PhD thesis, University of
    Warwick (1996).
Bradbury, Jonathan Paul, 'The 1929 Local Government Act: the formulation and
    implementation of the Poor Law (Health Care) and Exchequer grant reforms for
    England and Wales', PhD thesis, University of Bristol (1990).
Brooks, Jane, 'Visiting rights only: the early experience of nurses in higher education,
    1918–1960', PhD thesis, London School of Hygiene and Tropical Medicine (2005).
Kirby, Stephanie, 'The London County Council Nursing Service 1929–1948', PhD
    thesis, University of Nottingham (2000).
Miller, Carol Ann, 'Lobbying the League: women's international organisations and the
    League of Nations', PhD thesis, University of Oxford (1992).
Mortimer, Barbara, 'The nurse in Edinburgh c.1760–1860: the impact of commerce
    and professionalisation', PhD thesis, University of Edinburgh (2002).
Reinkemeyer, Sister Mary Hubert, 'The limited impact of basic university programs in
    nursing: a British case study', PhD thesis, University of California, Berkeley (1966).
Scott, Elizabeth J. C., 'The influence of the staff of the Ministry of Health on policies
    for nursing 1919–1968', PhD thesis, London School of Economics (1994).
Todd, Selina, 'Young women, employment and the family in interwar England', DPhil
    thesis, University of Sussex (2003).

Official reports

The Lancet Commission on Nursing. Final Report (London: The Lancet, 1932).

Ministry of Health and Board of Education, Inter-departmental Committee on Nursing Services. Interim Report [Athlone report] (London: HMSO, 1939).

Ministry of Information, Wartime Social Survey, The Attitudes of Women Towards Nursing, an Inquiry Made by the Regional Organisation of the Wartime Social Survey for Campaigns Division of the Ministry of Information, by Kathleen Box assisted by Enid Croft-White (London: July 1943).

Report of the Royal Commission on Equal Pay 1944–46, Cmd 6937 (London: HMSO, 1946).

Ministry of Labour and National Service, Nursing as a Career (London: HMSO, 1947).

Ministry of Health, Department of Health for Scotland, Ministry of Labour and National Service, Report of the Working Party on the Recruitment and Training of Nurses [Wood report] (London: HMSO, 1947).

Ministry of Health, Department of Health for Scotland, Ministry of Labour and National Service, Working Party on the Recruitment and Training of Nurses, Minority Report (London: HMSO, 1948).

The Nuffield Provincial Hospitals Trust, The Work of Nurses in Hospital Wards, Report of a Job-analysis (London: The Nuffield Provincial Hospitals Trust, 1953).

Ministry of Health, Department of Health for Scotland, the General Nursing Councils for England and Wales and Scotland, Report of the Committee Set Up to Consider the Function, Status and Training of Nurse Tutors (London: HMSO, 1954).

Department of Health for Scotland, Scottish Health Services Council, The State Enrolled Assistant Nurse in the National Health Service, Report by the Standing Nursing and Midwifery Advisory Committee (Edinburgh: HMSO, 1955).

Department of Health for Scotland, Scottish Health Services Council, The Work of Nurses in Hospital Wards, Report by the Standing Nursing and Midwifery Advisory Committee on the 'Job Analysis of the Work of Nurses in Hospital Wards' Prepared by the Nuffield Provincial Hospitals Trust (Edinburgh: HMSO, 1955).

International Labour Office, Employment and Conditions of Work of Nurses (Geneva: ILO, 1960).

Ministry of Health, Central Health Services Council, The Post-certificate Training and Education of Nurses, a Report by a Sub-committee of the Standing Nursing Advisory Committee (London: HMSO, 1966).

Ministry of Health, Scottish Home and Health Department, Report of the Committee on Senior Nursing Staff Structure [Salmon report] (London: HMSO, 1966).

National Board for Prices and Incomes, Report No. 60. Pay of Nurses and Midwives in the National Health Service, Cmnd 3585 (London: HMSO, 1968).

Department of Health and Social Security, Report of the Nurse Tutor Working Party (London: DHSS, April 1970).

Report of the Committee on Nursing, Chairman: Professor Asa Briggs [Briggs report] Cmnd 5115 (London: HMSO 1972).

Department of Health and Social Security, Report of the Committee of Inquiry into the Pay and Related Conditions of Service of Nurses and Midwives, Chairman: The Rt. Hon. The Earl of Halsbury, FRS [Halsbury report] (London: HMSO, 1974).

Standing Commission on Pay Comparability, *Report No. 3, Nurses and Midwives*, Chairman: Professor H. A. Clegg [Clegg report] Cmnd 7795 (London: HMSO, 1980).
Department of Health and Social Security, *NHS Management Inquiry Report* [Griffiths report] (London: DHSS, 1983).
Review Body for Nursing Staff, Midwives, Health Visitors and Professions Allied to Medicine, *First Report on Nursing Staff, Midwives and Health Visitors*, Chairman: Sir John Hedley Greenborough, Cmnd 9258 (London: HMSO, 1984).
Project 2000: a New Preparation for Practice (London: United Kingdom Central Council for Nursing, Midwifery and Health Visiting, 1986).

Reports sponsored by the Royal College of Nursing

Nursing Reconstruction Committee, *Report, Section I, the Assistant Nurse* [Horder report] (London: Royal College of Nursing, 1942).
Nursing Reconstruction Committee, *Report, Section II, Education and Training; Section III, Recruitment* [Horder report] (London: Royal College of Nursing, 1943).
Nursing Reconstruction Committee, *Report, Section IV, the Social and Economic Conditions of the Nurse* [Horder report] (London: Royal College of Nursing, 1949).
Working Party on Salary Structure, Accommodation for Nurses and Midwives, *Report of a Study of Accommodation Provided for Resident and Non-resident Nursing and Midwifery Staff in National Health Service Hospitals in England, Scotland and Wales, 1959. Studies in Nursing No. 1* (London: Royal College of Nursing, 1961).
Special Committee on Nurse Education, *A Reform of Nursing Education* [Platt report] (London: Royal College of Nursing and National Council of Nurses of the United Kingdom, 1964).
Administering the Hospital Nursing Service – a Review (London: Royal College of Nursing and National Council of Nurses of the United Kingdom, 1964).
Administering the Local Authority Nursing Service (London: Royal College of Nursing and National Council of Nurses of the United Kingdom, 1968).
New Horizons in Clinical Nursing, Report of a Seminar Held at Leeds Castle, Kent, October 1975 (London: Royal College of Nursing of the United Kingdom, 1975).
The Extended Clinical Role of the Nurse (London: Royal College of Nursing of the United Kingdom, 1979).
Standards of Nursing Care, a Discussion Document (London: Royal College of Nursing of the United Kingdom, 1980).
Towards Standards, a Discussion Document (London: Royal College of Nursing of the United Kingdom, 1981).
Standards of Nursing Care, Action to Safeguard Standards of Nursing Care (Belfast: Royal College of Nursing Northern Ireland Board, 1981).
To Teach or Not to Teach? That Is the Question (London: Royal College of Nursing of the United Kingdom, 1981).
A Structure for Nursing, Report of the Rcn Group on a Professional Nursing Structure for the NHS, a Discussion Document (London: Royal College of Nursing of the United Kingdom, 1981).

The Education of Nurses: a New Dispensation, Commission on Nursing Education [Judge report] (London: Royal College of Nursing of the United Kingdom, 1985).

Feeling Better: Getting Better, Why the Nursing Voice Must Be Heard (London: Royal College of Nursing of the United Kingdom, 1986).

In Pursuit of Excellence, a Position Statement on Nursing (London: Royal College of Nursing of the United Kingdom, 1987).

A Framework for Quality, a Patient-centred Approach to Quality Assurance in Health Care, RCN Standards of Care Project (London: Royal College of Nursing of the United Kingdom, 1989).

A Manifesto for Nursing and Health (London: Royal College of Nursing of the United Kingdom, 1990).

Published sources

Abel-Smith, Brian, *A History of the Nursing Profession* (London: Heinemann, 1960).

Abel-Smith, Brian and Richard H. Titmuss, *The Cost of the National Health Service in England and Wales* (Cambridge: Cambridge University Press, 1956).

Allen, Davina, *The Changing Shape of Nursing Practice: the Role of Nurses in the Hospital Division of Labour* (London and New York: Routledge, 2001).

Armstrong, Peter, *White Collar Workers, Trade Unions and Class* (London: Croom Helm, 1986).

Armstrong, Peter, Bob Carter, Chris Smith and Theo Nicols, *White Collar Workers, Trade Unions and Class Consciousness* (Oxford: Clarendon Press, 1989).

Bach, Stephen, 'Health sector reform and human resource management: Britain in comparative perspective', *International Journal of Human Resource Management* 11: 3 (2000), 925–42.

Bain, George Sayers, *The Growth of White-collar Unionism* (Oxford: Clarendon Press, 1970).

Balme, Harold, *A Criticism of Nursing Education* (London: Oxford University Press, 1937).

Baly, Monica E., *Nursing and Social Change*, 3rd edn (London: Routledge, 1995).

Beaumont, Catriona, 'Citizens not feminists: the boundary negotiated between citizenship and feminism by mainstream women's organisations in England, 1928–39', *Women's History Review* 9: 2 (2000), 411–29.

Beddoe, Deirdre, *Back to Home and Duty: Women Between the Wars 1918–1939* (London: Pandora, 1989).

Beishon, Sharon, Satnam Virdee and Ann Hagell, *Nursing in a Multi-ethnic NHS* (London: Policy Studies Institute, 1996).

Bendall, Eve and Elizabeth Raybould, *History of the General Nursing Council for England and Wales, 1919–69* (London: H. K. Lewis, 1969).

Beveridge, William, *Social Insurance and Allied Services* (London: HMSO, 1942).

Bowman, Gerald, *The Lamp and the Book: the Story of the Rcn, 1916–1966* (London: Queen Anne Press, 1967).

Bridges, Daisy C., *A History of the International Council of Nurses 1899–1964: the First 65 Years* (London: Pitman Medical, 1967).

Britten, Jessie D., *Practical Notes on Nursing Procedures* (Edinburgh: E. & S. Livingstone, 1957).

Brooks, Jane, 'Visiting rights only: the diplomas in nursing in the UK in the interwar period', *Nursing Inquiry* 13 (2006), 269–76.

Bruley, Sue, *Women in Britain Since 1900* (Basingstoke: Macmillan, 1999).

Brush, Barbara and Joan Lynaugh, *Nurses of All Nations: a History of the International Council of Nurses, 1899–1999* (Philadelphia: Lippincott, 1999).

Burchill, Frank, 'The Pay Review Body system: a comment and a consequence', *Historical Studies in Industrial Relations* 10 (Autumn 2000), 141–57.

Calder, Angus, *The People's War: Britain 1939–45* (London: Granada, 1982).

Carpenter, Mick, *Working for Health: the History of the Confederation of Health Service Employees* (London: Lawrence & Wishart, 1988).

Carter, Gladys Beaumont, *A New Deal for Nurses* (London: Gollancz, 1939).

———, *Reconsideration of Nursing: Its Fundamentals, Purposes and Place in the Community* (London: Nursing Mirror, 1946).

Castle, Barbara, *The Castle Diaries 1974–76* (London: Weidenfeld and Nicolson, 1980).

Charley, Irene Hannah, *The Birth of Industrial Nursing: Its History and Development in Great Britain* (London: Baillière, Tindall & Cox, 1954).

Clay, Trevor, in association with Alison Dunn and Neil Stewart, *Nurses: Power and Politics* (London: Heinemann Nursing, 1987).

Copelman, Dina M., *London's Women Teachers: Gender, Class and Feminism 1870–1930* (London and New York: Routledge, 1996).

Crossman, Richard, *The Diaries of a Cabinet Minister. Vol. 3, Secretary of State for Social Services, 1968–70* (London: Hamish Hamilton and Jonathan Cape, 1977).

Crowther, M. A., *The Workhouse System 1834–1929* (London: Methuen, 1983).

Cutler, Tony, '"A double irony": the politics of National Health Service expenditure in the 1950s', in Martin Gorsky and Sally Sheard (eds), *Financing Medicine: the British Experience Since 1750* (London and New York: Routledge, 2006), pp. 201–20.

Davies, Celia (ed.), *Rewriting Nursing History* (London: Croom Helm, 1980).

———, *Gender and the Professional Predicament in Nursing* (Buckingham: Open University Press, 1995).

Davies, Celia and Abigail Beach, *Interpreting Professional Self-regulation. A History of the United Kingdom Central Council for Nursing, Midwifery and Health Visiting* (London and New York: Routledge, 2000).

Davis, Gayle and Roger Davidson, '"Big White Chief", "Pontius Pilate", and the "Plumber": the impact of the 1967 Abortion Act on the Scottish medical community, c. 1967–1980', *SHM* 18 (2005), 282–306.

Dingwall, Robert, Anne Marie Rafferty and Charles Webster (eds), *An Introduction to the Social History of Nursing* (London: Routledge, 1988).

Dwork, Deborah, *War Is Good for Babies & Other Young Children: a History of the Infant and Child Welfare Movement in England 1898–1918* (London and New York: Tavistock, 1987).

Edwards, Elizabeth, *Women in Teacher Training Colleges, 1900–1960: a Culture of Femininity* (London: Routledge, 2000).

Evans, Joan, 'Men nurses: a historical and feminist perspective', *Journal of Advanced Nursing* 47: 3 (2004), 321–8.

Finlayson, Louise R. and James Y. Nazroo, *Gender Inequalities in Nursing Careers* (London: Policy Studies Institute, 1997).

Gilbert, Bentley B., *British Social Policy 1914–1939* (London: Batsford, 1970).

Glick, Daphne, *The National Council of Women of Great Britain. The First One Hundred Years* (London: NCW, 1995).

Gorsky, Martin, John Mohan and Martin Powell, 'British voluntary hospitals, 1871–1938: the geography of provision and utilisation', *Journal of Historical Geography* 25: 4 (1999), 463–82.

——, 'The financial health of voluntary hospitals in interwar Britain', *Ec.H.R.* 55: 3 (2002), 533–57.

Gorsky, Martin and Sally Sheard (eds), *Financing Medicine: the British Experience Since 1750* (London and New York: Routledge, 2006).

Hardy, Anne, *Health and Medicine in Britain Since 1860* (Basingstoke: Palgrave, 2001).

Hart, Christopher, *Behind the Mask: Nurses, Their Unions and Nursing Policy* (London: Baillière Tindall, 1994).

——, *Nurses and Politics: the Impact of Power and Practice* (Basingstoke: Palgrave Macmillan, 2003).

Humphreys, John, 'English nurse education and the reform of the National Health Service', *Journal of Education Policy* 11: 6 (1996), 655–79.

Innes, Sue, 'Constructing women's citizenship in the interwar period: the Edinburgh Women Citizen's Association', *Women's History Review* 13: 4 (2004), 621–47.

Jones, Helen, *Health and Society in Twentieth Century Britain* (New York: Longman, 1994).

Kirby, Stephanie, 'Reciprocal rewards: British Poor Law nursing and the campaign for state registration', *International History of Nursing Journal* 7 (2002), 4–13.

——, 'Splendid scope for public service: leading the London County Council Nursing Service, 1929–1948', *Nursing History Review* 14 (2006), 31–57.

Lewis, Jane, *The Politics of Motherhood: Child and Maternal Welfare in England, 1900–1939* (London: Croom Helm, 1980).

——, *Women in England 1870–1950: Sexual Divisions and Social Change* (New York and London: Harvester Wheatsheaf, 1984).

——, *Women in Britain Since 1945: Women, Family, Work and the State in the Post-war Years* (Oxford: Blackwell Publishing, 1992).

Loudon, Irvine, *Death in Childbirth: an International Study of Maternal Care and Maternal Mortality, 1800–1950* (Oxford: Clarendon Press, 1992).

Lowe, Rodney, 'Hours of labour: negotiating industrial legislation in Britain 1919–39', *Ec.H.R.* 35 (1982), 254–72.

Maggs, Christopher J., *The Origins of General Nursing*, 1985 edn (London and Dover, NH: Croom Helm, 1983).

McGann, Susan, *The Battle of the Nurses: a Study of Eight Women Who Influenced the Development of Professional Nursing, 1880–1930* (London: Scutari Press, 1992).

——, 'The wind of change is blowing', *Nursing History Review*, 10 (2002), 21–32.

——, 'Collaboration and conflict in international nursing 1920–1939', *Nursing History Review* 16 (2008), 29–57.

Mortimer, Barbara and Susan McGann (eds), *New Directions in the History of Nursing: International Perspectives* (London: Routledge, 2005).

Newstead, Betty, 'Industrial relations and the nurse', *Nursing Mirror* 134 (1972), 14–16.

NLD [Nan Dorsey] and MMK [Marjorie Kilby], *The Lamp Radiant, the Story of an Association of Nurses from Many Lands, by Two of Its Members* (London: privately published, 1955).

Nottingham, Chris (ed.), *The First Fifty Years of the N.H.S. in Scotland* (Aldershot: Ashgate, 2000).

———, 'The rise of the insecure professionals', *International Review of Social History* 52: 3 (2007), 445–75.

Nutting, M. A. and L. Dock, *A History of Nursing: the Evolution of Nursing Systems from the Earliest Times to the Foundation of the First English and American Training Schools for Nurses* (New York and London: G. P. Putnam and Sons, 1907).

Oram, Alison, *Women Teachers and Feminist Politics 1900–1939* (Manchester: Manchester University Press, 1996).

Pelling, Henry, *A History of British Trade Unionism*, 5th edn (Basingstoke: Macmillan, 1992).

Perkin, Harold, *The Rise of Professional Society: England Since 1800* (London: Routledge, 1989).

Pickstone, John, *Medicine and Industrial Society: a History of Hospital Development in Manchester and Its Region 1752–1946* (Manchester: Manchester University Press, 1985).

Pugh, Martin, *Women and the Women's Movement in Britain, 1914–1959* (Basingstoke: Macmillan, 1992).

Purvis, June, *Women's History: Britain, 1850–1945: an Introduction* (London: UCL Press, 1997).

Quinn, Sheila, *A Dame Abroad* (Stanhope: Memoir Club, 2004).

Rafferty, Anne Marie, 'Internationalising nurse education', in Paul Weindling (ed.), *International Health Organisations and Movements 1918–1939* (Cambridge: Cambridge University Press, 1995), pp. 266–82.

———, *The Politics of Nursing Knowledge* (London: Routlege, 1996).

Rafferty, Anne Marie, Jane Robinson and Ruth Elkan, *Nursing History and the Politics of Welfare* (London: Routledge, 1997).

Reid, Alastair J., *United We Stand: a History of Britain's Trade Unions* (London: Allen Lane, 2004).

Robb, Barbara, *Sans Everything: a Case to Answer* (London: Nelson, 1967).

Runciman, W. G., 'Explaining union density in twentieth-century Britain', *Sociology* 25 (1991), 697–712.

Salvage, Jane, *The Politics of Nursing* (London: Heinemann Nursing, 1985).

Simpson, H. Marjorie, 'The Royal College of Nursing of the United Kingdom 1916–1976: role and action in a changing health service', *Nursing Mirror* 143 (2. Dec. 1976), 39–41.

Sked, Alan and Chris Cook, *Post-War Britain: a Political History*, 3rd edn (London: Penguin, 1990).

Slaney, B. M., *Nursing at Work: the Direction and Development of Occupational Health Nursing 1947–1984* (Bushey: B. M. Slaney, 2000).

Smith, Harold L., 'The problem of "equal pay for equal work" in Great Britain during World War II', *Journal of Modern History* 53 (1981), 652–72.

———, 'The politics of Conservative reform: The equal pay for equal work issue, 1945–1955', *Historical Journal* 35 (1992), 401–15.

———, 'British feminism and the equal pay issue in the 1930s', *Women's History Review* 5 (1996), 97–110.

Smith, Jennifer, *1896–1996: a History in Health. Health Visitors' Association 100 Years* (London: Health Visitors Association, 1996).

Spoor, Alec, *White-collar Union: Sixty Years of NALGO* (London: Heinemann, 1967).

Starns, Penny, *March of the Matrons: Military Influences on the British Civilian Nursing Profession 1939–1969* (Peterborough: DSM, 2000).

Stewart, Isabel Maitland, *The Education of Nurses: Historical Foundations and Modern Trends* (New York: Macmillan, 1944).

Stewart, John, *The Battle for Health: a Political History of the Socialist Medical Association, 1930–51* (Aldershot: Ashgate, 1999).

———, 'Angels or aliens? Refugee nurses in Britain, 1938 to 1942', *Medical History* 47: 2 (2003), 149–72.

Strong, Phil and Jane Robinson, *New Model Management: Griffiths and the NHS*. Nursing Policy Studies 3 (University of Warwick: Nursing Policy Studies Centre, 1988).

———, *The NHS – Under New Management* (Milton Keynes and Philadelphia: Open University Press, 1990).

Sweet, Helen M. and Rona Dougall, *Community Nursing and Primary Healthcare in Twentieth-century Britain* (London: Routledge, 2008).

Tavistock Institute of Human Relations, *An Exploratory Study of the Rcn Membership Structure* (London: Royal College of Nursing, 1973).

Taylor, Robert, *The Trade Union Question in British Politics: Government and the Unions Since 1945* (Oxford: Blackwell, 1993).

Thane, Pat, 'Towards equal opportunities? Women in Britain since 1945', in Terry Gourvish and Alan O'Day (eds), *Britain Since 1945* (London: Macmillan, 1991), pp. 183–208.

———, *Foundations of the Welfare State* (Harlow: Longman, 1996).

———, *Old Age in English History: Past Experiences, Present Issues* (Oxford: Oxford University Press, 2000).

———, 'What difference did the vote make? Women in public and private life in Britain since 1918', *Historical Research* 76 (2003), 268–85.

Todd, Selina, *Young Women, Work and Family in England 1918–1950* (Oxford: Oxford University Press, 2005).

Tooley, Sarah, *The History of Nursing in the British Empire* (London: S. H. Bousfield, 1906).

Webster, Charles, *The Health Services Since the War. Vol. 1* (London: HMSO, 1988).

———, *The Health Services Since the War. Vol. 2, Government and Health Care: the National Health Service 1958–1979* (London: HMSO, 1996).

————, *The National Health Service: a Political History* (Oxford and New York: Oxford University Press, 1998).

Weir, Rosemary I., *A Leap in the Dark, the Origins and Development of the Department of Nursing Studies, the University of Edinburgh* (Penzance: Jamieson Library, 1996).

————, *Educating Nurses in Scotland: a History of Innovation and Change: 1950–2000* (Penzance: Hypatia, 2004).

White, Geoff, 'The Pay Review Body system: its development and impact', *Historical Studies in Industrial Relations* 9 (Spring 2000), 71–97.

White, Rosemary, 'The development of the Poor Law Nursing Service 1848–1948. A discussion of the historical method and a summary of some of the findings', *International Journal of Nursing Studies* 14 (1977), 19–27.

————, *The Effects of the NHS on the Nursing Profession: 1948–1961* (London: King Edward's Hospital Fund for London, 1985).

———— (ed.), *Political Issues in Nursing: Past, Present and Future* (Chichester: John Wiley, 1985).

Wivel, Ashley, 'Abortion policy and politics on the Lane Committee of Enquiry, 1971–1974', *SHM* 11: 1 (1998) 109–35.

Index

Page numbers in **bold italic** refer to illustrations; n. denotes note on that page.

abortion 267, 269–71
Abortion Act (1967) 269–70
Actresses' Franchise League 20
Addison, Christopher 30, 63
AIDS nursing course 307
Aitken, Janet 183
Altschul, Annie 186
American Federation of Women's
  Clubs 109
American Nurses' Association 267
American Oncology Nursing
  Society 259
ancillary workers 244, 245, 251, 272, 285,
  296
Annual Meetings 48, 207
anti-smoking stance 316
Appointments Bureau 57, 82n.33
Archer, Jeffrey 232
Area Nurse Training Committees 142,
  180
Armstrong, Katherine 190
Association of Health Visitors 270
Association of Hospital Matrons 47,
  110, 117, 145, 163, 198–9, 218
Association of Hospital Officers 62
Association of Male Nurses 153
Association of Nurse Education 301
Association of Nurses 95, 97, 101,
  122n.20, 146
Association of Poor Law Unions 28
Association of Supervisors of
  Midwives 145
asylum nurses 29

Athlone Committee and reports 79, 86,
  99–100, 101–4, 109, 112
Auld, Margaret 302

Baggallay, Olive 141, 187
Baldwin, Stanley 65
Balme, Harold 101, 117
Baly, Monica 174, 206, 229, 272
Barker, Dennis 219
Barton, Eleanor 17
Bedford College for Women 50, 52, 53,
  72
Bennett, Bethina 141
Bennett, Louie 26
Berkeley, Sir Comyns 13, 17
Bevan, Aneurin 120, 121, 126–7, 131,
  141–2, 143, 146
Beveridge Committee and report 117
Bevin, Ernest 93, 94, 108, 110, 122n.15,
  145
Birmingham and Three Counties Trust
  for Nurses 180
Birmingham Education Centre 180, 308
Blair-Fish, Hilary (*née* Heaton) **88**, 128,
  138, **181**
Blakeley, Mary 228
Bocock, Joan 182
Bowley, Marion 175
Branches Standing Committee 24, 44,
  48, 49, 190, 206
Bridger, Harold 254
Bridges, Daisy 137, **162**
'Bridge that gap' campaign 286

Briggs report 239–40, 246, 251, 244, 260, 267, 274–5, 276, 277, 303
British College of Nurses 44, 46, 47
British Council 178
British Federation of Business and Professional Women 153
British Federation of University Women 152
British Geriatrics Society 309
British Hospitals Association 62, 110, 132
British Journal of Nursing 14, 44, 190
British Medical Association (BMA) 3, 24, 79, 127, 147–8, 174, 215, 219, 226, 262
British Medical Journal 46
British Psychological Society 309
British Red Cross Society 5, 10, 14, 17, 53
British Women's Hospital Committee 20, 21, 22
Brockington, Fraser 188
Brockway, Fenner 60
Brook, Iris 97
Brown, (Alfred) Ernest 109, 110, 118
Bulletin 24, 44
Burdett, Sir Henry 35

Cadbury family 180
Callaghan, James 212, 284
Canada: nurse education 53, 55, 181
cancer nursing 259
Cancer Nursing Society 280n.67
Carling, Esther 76
Carling, Sir Ernest Rock 166–7
Carpenter, Mary 138, 178–9, *181*, 183, 254, 260
Carr, Robert 242
Carter, Gladys 135–6, 139, 169, 184, 187
Castle, Barbara 231, 242, 245, 246, 290, 309
Central Advisory Board 106, 123n.59
Central Committee for the State Registration of (Trained) Nurses 13, 30
Central Council of Midwives 202
Central Emergency Committee for Nurses 104, 105
Central Health Services Council 119, 126, 127
Central Midwives Board (CMB) 17, 54

Central Sectional Committee of RCN 49, 205
Chamberlain, Neville *43*, 44, 75
CHANNEL project 274
Charley, Irene 72–3, 107, 187
Chartered Society of Massage and Medical Gymnastics 96
Chief Officers' Committee 254
Churchill, Winston 117, 121, 152
City University: diploma course 306
Civil Nursing Reserve (CNR) 104, 105, 106, 109, 118, 123n.59, 130, 131
Clark, Dame June 202, 227, 277
Clarke, Kenneth 291, 292, 293, 294–5, 317
class issues 3, 9, 12, 14, 18, 32, 33, 203
Clay, Trevor 233, 253, **289**, 295, 297, 299, 300, 302, 304, 313, 314, 316
   character, background 288–9
   relations with government 294
Clegg report 279n.35, 284–6, 301
clinical grading 299–300
clinical practice movement 311
coat of arms (RCN) 161, 314
Cockayne, Dame Elizabeth 137, 142, 173
Code of Professional Conduct 266–7, 327
'Cogwheel' report 226, 237n.116
Cohen, John 137, 140–1
College of Midwives 115, 116, 148
College of Nursing (later RCN) 16, 46, 47
   Articles of Association 16
   council 17–18, 20
   founding principles 1, 2, 3, 9, 10, 11, 14, 16, 325
   see also Royal College of Nursing
College Salaries Committee 57
Colonial Nursing Service 134
Colonial Office 178, 271
Commission for Racial Equality 276
Commission on Industrial Relations 249
Commission on Nursing Education 302
Committee for Imperial Defence 104
Committee for Northern Ireland 209
Committee on Social Insurance and Allied Services *see* Beveridge Committee
committee on standards of nursing care 309–10

Commonwealth Immigrants Act
    (1962) 272
Commonwealth Immigration Act 274
Commonwealth nurses 109, 214, 271,
    272, 273, 274
    see also overseas nurses
Community Nursing Association 306
Confederation of Health Service
    Employees (COHSE) 4, 150, 201,
    211, 212, 213, 214, 215, 219, 228,
    238n.142, 242, 244, 245, 246, 247,
    300, 327
Congress (RCN) 48, 207, 314, **315**
Conservative Party 155, 213
Consultative Committee of Women's
    Organisations 70
contraception 42, 269, 270
convalescent homes 143
Cooper, Sir Edwin 44
Council for the Training of Health
    Visitors 202
Council of Women Civil Servants 152
County Councils' Association 117
Coward, Amy 73–4
Cowdray Club 42, 44, 73, 74, 201, 305
Cowdray, Lady (Annie Pearson, Lady
    Cowdray) 21, 22, 42, *43*, 44, 55,
    67
Cowdray, Lord (Weetman Pearson,
    Viscount Cowdray) 21, 22, 42
Cowlin, Gertrude 18, 31, 39n.33, 55, 76,
    88, 99
Cox-Davies, Rachael 5, 6, 11, 17, 25, 31,
    36, 54–5, *67*, 78, 91
Crew, Albert Francis 184
Crossman, Richard 229, 231, 239, 248,
    263
Crouch, Herbert C. 56, 57

Dalton, Hugh 154
Dan Mason Medical Research Trust
    175
Daphne Heald Research Unit 312
Davies, Mary 207–8, 235n.51
Davies, Mary Elizabeth (Betty) see
    Newstead, Betty
de Cent, Lt. Colonel Douglas 205,
    206–7, 229, 313
Denman, Lady (Gertrude Mary
    Denman, Lady Denman) 42

Department of Nursing Policy and
    Practice 309
Derbyshire, Ruth 76
diamond jubilee 262
district nurses 91, 202, 263–4, 297
    see also Queen Victoria's Jubilee
    Institute for Nurses
District Nursing Association 307
domiciliary nursing 7, 125n.102, 119
drug errors 266
Duff Grant, Lucy *162*
Dunn, Alison 313, 314, 315
Dunsford, Sister Dorothy 229
Dynamic Quality Improvement
    Programme 312
Dynamic Standard Setting System
    (DySSSy) 311

education/training see nursing
    education/training
Education Act (1944) 130, 133, 152
Education Bill (1943) 115
Education Department 54, 72, 176–80,
    183, 250
Educational Appeal Fund 177–8
EEC Permanent Liaison Committee on
    Nurses 263
Elizabeth, Queen (the Queen
    Mother) 176, 262
Elizabeth II 143, *147*, 176, 177, 178, 262
Emergency Medical Services 108
Emergency War Committee 106
Employment Protection Act (1975) 249
English National Board 303
Ennals, David 251, 252, 291
equal pay 151–5, 156, 225, 328–9
Equal Pay Campaign Committee 152,
    153, 154–5
ethical issues 266–7, 269–70
Evans, Olwen Caradoc 208, 235n.51

Factories (Medical and Welfare)
    Order 107
Federated Superannuation Scheme for
    Nurses and Hospital Officers 47,
    62, 78, 83n.50
Fellowships 262
Fenwick, Ethel Bedford 8–9, 13–14, 17,
    18, *19*, 21, 23, 31, 44, 57, 60, 100,
    103, 188–9

fever nurses 29, 31
First World War 5, 9, 10, 11, 14, 21, 29,
  36, 37, 41
Fowler, Norman 286, 288, 291, 292, 294,
  295

gender issues 1, 2, 3, 7, 8, 16, 247–8, 326,
  328–9
  see also equal pay; male nurses
General Infirmary, Leeds: Diploma in
  Nursing 50
General Medical Council 14, 47
General Nursing Council for England
  and Wales (GNC) 4, 25, 30,
  31–2, 49, 78, 79, 130
  Briggs report 239
  educational requirements for
    nurses 185, 186
  hostility to Platt report 219, 220
  relations with government 117
  roll of assistant nurses 114, 123n.82
  syllabus 172, 173
  views on Hours of Employment
    Bill 60
General Nursing Council for Ireland 27,
  31, 49, 79, 130, 185, 239
General Nursing Council for
  Scotland 31, 49, 78, 79, 114, 130,
  185, 239
geriatric nursing 258, 276, 309
Gibson, George 95
Gill, Annie 11
Godber, Sir George 237n.116
Goddard, H. A. 165, 166, 167
golden jubilee 224
Goodall, Frances 88, 89, 100, 110, 116,
  127, 134, 162, 181, 212
  appointment, appearance and
    character 87, 89–90
  New Deal 132
  NHS White Paper 118, 120
  Nuffield report 169
  relations with
    male nurses 151–2, 200
    NCN 190
    trade unions 145–6, 148, 163
    TUC 93, 116, 145
  retirement 196
  role and title 116
  Wood report 138

Goodenough report 119
Gough, Miriam 208, 235n.51
Gould, Marion 182
Green, Margaret 256, 304
Greenborough, Sir John Hedley 292, 293
Greenwood, Arthur 68
Griffiths report 293–7, 298, 301, 310, 318,
  319
Grimond, Jo 213
Guild of Nurses 97, 122n.26, 137, 146,
  158n.53
Guillebaud report 169
Gunter, Ray 212

haemodialysis nursing 258
Hall, Dame Catherine Mary 198, 213,
  214, 216, 219, 220, 221, 225, 228,
  229, 230, 231, 241, 242, 243, 251,
  267, 269–70, 276, 277, 288,
  289–90, 329
  appointed to Industrial Relations
    Commission 242
  appointment, character, training and
    appearance 196–7
  attitude to male nurses 200, 201
  negotiations with TUC 253
  sits on Merrison Committee 243
  tributes 290
Hallowes, Ruth 55
Halsbury inquiry and report 246,
  248–9, 250
Hamilton, Willie 212
Hancock, Christine 239, 290, 316, 317
Haughton, Louisa 11, 12, 14, 17
Hayhoe, Barney 295
Health and Munitions Workers'
  Committee 72
Health and Safety at Work Act
  (1974) 249
health visitors 66, 68, 202
  eligibility for College membership
    68
  salary 68, 69, 70, 71
  trade union membership 70
  training 68, 71, 187–8
Health Visitors' Association 306–7
Heath, Edward 241, 245, 286
Heaton, H. see Blair-Fish, Hilary
higher education funding
  changes 307–8

Hill, Graham 230
Hill, Muriel 186
Hillman, David 314
HIV/AIDS 307
Holder, Stanley 273
Hopkins, Hetty 208, 235n.51
Horder, Lord (Thomas Jeeves Horder,
    Lord Horder) 106, 112, *113*
Horder Committee and reports 112, *113*,
    115, 116, 121, 124n.86, 139, 216, 219,
    277
Horsbrugh, Florence (Baroness
    Horsburgh) 106
hospital management 224, 225, 226, 294,
    295–6, 297
Hospital Nurses' Charter 131
Hospitals and Welfare Services
    Union 146
Hours of Employment Bill 25, 58–60

Inch, Thomas 137
indemnity insurance 62–3, 209, 235n.56,
    256, 258
Industrial Disputes Council 162
Industrial Disputes Order (1951) 162,
    163
industrial nurses 72–3, 107–8
industrial relations 161–4, 241–53, 276
Industrial Relations Act (1971) 242, 243,
    244, 245, 249
Industrial Relations Bill (1970) 241
Industrial Relations Committee 213
Industrial Welfare Society 72
Innes, Euphemia 50
Institute of Advanced Nursing
    Education (IANE) 254, 305, 306,
    307–8
Institute of Hospital Administrators 172
Institute of Hospital Almoners 96
Institute of Industrial Welfare
    Workers 72
Institute of Medical Psychology 54
Institute of Nursing 311–12
intensive care nursing 258
Interdepartmental Committee on
    Nursing Services *see* Athlone
    Committee
International Council of Nurses
    (ICN) 14, 18, 54, 189–90, 209,
    216, 261, 271

International Council of Women 189
International Department 209
Irish Board (College of Nursing) 23,
    25–7
Irish Matrons' Association 26
Irish Nurses' Association 26, 39n.40
Irish Nurses' Organisation 39n.40
Irish Nurses' Union 26, 27
Irish Nursing Board (independent
    board) 26, 27
Irish Women Workers' Union 26,
    39n.40

Jepson, Jack 211, 219
Jewish women refugees 98, 105
Joint Emergency Committee of the
    Professions 148
Joseph, Sir Keith 242, 245
Judge Committee and report 302–3,
    304, 305

Kelley, Richard 232
Kendall, Helen 311
Kettle, Marguerite 76
King's College for Household and Social
    Science 53, 82n.24
King's College for Women 50, 52, 53,
    81n.18
Kitson, Alison 311, 312
Knight, Marion *181*
Knutsford, Lord (Sydney George
    Holland, Lord Knutsford) 12–13,
    59

Labour Party 36, 58, 60, 64, 212
labour relations 2
Labour Relations Department 209, 244,
    259
Lamb, Margaret 168, 182, 183, 184
Lancet, The 129
Lancet Commission 75–9, 98
Lane Committee 269, 270
Lansbury, George 97
Lawson, Mabel 190, 191, 218
League of Red Cross Societies 53
Leeds General Infirmary: diploma in
    nursing 50
legal issues 172, 173, 267, 270–1
Leggett, Sir Frederick 209, 235n.54
library 143, *144*, 179–80, 254, 312–13

Limitation of Hours Bill (1937) 159n.57
Lloyd George, David 30, 63
Lloyd Still, Dame Alicia 11, 17, *19*, 31,
    40n.68, *67*
Local Authorities' Nursing Services
    Joint Committee 109, 110, 111
local authority nursing 63, 64, 65
Local Government Act (1929) 75, 97
Local Government and Other Officers
    Superannuation Act (1922) 61
logo (linked hands) 314, *315*
London Childhood Guidance
    Council 54
London County Council (LCC) 77,
    97
London County Council Nursing
    Service 69
Loughlin, Dame Anne 159n.71
Luckes, Eva 12, 13
Lyle, Leonard 61

MacCallum, Maude 33, 34, 35
McCarthy, Dame Maud 40n.68, *67*
Macdonald, Isabel 34
McFarlane, Jean, Baroness McFarlane of
    Llandaff 180, 254
Macleod, Iain 174
MacManus, Emily 139, 140, 152
male nurses 7, 31, 89–90, 92, 108, 151–5,
    160, 197–203, 233n.16
    first admitted members 2, 14, 197–8,
        200
    Salmon reforms 227
male tutors 81n.17
Margaret, Princess 204, 208, 231
married nurses 127, 130, 132–3, 248, 258,
    328, 329
Mary, Queen 22, 43, 44, 86, 176, 178
Maternity and Child Welfare Act
    (1918) 68
Matheson, Vera 25
matrons 12, 15, 16–17, 37, 80, 137, 139–40,
    224, 295, 297
Matrons' Council of Great Britain and
    Ireland 46, 47
Medical Defence Union 172, 174
Medical Women's Federation 96
membership 10–11, 14–15, 22–3, 28, 161,
    196, 197, 201, 234n.29, 242–3, 247,
    254, 255–6, 259–60, 312, 316

current 325–6
life membership 81n.14
Mental Handicap Nursing Society 259
Mental Hospital and Institutional
    Workers' Union 93, 95, 158n.53
mental hospitals 7, 197, 198, 199, 276
mental nurses 31, 108, 197
    see also psychiatric nurses
Merrison Committee 243
midwives 53
Midwives' Institute 54, 96
Ministry of Health: Division of
    Nursing 111, 119
    and public health 66, 68, 69, 70, 71
    relations with College 46, 55–6, 63–6,
        80
Ministry of Overseas Development 178
Monckton, Sir Walter 162, 163
Morgan, David 208
Mothers' Union 41
motto (RCN) 161
Mountbatten, Lady (Edwina
    Mountbatten, Countess
    Mountbatten) *162*, 177, 184
Muir, Joseph 36
Murray, Len 253
Musson, Dame Ellen 17, 31, 40n.68, *67*,
    78, 99

Nation's Fund for Nurses 21, 22, 34, 55
Nation's Nurses and Professional
    Women's Clubs 42
'Nation's Nurses' conferences 142–3
National Advisory Council on Nurses
    and Midwives 129, 130, 148
National Association of Assistant
    Nurses 114, 124n.84
National Association of Local
    Government Officers (later
    National and Local Government
    Officers Association)
    (NALGO) 70, 75, 92, 111, 145,
    152, 163, 246, 327
National Association of State Enrolled
    (Assistant) Nurses (NASEN) 4,
    124n.84, 203, 215
National Asylum Workers' Union 33
National Consultative Council on the
    Recruitment of Nurses and
    Midwives 271

National Council of Nurses of Great
    Britain and Ireland (NCN) 4, 18,
    188–91, 200, 261
National Council of Women
    (NCW) 41, 56–7, 78, 96, 152
National Federation of Women's
    Institutes 41, 42
National Health Service (NHS) 2, 117,
    126–8, 133, 142, 145, 149, 156
  Bevan's proposals 120, 121
  Guillebaud report on costs 169
  in Scotland 241
  restructuring 239
  student nurses' protest 149–51, **150**
  White Paper (1944) 118–20, 135
National Health Service Act (1946)
    126
National Insurance 56, 58, 62, 117
National Insurance Act (1911) 61, 63
National Union of County Officers 93,
    97, 158n.53
National Union of General and
    Municipal Workers 93, 158n.53
National Union of Public Employees
    (NUPE) 4, 93, 146, 158n.53, 246,
    252, 327
National Union of Societies for Equal
    Citizenship 41
National Union of Students 214
National Union of Teachers 148
National Union of Women
    Teachers 152
National Union of Women Workers 56,
    70
Nettlefold, Lucy 159n.71
'New Deal for Nurses' 131–2
Newstead, Betty (*née* Mary Elizabeth
    Davies) 209, 213, 229, 230, 242,
    246, **247**
Newstead, Keith 209, 235n.55
Nightingale tradition 77, 181, 186, 329
Nightingale Training School 182, 187
Nightingale, Florence 1, 5, 6, 8, 17, 87,
    111–12, 167, 294, **298**, 326, 329
  The Lady with the Lamp 177
North America: nurse education 53, 55,
    181
Northern Ireland Board 27, 209
Northfield, Colonel E. W. 143, 144
Norton, Doreen 176

no-strike policy 251, 252, 288, 290, 291,
    299, 327
Notification of Births Acts (1907
    and 1915) 68
nuclear war 297, 299
Nuffield Provincial Hospitals Trust 108,
    164, 166, 175
Nuffield report 164–70, 171–2, 174, 175,
    192, 217
'Nurse Alert' strategy 296, 299, 309, 318
nurses
  accommodation 248, 260, 296
  education *see* nursing education/
    training
  emigration 271, 275, 282n.113
  image 3, 8, 15, 161, 213, 246, 247–8,
    291, 299, 327
  nurse managers 224–5, 226–7
  nurse practitioners 306–7
  nurse specialists 267–8
  nurse tutors 81n.17, 182, 183–4, 186,
    222–3, 301; *see also* sister tutors
  pay and conditions 2, 32–6, 55–61,
    75–9, 92–3, 109–11, 210–15, 212,
    227–8, 231–2, 284, 291–2, 293, 299
  shortages 76–8, 79, 93, 95, 97–104,
    128–33, 135, 137, 160, 170, 212, 213,
    214
  status 1, 7, 9, 10, 12, 17, 23, 32, 133, 161,
    171, 188
  unemployment insurance 61–3
  working hours 29, 33, 57, 58–60, 64,
    77, 78, 93–4, 95, 97, 101, 103, 111,
    132, 138, 214, 249, 250, 284, 285,
    293, 301
  see also equal pay; named reports and
    Commissions; overseas nurses
    and types of nurse
Nurses Act (1919) 2
Nurses Act (1943) 114
Nurses Act (1949) 142, 197
Nurses Act (1957) 197
Nurses and Midwives Whitley
    Council 145, 158n.53, 163, 165,
    209, 212, 213, 214, 228, 285, 291–2
Nurses' Appeals Committee, Wales 208
Nurses Bill, draft proposals (1948) 141–2
Nurses, Midwives and Health Visitors
    Act (1979) 239, 276, 277, 302
Nurses Registration Acts 31

Nurses' Salaries (Rushcliffe)
    Committee 110, 111, 132, 149, 151,
    152, 153
Nurses (Scotland) Bill 114
Nursing and Midwifery Staffs
    Negotiating Council 293
nursing agencies 7, 73, 74–5, 92, 114, 272,
    273, 326, 327
nursing assistants 316, 317
nursing as vocation 1, 8, 12, 14, 35, 192
nursing bibliography 135, 312–13
nursing care standards 309–12
nursing duties 172, 173, 174, 265–6
nursing education/training 1, 8, 9, 12,
    32, 49–55, 215–27, 240, 260, 301–8
    founding aims of College 14, 49
    further education 181–8
    in mental hospitals 7
    in poor law hospitals 6–7, 28
    in voluntary hospitals 6
    see also named reports
Nursing Mirror 44, 81n.10, 210, 315
nursing practice, changes in 258, 268
Nursing Reconstruction Committee *see*
    Horder Committee
nursing research 174, 175–6, 188, 312
    first fellowship 175–6
Nursing Services' Joint Committee 109,
    110, 111
nursing skills 1, 164–6
Nursing Standard 210, 314, 315–16
Nursing Times 46, 313, 314, 315, 316
    official RCN journal 44
    quoted on
        Athlone report 102–3
        changes in 1960s 209–10
        College policy and trade
            unionism 96
        GNC and social class 32
        Lancet Commission report 78–9
        Nuffield report 166
        RCN membership criteria 30
    wartime articles on nursing 108–9
Nuttall, Peggy 210

occupational health courses 258, 306
Occupational Health Nurses'
    Section 205
Oncology Nursing Society 280n.67
ophthalmic nursing 268

overseas nurses 178, 185, 214, 271–6, 306,
    327
overtime pay 214–15

Paediatric Nursing Society 259
Parliamentary Committee 60
Pavitt, Laurence 212
'Pay not peanuts' campaign 251, **252**
Pay Review Body 292
Pearce, Evelyn 135–6, 141
Pearson, Alan 311
Pecker, Ruth **88**, 100
Pembrey, Sue 311
pensions 61, 62, 91–2
Perry, Sir Cooper 11, 15, 17, 44, 50, 53, **67**
Platt Committee and report 216, 217–23,
    225, 235n.78 and n.80, 263, 302
poor law
    abolition 126
    infirmaries 7, 12, 35, 63, 63–4, 75
    nurses 7, 12, 23, 28, 35, 36, 64, 65, 316
Poor Law Association 17
Poor Law Infirmary Matrons'
    Association 47
Poor Law Officers' Association 35, 46
Poor Law Workers' Trade Union 35
Powell, Enoch 210–11, 212, 213, 214, 216,
    273
Prentice, Dame Winifred **243**, 245
Press and Public Relations
    Department 313–5
Prices and Incomes Board 222–3, 225
primary health care nursing 258
private nurses 52, 73–5, 91, 272, 326
Private Nurses' Committee 73, 74
Private Nurses' Section 75, 80, 205
private patients 266
Professional Nursing Department 255,
    257, 258, 259, 308–9
Professional Union of Trained
    Nurses 35, 46, 47, 60
Project 2000 303–5, 317, 322n.68 and
    n.80
psychiatric nurses 245, 258, 265
public health 66–73, 106–7
public health nurses 52, 66–73, 106–76,
    108, 187–8, 192
Public Health Section 69, 70, 71, 72, 80,
    107, 205, 274
    Second World War 106–7, 264

public relations 204–5, 206, 313
pupil nurses 171, 203

Queen Alexandra's Imperial Military
      Nursing Service Reserve 105
Queen Victoria's Jubilee Institute for
      Nurses 7, 17, 49, 91, 263
Quinn, Dame Sheila **255**, 296, 309, 311

Race Relations Acts (1965 and 1968) 273
racism 273–4, 276
RADNO Group 281n.79
'Raise the Roof!' campaign 227–32
Ramsden, Gertrude 175
Rathbone, Eleanor 91
Raven, Dame Kathleen 223, 239
Rayner, Claire 269
Red Cross *see* British Red Cross Society,
      League of Red Cross Societies
      and Red Cross Societies
Red Cross Societies 53, 54
Rees, Eileen M. 208, 235n.51
registration of nurses 7, 8–9, 13, 30–2,
      197, 200
reorganisation of RCN 204–210, 254–60
Research Discussion Group 175–6, 258
Research Society 175, 312
Review Body for Nursing Staff,
      Midwives, Health Visitors and
      Professions Allied to
      Medicine 292
Rhondda, Lady (Margaret Haig
      Thomas, Lady Rhondda) 100–1
Rice, Frank 273
Robbins report 216–17, 218
Robinson, Kenneth 213, 220, 221, 263
Rockefeller Foundation scholarships
      and grants 55, 179, 184
Royal Army Medical Corps 199
Royal British Nurses' Association
      (RBNA) 9, 13, 16, 30, 34, 46, 47
Royal Charter 66
   granted 47, 80, 103
   amended 250, 288
Royal College of Midwives 145, 162, 270
Royal College of Nursing and National
      Council of Nurses of the United
      Kingdom (Rcn) (1963) 191
Royal College of Nursing Charitable
      Trust 250

Royal College of Nursing Development
      Trust 260, 280n.72
Royal College of Nursing of the United
      Kingdom (RCN)
   becomes trade union 2, 242, 250, 327
   founding aims 1, 2, 3, 9, 10, 11, 14, 16,
      49, 325
   headquarters 10, 14, 21, 22, 42, 44, **45**,
      46
   name changes 188–91
   prefix first used 48, 86
   public image 3, 89
   Royal Charter 47, 66, 80, 103
   see also College of Nursing
Royal College of Nursing Representative
      Body (RRB) 202, 206–7, 251,
      255
Royal College of Nursing v. the
      Department of Health and Social
      Security 270
Royal College of Psychiatrists 309
Royal College of Surgeons of Ireland 26
Royal Commission on Equal Pay 152,
      153–4, 159n.71
Royal Commission on the Health
      Service (1977) 226
Royal Holloway College: training
      courses for nurses 52
Royal Naval Nursing Service 33
Royal Sanitary Institute 69, 70, 71
Rucker, Sir Arthur 119
'Rule 12' 252, 288, 292, 300, 328
Rundle, Mary 18, **20**, 22, 25, 27, 36, 46,
      50, 59, 61, 64, **67**, 69, 87, **88**, 89
Rushcliffe Committee *see* Nurses'
      Salaries Committee
Rye, David 308, 311

Salmon Committee and report 223,
      224–7, 263
Sanitary Inspectors' Association 84n.73
Scottish Board 23, 184, 105, 114, 119, 184,
      202, 218
Scottish General Nursing Council 218
Scottish Home and Health
      Department 218, 295–6
Scottish Matrons' Association 114, 145
Scottish Nurses' Association 46
Scutari Projects Ltd 314, 315, 316
Second World War 86, 104–9, 143, 202

Serota, Baroness (Beatrice K. Serota, Baroness Serota) 207
Sex Discrimination Act (1975) 203
Shackleton, Sir David 59
sick children's nurses 31
silver jubilee 111
Silverthorne, Thora 95, 100, 146
Simpson, Marjorie 175, 187, 268
Sister and Charge Nurses Section 202
sister tutors 50, 52, 80, 81n.17, 182–5, 186–7
Sister Tutor Section 52, 175, 183, 186, 205
Smith, Dorothy M. 99
Socialist Medical Association (SMA) 95, 157n.22
    views on nurses 135
Society of Medical Officers of Health 69, 96, 127, 172
Society of Nursing Research 258
Society of Registered Male Nurses 200, 201
Sparshott, Dame Margaret 24, 25, 31, **94**
Special Committee on Salaries and Conditions of Employment for Nurses 57
Standards of Care Project 311–12
Standing Conference of Women's Organisations 155
Standing Nursing Advisory Committee (SNAC) 126, 127, 175
Standing Nursing and Midwifery Advisory Committee (Scotland) 127, 168–9
Stanley, Sir Arthur 5, 6, 8, 9, **10**, 10, 11, 13, 14–15, 16, 17, 20, 23, 25, 28, 29, 30, 31, 34, 35–6, **43**, 44, 47–8, 57, **67**, 143, 318, 330
Stanley, Lord Edward 5
Star and Garter Fund 21
state enrolled nurses (SEN) 4, 114, 170, 171, 186, 203–4, 215, 217–18, 273
    in Scotland 114
    admitted members 203
State Nurses' Guild 35
state registered nurses (SRN) 4, 114, 130, 166, 186
Stewart, Isla 189
Stewart, Neil 313, 315
stoma care nursing 268

student nurses 24, 36, 90–1, 167–8, 149–51, **150**, 185–6, 203–4, 214, 215
Student Nurses' Association 36, 48, 49, 102, 111, **147**, 151, 204, 258, 273
Student Nurses' Section 252, 258
subscriptions 18, 256, 259–60
support workers 317–18, 326
Swift, Dame Sarah 5, **6**, 6, 8, 9, 10, 11, 14, 17, 23, 30, 40n.68, **43**, 44, **67**, 87, 330

Tavistock Institute reports 254, 256–8
Territorial Army Nursing Service 105
Thatcher, Margaret 277, 285, 286, **287**, 291, 296, 300, 327
Thomson, Alice 179, 180
Time and Tide
    articles on nursing 100–1
    on Athlone report 103–4
Trade Disputes and Trade Unions Act (1927) 148
Trades Union Congress (TUC) 3–4, 70, 93–5, 111, 112, 120, 159n.57, 242, 250, 253, 291
Trade Union Act (1913) 162
Trade Union and Industrial Relations Act (1974) 249
trade unionism and RCN 33–4, 36, 37, 64, 65, 80, 92–7, 145–51, 203, 277, 327
    becomes trade union 250
    considers affiliation to TUC 252–3, 288, 292
    registers as independent union 249
    registers as professional association under Industrial Relations Act 242
training *see* nursing education/training
Transport and General Workers' Union (TGWU) 93
Trenchard, Hope 251
Tynemouth poor law union 12

Udell, Florence **88**, 96, 100, 114, 134, 190, 191, 271
UK Central Council for Nursing, Midwifery and Health Visiting (UKCC) 240, 276, 302, 303, 304, 305
UK Education Committee 254

Unemployment Act (1922) 61
unemployment insurance 61–3
UNISON 327
United Nations Relief and
        Rehabilitation Administration
        (UNRRA) 134
United Nurses' Association 228
university education
    first university department in UK 52,
        82n.21
    first chair in UK 52, 82n.21
    see also nursing education/training
University of Birmingham 72, 187
University of Edinburgh 52, 82n.21, 175,
        184, 187
    Department of Nursing Studies 185
    Nurse Teaching Unit 184–5
University of Leeds: Diploma in
        Nursing 50
University of London 50, 52, 53, 182,
        183, 184, 306
University of Manchester 82n.21, 180,
        187–8, 306
University of Southampton: health
        visitor training 187
University of Surrey: occupational
        health degree 306
USA: nurse education 53, 55, 181, 219

Vaughan, Dame Janet 159n.71
Veal, Patricia 228
Vergebovsky, Tatiana 263
violence against nurses 265
Voluntary Aid Detachment workers
        (VADs) 14, 15, 32, 130, 131, 318
voluntary hospitals 7, 12, 28, 63–4, 316
Voluntary Hospitals Commission 96

Wakeford, Frances 99–100
Walsh, Susan 275

Ward, Dame Irene 89, 163, 211
Ward and Departmental Sisters'
        Section 147, 205
Watt, Katherine 111, 115, 118
Welfare Advisory Service 209
Welsh Board 207–8
Welsh Hospitals and Health Services
        Association 208
West Derby Union poor law
        union 28–9, 33
Wetenhall, J. P. 110
Whitley Councils 94, 110, 122n.16, 151,
        163, 292
    see also Nurses and Midwives Whitley
        Council
Whittamore, Albery Verdun 200
Whitty, Dame May 20, 57
Wilkie, Elaine 178, 187
Williams, Gertrude 167
Williams, John 108
Williams, Margaret 176
Willink, Sir Henry 116, 118
Wilson, Harold 227, 249
Women Public Health Officers'
        Association 93, 145, 152,
        158n.53
Women Sanitary Inspectors and Health
        Visitors Association
        (WSIHVA) 70, 71, 84n.73
women's suffrage 9, 16, 21, 41
Women's Trade Union League
        70
Wood, Sir Kingsley 96–7
Wood, Sir Robert 136–7, 143
Wood report 136–42, 218, 325
Woodman, Ada 138, *162*, 187
World Health Organization 54, 178–9,
        187, 189, 311

Yapp, Charlotte Seymour 34